Pediatric and Postpartum Home Health Nursing

Assessment and Care Planning

D1569434

Pediatric and Postpartum Home Health Nursing

ASSESSMENT AND CARE PLANNING

KATHYRN A. MELSON, RN, MSN

Private Practice,
El Paso, Texas

MARIE S. JAFFE, RN, MS†

Formerly Nursing Faculty,
University of Texas at El Paso,
College of Nursing and Allied Health,
El Paso, Texas

†Deceased.

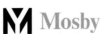

St. Louis Baltimore Boston Carlsbad Chicago Naples New York
Philadelphia Portland London Madrid Mexico City Singapore
Sydney Tokyo Toronto Wiesbaden

Vice President and Publisher: Nancy L. Coon
Executive Editor: N. Darlene Como
Senior Developmental Editor: Laurie Sparks
Project Manager: Patricia Tannian
Senior Production Editor: Suzanne C. Fannin
Book Design Manager: Gail Morey Hudson
Manufacturing Manager: David Graybill
Cover Designer: Teresa Breckwoldt

Copyright© 1997 by Mosby–Year Book, Inc.

Printed in the United States of America
Composition by Graphic World, Inc.
Printing/binding by R.R. Donnelley & Sons Company

Mosby–Year Book, Inc.
11830 Westline Industrial Drive
St. Louis, Missouri 63146

Library of Congress Cataloging in Publication Data

Melson, Kathryn A.
  Pediatric and postpartum home health nursing: assessment and
care planning/Kathryn A. Melson, Marie S. Jaffe.
      p.   cm.
  Includes bibliographical references and index.
  ISBN 0-8151-4876-3
  1. Pediatric nursing.   2. Postnatal care.   3. Obstetrical
nursing.   4. Home care services.   5. Child health services.
I. Jaffe, Marie S.   II. Title.
  [DNLM: 1. Home Care Services – United States.
2. Pediatric Nursing – methods.   3. Child Care – methods –
nurses' instruction.   4. Postnatal Care – methods – nurses'
instruction. WY 115 M528p 1997]
RJ245.M45 1997
610.73′62 – dc20
DNLM/DLC   96-25620
for Library of Congress   CIP

96 97 98 99 00 / 9 8 7 6 5 4 3 2 1

DIRECTIONS FOR ADMINISTRATION

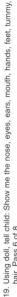

1. Try to get child to smile by smiling, talking or waving. Do not touch him/her.
2. Child must stare at hand several seconds.
3. Parent may help guide toothbrush and put toothpaste on brush.
4. Child does not have to be able to tie shoes or button/zip in the back.
5. Move yarn slowly in an arc from one side to the other, about 8" above child's face.
6. Pass if child grasps rattle when it is touched to the backs or tips of fingers.
7. Pass if child tries to see where yarn went. Yarn should be dropped quickly from sight from tester's hand without arm movement.
8. Child must transfer cube from hand to hand without help of body, mouth, or table.
9. Pass if child picks up raisin with any part of thumb and finger.
10. Line can vary only 30 degrees or less from tester's line.
11. Make a fist with thumb pointing upward and wiggle only the thumb. Pass if child imitates and does not move any fingers other than the thumb.

12. Pass any enclosed form. Fail continuous round motions.

13. Which line is longer? (Not bigger.) Turn paper upside down and repeat. (pass 3 of 3 or 5 of 6)

14. Pass any lines crossing near midpoint.

15. Have child copy first. If failed, demonstrate.

When giving items 12, 14, and 15, do not name the forms. Do not demonstrate 12 and 14.

16. When scoring, each pair (2 arms, 2 legs, etc.) counts as one part.
17. Place one cube in cup and shake gently near child's ear, but out of sight. Repeat for other ear.
18. Point to picture and have child name it. (No credit is given for sounds only.) If less than 4 pictures are named correctly, have child point to picture as each is named by tester.

19. Using doll, tell child: Show me the nose, eyes, ears, mouth, hands, feet, tummy, hair. Pass 6 of 8.
20. Using pictures, ask child: Which one flies?...says meow?...talks?...barks?...gallops? Pass 2 of 5, 4 of 5.
21. Ask child: What do you do when you are cold?...tired?...hungry? Pass 2 of 3, 3 of 3.
22. Ask child: What do you do with a cup? What is a chair used for? What is a pencil used for?
    Action words must be included in answers.
23. Pass if child correctly places and says how many blocks are on paper. (1, 5).
24. Tell child: Put block on table; under table; in front of me, behind me. Pass 4 of 4. (Do not help child by pointing, moving head or eyes.)
25. Ask child: What is a ball?...lake?...desk?...house?...banana?...curtain?...fence?...ceiling? Pass if defined in terms of use, shape, what it is made of, or general category (such as banana is fruit, not just yellow). Pass 5 of 8, 7 of 8.
26. Ask child: If a horse is big, a mouse is ___? If fire is hot, ice is ___? If the sun shines during the day, the moon shines during the ___? Pass 2 of 3.
27. Child may use wall or rail only, not person. May not crawl.
28. Child must throw ball overhand 3 feet to within arm's reach of tester.
29. Child must perform standing broad jump over width of test sheet (8 1/2 inches).
30. Tell child to walk forward, ⟳⟳⟳⟳ heel within 1 inch of toe. Tester may demonstrate.Child must walk 4 consecutive steps.
31. In the second year, half o' normal children are non-compliant.

OBSERVATIONS:

Consultants

The authors wish to thank the following individuals for their assistance in reviewing the manuscript:

Jill Brusiloff, RNC
Maternal/Child Care Services
Private Duty Department
Visiting Nurse Association
El Paso, Texas

Debra Ann Davis, RN, BSN
Pediatric Nurse
Sierra Medical Center
El Paso, Texas

Mary Lou Ende, RN, MNEd
Formerly Director of Pediatric/Maternal-Child
    Health Nursing
South Hills Health System
Home Health Agency
Homestead, Pennsylvania

Cheryl A. Grande, RN, BSN
Staff Nurse
VNA Health Care, Inc.
Waterbury, Connecticut

Katherine Porpora, RN, MSN
Private Practice, Pediatric Home Care
Westchester, New York

To the memory and spirit of
Marie S. Jaffe

Preface

Concern with escalating hospital and health care costs, emphasis on managed care systems, and shortened hospital stays have resulted in the discharge of patients who are stable but still acutely ill. This has led to an increasing call for home health services, frequently delivered and coordinated by the home health nurse. Although the nursing skills are similar to those found in the acute care setting, the home health nurse needs to be flexible for several reasons: differences in client and family needs; location of practice; need to work cooperatively and independently with patient, family, and other members of the health care team; and regulatory requirements to control costs.

The focus of this book is to assist the nurse by providing a broad framework of process, within which tasks to be completed are outlined and outcomes defined. In doing so, the nurse is assisted in the delivery of direct care and helps families/clients through instruction, assistance, and support. This provides direction for ongoing care rendered by the family, aids independence, and helps in family coping with the psychologic stressors of illness.

This book is intended to be a handbook containing concise, accurate, and practical material of use to those providing nursing care in the home and community. It is useful to nurses already in practice as well as to student practitioners and others in the home care setting. A knowledge of basic nursing concepts and competency in technical nursing skills are prerequisite to is use.

The book is unique in that it is among the first to address the need of the pediatric client at home. It is both family and client oriented. It includes psychosocial and physical components of care. There is a focus on health maintenance, prevention of illness, facilitation of growth and development, as well as specific illness needs. New information on the treatment of pediatric acquired immunodeficiency syndrome and critical care pathways is included.

Kathryn A. Melson
Marie S. Jaffe

Guidelines for the use of this book

The following outline presents the format of this book and briefly describes its content.

ASSESSMENTS

Assessment is the first step in the nursing process. It provides a database for problem identification, goal setting, treatment planning, and implementation. Included are client history, review of systems, and physical assessment by body system. The standardized examination sequence of inspection, palpation, percussion, and auscultation is used. Psychosocial assessment includes client reports and the nurse's observations of the client's developmental status and psychologic stage, family profile, and environmental and financial considerations. Assessments are referenced in the individual nursing care plans (NCP) because they are important to data collection.

NURSING CARE PLANS

Nursing process is used so sequencing is logical. A continuous feedback system permits easy modification of pathways. Care plans are grouped by body systems, and conditions and disorders, which are frequently in the home care setting, are presented. Each NCP includes the following information:

1. An introductory passage that includes a definition, its clinical manifestations, etiology, medical implications, and nursing focus.
2. Nursing diagnosis derived from the 1994 revised index of official nursing diagnoses as presented by the North American Nursing Diagnosis Association (NANDA). Selection of nursing diagnoses is based on those most frequently associated with the given disorder. Additional, supplemental diagnoses may be used based on client need. A complete listing is found in the Appendix.
3. Related factors such as physical and psychosocial elements that render a specific diagnosis. They may in-

clude physiologic processes, risk factors, genetic predisposition, and responses.

4. Defining characteristics such as signs and symptoms
   or other phenomena associated with the condition.
   The composite of nursing diagnosis, related factors, and defining characteristics provides a knowledge
   base for appropriate nursing care.

5. Outcomes, or patient-centered statements that define a
   course of action to stabilize or remediate problems
   identified in the diagnosis. They are specific, measur-
   able, and time referenced as short-term and long-term.

6. Interventions, those activities that assist in the achievement of defined goals. Nursing interventions are in the
   purview of the home health care worker include assessment, instruction, provision of physical nursing care,
   and referrals to other disciplines. Caregiver/client and
   family interventions are activities performed by the
   family. They refer to persons responsible for care and
   not necessarily the biologic parent. Caregiver interventions may result from direct nursing instruction or referral or they may be self-generated as a result of professional support and assistance. Each nursing intervention includes a flexible time frame to meet client
   needs as well as to conform with agency policy and insurance directives. Instruction is always given in a manner that is age suitable and culturally, educationally,
   and linguistically appropriate.

The NCP is a guide to care. It is process oriented and
may be modified at any point because of changing client status and needs. As with any NCP, it must be adapted to the
individual client's specific needs.

APPENDICES

Appendices contain supplementary resource information.
These include a list of the NANDA-approved nursing diagnoses, cardiopulmonary resuscitation guidelines, universal
precautions, recommended immunization schedule, recommended energy intake and water requirements, vital
signs, guidelines for medication administration and specimen collection, and a sample clinical pathway documentation guidelines.

Contents

APPENDICES

Assessments

Strategies for Examining the Infant/ Child

Strategies are presented as guidelines. They should be adapted to the needs of the individual and family.

- Schedule home visit to facilitate family's routine when visit is least likely to be disruptive or cause multiple interruptions.
- Bring adequate supplies that are in good working order such as extra batteries for lighted instruments. Have available a supply of toys that are colorful, nonbreakable, easily cleaned, and that have no removable parts.
- Establish and maintain rapport and trust. Be mindful that nurse is guest in home.
- Before physical examination of child, assess general states of health and nutrition, mood, displayed developmental skills, activity selection and tolerance, color, respirations, cry, caregiver's response, and child-caregiver interactions.
- Explain purpose and extent of visit. Ask if there are questions or concerns.
- Be direct, confident, and positive in approach. Speak to child as well as to caregiver. Be sensitive to cultural nuances of role, touch, and space.
- Perform examination/procedure in most appropriate place. Consider child's safety, security, family preference, privacy, ambient temperature, and equipment on which child is dependent.
- Take out only supplies and equipment that are essential for examination. Offer child's favorite toy, blanket, or pacifier. Use distractors as necessary (e.g., flashlight).
- Explain clearly and simply what will be done. Involve child. Acquaint child with examining instruments. Allow child to use stethoscope on self. Demonstrate examination on self or toy animal.
- Place child in position of comfort, whether seated or on caregiver's lap. Proceed in an orderly, unrushed manner. Use smooth, efficient movements. Incorporate play and games into examination.

- State directions firmly. Set limits on choices given to child.
- Keep infant diapered as long as possible. Undress child only as necessary for examination. Maintain warmth and privacy.
- Allow ticklish child to place hand under examiner's hand to facilitate abdominal examination.
- Perform anticipated painful procedures last.
- Demonstrate sensitivity to child's responses. Listen. Praise. Encourage.
- Provide closure. Discuss results of examination. Query for concerns. Give child age-appropriate reward.

Health History

Information in the health history is inclusive. It may be elicited from the caregiver or other family members or may be obtained from medical records. Modifications may be necessary to adapt to client and family needs and abilities.

IDENTIFYING INFORMATION

Date of interview, informant/complainant, source of referral
Name (of child), including nickname
First names of parents and last names, if different; their ages, occupations, educational levels
Others in household; their names, ages, relationships with client
Address
Home and work telephone numbers
Age, date of birth
Sex, race, religion, nationality, place of birth
Language ability (age appropriate), preference, need for translator
Community agencies used, telephone numbers
Support systems, telephone numbers

CURRENT ILLNESS

1. Chief complaint or reason for visit (in client's or caregiver's words)

2. Profile of illness, using PQRST mnemonic:
    P— prodromal, precipitating factors
    Q—qualitative, quantitative factors
    R—region, radiation
    S— severity (on a scale of 1 to 10)
    T— timings (date, onset, manner)
3. Progression of illness and effect of therapy

HISTORY

1. Perinatal history
    a. Health of mother before, during pregnancy
        Maternal age, length of pregnancy, gravida and parity, extent of prenatal care
        Illnesses, medical conditions, exposure to communicable disease, complications relating to pregnancy, blood type
        Medications used and prescribed, exposure to toxins or chemicals
        Responses to pregnancy
    b. Duration, nature, severity of labor; use of sedatives, analgesics
        Type, date, location of delivery
        Procedures performed
        Complications
    c. Infant status, health at birth; Apgar score
        Weight, length, estimated gestational age
        Congenital anomalies, birth injuries
2. Developmental history
    Age, height, weight, dentition
    Performance of age-related developmental tasks, observed and recounted (see "Growth and Developmental Assessment," p. 31), periods of delayed or accelerated growth, comparison with siblings, parental perceptions
    Grade expected and attained, quality of schoolwork
    Extracurricular activities, play
    Family/social relationships
3. Activity/performance history
    General disposition, personality, temperament
    Rituals, behaviors, responses to discipline or frustration
    Play and diversional activities, amount and type of exercise

Eating patterns, food intake (see "Gastrointestinal System Assessment and Nutritional Assessment," pp. 16-17), alternative feeding management

Sleep/nap patterns, duration, disturbances, aggravating and alleviating factors

Urinary/bowel control, patterns, problems, remedies

Sexual maturity, activity, concerns

Drug use/abuse

4. Childhood diseases

Type, age, severity, complications, sequelae

5. Immunizations

Type, date, dosage, boosters, unusual reactions

Presence of written record

6. Medications

Over-the-counter, prescribed, borrowed; home remedies

Type, condition being treated, dose, frequency, duration, form, side effects; medication label, directions, pill count, as appropriate

Safe, accurate administration by observation, child-proofing measures

7. Allergies

Hypersensitivity to foods, drugs, animals, insects, plants

Hay fever, asthma, allergic rhinitis, eczema, urticaria

8. Serious illness

Illness, injury, accidents: date, symptoms, family prevalence, course, pattern, recurrence, complications, sequelae

Dates and descriptions of hospitalizations, surgeries

Dates and results of special procedures, tests, screening panels

Presence of indwelling, central venous or peripheral catheters, tracheotomy; competence with use, maintenance

9. Family medical history

Age, sex, health status of family members

Genogram child's biologic maternal/paternal grandparents, parents, offspring, aunts, uncles, first cousins; indicate age, health status/problems, cause of death; include stillbirths, miscarriages, abortions

Familial illnesses, conditions, anomalies (e.g., cardiovascular disease, hypertension, cerebrovascular accidents, cancer, diabetes, any condition currently suspected or diagnosed in client)

Lifestyle choices (e.g., substance use/abuse, sedentary behaviors) (see "Family Assessment," p. 41)
10. Psychosocial history
    Family structure, roles and functions, cohesiveness
    Family expectations, attitudes, outlook, bonding behaviors
    Language spoken at home, communication patterns
    Marital status, relationships, significant others
    Educational levels, current and past employment, socioeconomic status, caregivers' work schedules
    Home environment adequacy, safety
    Ethnic, cultural, religious milieu
    Lifestyle, health care beliefs; recreation, perceived stressors, health care concerns
    Relationships with peers, employer, coworkers, schoolmates, community
    Support systems, coping capacity of caregiver, resources

 # Review of Systems

GENERAL

General state of health, ability to perform age-dependent activities of daily living, unexplained weight change, fever, fatigue, constitutional symptoms, serious illness

PULMONARY SYSTEM

Shortness of breath (at rest, on exertion, positional), wheezing, stridor, frequent colds, infections, cough, hemoptysis, sputum production, date and results of last tuberculin skin testing and chest x-ray examination, use of ventilatory aids/devices

CARDIOVASCULAR SYSTEM

History of familial cardiac anomalies, congenital defects, heart murmurs, anemia, unexplained or disproportionate fatigue, activity intolerance, failure to gain weight, delayed growth/development, marked pallor, cyanosis, orthopnea or preference for squatting position, tachypnea, tachycardia, edema, dates and results of latest hematologic examination, electrocardiogram, echocardiogram

NEUROLOGIC SYSTEM

Maternal drug use, birth injury or anomaly, prematurity, trauma, delayed development, use of ototoxic drugs, tremors, spasms, seizures, ataxia, paresis, paresthesias, paralysis, any abnormal involuntary movement, difficulties with balance or coordination, difficulty swallowing, sensory defects or disturbances, delayed language development/ speech problems, learning difficulties, altered level or loss of consciousness, memory loss, change in cognitive ability, behavior, affect

GASTROINTESTINAL SYSTEM

Appetite, dietary intake, food intolerances, difficulty swallowing, weight change, anorexia, nausea, regurgitation, vomiting, pain, bowel control/habits, excessive eructation or flatulence, diarrhea, constipation, change in color/ appearance of stools, infection, rectal pain/bleeding

ENDOCRINE SYSTEM

Changes in weight, skin texture, hair distribution, pigmentation; weakness; fatigue; temperature intolerance; delayed/accelerated growth and development; polydipsia; polyphagia; polyuria; delayed/accelerated sexual maturation; personality changes; headache; visual disturbances

HEMATOLOGIC SYSTEM

Local to generalized bleeding from any site (spontaneous or disproportionate to injury); petechiae; epistaxis; bruises; hyperbilirubinemia; anemias; fatigue; activity intolerance; weakness; pallor; exposure to/ingestion of chemicals, drugs, toxins; recent and past infections; chronic disease; transfusion history

MUSCULOSKELETAL SYSTEM

Strength, coordination, gait, ability to perform age-dependent activities of daily living, spinal curvature, back pain, movement limitations, fractures, deformities; muscle weakness, cramping, pain; joint stiffness, erythema, edema, pain; assistive/prosthetic devices

RENAL/URINARY SYSTEMS

Renal and nonrenal congenital anomalies, past infections, fever, trauma, exposure to nephrotoxic drugs or heavy metals, bladder control/habits, number of wet diapers, changes in color/odor of urine, force of stream, oliguria, polyuria, dysuria, hematuria, frequency, urgency, hesitancy, nocturia, enuresis, back or flank pain, anemia

REPRODUCTIVE SYSTEM

Sexual maturity and activity; genital discharge; pruritus; lesions; rashes; breast pain, masses, discharge; measures to prevent pregnancy, sexually transmitted diseases

- Female: menarche, last menstrual period, menstrual pattern, date and results of last Papanicolaou smear, performance of breast self-examination
- Male: descended testicles, circumcision, scrotal swelling, lesions, masses, performance of testicular self-examination

INTEGUMENTARY SYSTEM

Pruritus; jaundice; rashes; moles; birthmarks; congenital anomalies; scarring; petechiae; lesions; acne; ecchymoses; excessive oiliness or dryness; changes in amount/texture of hair; changes in appearance, configuration/color of nails; lice infestation; insect bites; exposure to drugs, plants, environmental toxins; recent travel

EYE, EAR, NOSE, AND THROAT

- Eye: infection, discharge, excessive tearing, itching, photosensitivity, pain, edema of lids, yellowing of sclera, blurred or double vision, changes in vision, strabismus, use of corrective lenses, date and results of last eye examination
- Ear: infection, discharge, earache, tinnitus, change in hearing, vertigo, delayed speech development, date and results of latest auditory examination
- Nose: obstruction, stuffiness, discharge, sneezing, allergies, sinus pain, epistaxis, altered sense of smell
- Throat: difficulty chewing/swallowing, tongue soreness, sore throat, change in color/integrity of mucosa, hoarseness, voice aberrations, dentition, toothache, caries, gum swelling/bleeding, abscesses, pattern of dental hygiene, date and results of last dental examination

PSYCHOLOGIC

Facial expressiveness; body posture; grooming, personal hygiene; speech, language usage; mood; affect; tension; memory; cognitive function; performance of developmental tasks; activity patterns; coping abilities; relationship with family, peers, schoolmates, authority figures; school performance

---

 # *Pulmonary System Assessment*

INSPECTION

- Vital signs, including blood pressure
- Respiratory rate (to be taken for 1 minute): approximately 40 breaths per minute in infant, decreasing to adult levels (16 to 20 breaths per minute) as child matures
- Respiratory depth, pattern, inspiratory/expiratory duration ratio
- Ease of respiration: typically quiet and effortless; diaphragmatic breathing in younger child, thoracic breathing in older child
- Chest configuration: typically barrel-shaped with increases in lateral growth as child matures; anatomic landmarks, symmetry, expansion, delayed/impaired movement
- Structural deformities or deviations such as pigeon breast (pectus carinatum), funnel chest (pectus excavatum), tracheal deviation from midline, spinal alterations
- Color of buccal mucosa, lips, ears, nails, skin; clubbing of nails
- Sputum production, color, amount
- Gagging, hoarseness, coughing, wheezing, grunting, any difficulty breathing, stridor; chest wall retractions, nasal flaring, pain
- Difficulty feeding, listlessness, apprehension, diaphoresis, preference for upright position, fatigue, exertional dyspnea

PALPATION

- Chest for pain, deviations noted on inspection
- Symmetry of chest expansion
- Location and character of tactile fremitus; increases, decreases, absence; crepitus, pleural friction rub

PERCUSSION

- Thoracic field: intensity, pitch, duration (assess anteriorly and posteriorly, with bilateral comparison)
- Generally, resonance is heard over air-filled lung tissue; dullness, fluid or solid tissue; flatness, solid tissue; hyperresonance, hyperinflated air-filled tissue; tympany, air-filled stomach

AUSCULTATION

- Elicited during quiet time when child is not crying and is cooperative or being distracted
- Normal breath sounds: location, intensity, pitch, quality, inspiratory/expiratory duration ratio; vesicular sounds heard over most of lung; bronchovesicular sounds over main bronchi (i.e., first and second intercostal spaces anteriorly and between scapulas posteriorly); bronchial sounds over trachea
- Breath sounds in uncharacteristic area, absent/diminished sounds
- Adventitious sounds: crackles, wheezes, rhonchi, pleural friction rub; note description, position in lung (½, ¼, bases), duration, timing
- Voice sounds generally muffled; note loudness, clarity, distortion

---

 Cardiovascular System Assessment

INSPECTION

- Chest pulsations, asymmetry, bulging, retractions, heaves
- Posture and positions of comfort
- Respirations: rate, depth, ease, relation to position and activity, presence of stridor or dyspnea; integrate with data from pulmonary system assessment
- Cyanosis of lips, lobes, nails, buccal mucosa
- Edema of face, eyelids, extremities, spinal base; reported rapid weight gain
- Tiring, avoidance pattern
- Sweating during activity/exertion; head, arms, torso concurrently cold feel

- Venous pulses in older child
- Clubbing of fingers, generally seen after 1 year of age

PALPATION

- Apical impulse for location, quality; point of maximum intensity
- All pulses bilaterally for carotid, radial, brachial, femoral, popliteal, posterior tibial, dorsalis pedis pulses; note rate (normally rapid with wide fluctuations), rhythm (regular), amplitude (full)
- Cardiac thrills, aortic bruit, pericardial friction rubs; note location and timing of thrills
- Rapid capillary refill time normally for 3 seconds or less

PERCUSSION

- Heart, lung, liver, spleen (location of each)

AUSCULTATION

- Elicited during quiet time when child is not crying and is cooperative or being distracted
- Brachial blood pressure, noting Korotkoff (K) sounds K1, K4, K5; take popliteal blood pressure one time
- Heart sounds in each auscultatory area (aortic, pulmonic, tricuspid, mitral): S1 and S2, splitting, other heart sounds (S3 and S4); note rate, rhythm, intensity
- Murmurs for location, timing in cardiac cycle, sound distribution, quality
- Ejection clicks, snaps, gallops, hum, friction rub

 # *Neurologic System Assessment*

INSPECTION

General
- Vital signs, including temperature
- Shape of head, head circumference, status of fontanels, transillumination of skull (generally a 2-cm flashlight halo over frontal and parietal areas, 1-cm halo over occipital area)
- Level of alertness, cry, behavior

- Facial expression, characteristics
- Pupil size, equality, reactivity, movement
- Body symmetry, muscle mass, position; spontaneous, induced, and adventitious movements
- Breathing pattern, rate, rhythm
- Condition of skin, hair, nails
- Soft signs such as clumsiness, short attention span

Motor function: bilateral and upper/lower comparison
- Muscular strength; movement of each joint through full range of motion, noting tone, spasticity, rigidity, flaccidity; degrees of resistance with active and passive exercises
- Posture, ability to support head and body weight; body tone
- Gait, coordination, balance
- Ability to crawl, walk, run, rise from supine position
- Gross and fine motor movements; progression through age-specific developmental tasks (see "Growth and Developmental Assessment," p. 31)

Sensory function
- Awareness of environment and reaction to/withdrawal from auditory and visual stimuli
- Uniformity of skin color, temperature
- Hearing, vision, temperature discrimination
- Ability to participate in testing for joint position, light touch and pain sensation, vibration, proprioception, tactile localization and discrimination after age 4 to 5 years

Mental function
- State of alertness or consciousness, reaction to stimuli
- Orientation, attention span
- Memory, cognition
- Judgment, mood, affect
- Handedness
- Progression through age-specific developmental tasks (see "Growth and Developmental Assessment," p. 31)

INFANT REFLEXES

The following reflexes are tested in each newborn:

- Rooting reflex: stroking infant's cheek at or near corners of mouth results in infant opening mouth and turning

head toward stroking. Upper lip stimulation results in head extension; lower lip, jaw drop. Reflex disappears at age 3 to 4 months.
- Palmar grasp reflex: placing of fingers or objects in infant's hand results in finger flexion and grasping of object. Reflex disappears at age 3 to 4 months.
- Moro's (startle) reflex: sudden loud noise or jarring results in abducting and extending of arms, opening of hands with finger flexion, and slight flexing and abducting of legs. Subsequent flexing and adducting of arms and crying. Reflex disappears at age 4 months.
- Tonic neck reflex: turning supine infant's head to one side over the shoulder results in fencing posture (extending of arm and leg to turned side while flexing opposing side). If not present at birth, reflex develops at age 2 months and disappears at age 4 to 6 months.

CRANIAL NERVE INNERVATION

I. Olfactory (smell): odor identification of familiar aroma such as peanut butter or coffee

II. Optic (vision): optic disc and retina examinations; visual fixation of light, letter, or symbol visual acuity test; peripheral vision

III. Oculomotor (pupillary reactions, extraocular movements): pupillary size and reactivity to light, accommodation, flow of eye movements, visual recognition, following of familiar objects, six cardinal fields of gaze

IV. Trochlear (extraocular movement): downward and inward movement of eyes

V. Trigeminal (jaw movement, facial sensation, corneal reflexes): chewing; ability to open and close jaw; grimacing in response to nostril stimulation with cotton tip; response to light touch of face, scalp, nasal and buccal mucosa; eye closure in response to touching cornea with cotton wisp

VI. Abducens (eye abduction): eye movement to temporal side; check for disconjugate gaze

VII. Facial (facial expressions, taste): symmetric smile, frown, eyebrow raising, taste discrimination of salt and sweets

VIII. Acoustic (hearing and balance): recognition and response to sound, Weber and Rinne tests for air and bone conduction, equilibrium

  IX. Glossopharyngeal (pharynx, posterior tongue): gag response to stimulation of posterior pharynx, taste at posterior tongue

   X. Vagus (pharynx, larynx, palate): check voice for hoarseness, gagging when back of throat is stimulated, midline rise of uvula when saying "oh," ability to swallow

  XI. Accessory (sternocleidomastoid and trapezius muscles): shoulder shrugging against mild resistance on command; turning head against resistance

 XII. Hypoglossal (tongue): child is asked to move tongue from side to side and to stick out tongue; note strength, symmetry of movement, deviation from midline

PALPATION

- Contour, symmetry, integrity of skull
- Size, bulging, concavity of fontanels (usually slightly depressed, pulsating)
- Closure of cranial sutures (anterior fontanel closes at approximately 18 months of age; posterior fontanel closes at approximately 6 to 8 weeks of age)
- Spinal contour, tenderness
- Commonly tested reflexes and responses

  Biceps (C5, C6)
  Patellar (L2, L3, L4)
  Achilles tendon (S1, S2)
  Plantar (L5, S1)

- Other reflexes

  Brudzinski's and Kernig's signs: suspected meningeal irritation
  Anal reflex: suspected spinal cord lesion

AUSCULTATION

- Blood pressure
- Intracranial, intraspinal bruits (generally benign in younger child)

Gastrointestinal System Assessment

INSPECTION

- Height, weight (use same scale and clothing at same time of day); relate to age, sex, frame
- Nutritional status, ease of feeding, normal regurgitation, vomiting and amount, characteristics; visible peristalsis; food diary
- Feeding: breast, bottle, self
- Integrity of oral cavity, defects, clefts, odor, dentition, caries, malocclusion, bleeding, stomatitis
- Skin turgor, pigmentation (including jaundice), ecchymosis, scarring, striae, expected superficial venous pattern, unusual hair distribution
- Abdominal size, symmetry, contour (usually protuberant when standing), tone
- Umbilical location, degree of stump healing in newborn, protrusion or herniation, inflammation, fistulas
- Abdominal distention, ascites, herniation, lesions, masses, organomegaly
- Aortic pulsations in epigastrium
- Presence of abdominal reflexes after 6 to 12 months of age (upper, T8, T9, T10; lower, T10, T11, T12)
- Stools, including amount, color, consistency
- Anal itching, inflammation, tearing, bleeding

AUSCULTATION

- Active bowel sounds in all four quadrants, including frequency (generally 10 to 30/min), pitch, loudness, characteristics such as rushing, tinkling, swishing, gurgling
- Suspect bowel sounds including hyperactivity, hypoacuity, bruits, hums, peritoneal friction rub

PERCUSSION

- Liver size and span
- Spleen size and span
- Shifting dullness of ascites
- Uterus in pregnant adolescent female

PALPATION

- Skin turgor
- Major organ sites for liver approximately 1 to 2 cm below right costal margin; spleen approximately 1 to 2 cm below left costal margin; kidneys may be palpable (tip of right kidney on inspiration)
- Light palpation for areas of tenderness (note change in facial expression, anticipatory guarding, pitch of cry), tone, rebound tenderness, fluid, masses
- Shifting dullness or fluid waves of ascites
- Deep palpation for masses, noting location, size, shape, mobility, consistency, tenderness
- Aortic pulsations and femoral pulses

 Nutritional Assessment

DIETARY HISTORY

Infant
- Estimated, actual birth dates
- Presence of rooting, sucking, swallowing, gag reflexes
- Birth weight, time to double and triple birth weight
- Caregiver's perception of infant's appetite
- If breast-fed:

  Frequency, interval, duration of feedings, latching on
  Degree and duration of infant satiety
  Use of complementary/supplementary feedings
  Use of iron supplementation
  Age at and duration of weaning

- If bottle-fed:

  Type and concentration of formula; observation of formula mixing
  Number of feedings per day, ounces consumed per feeding
  Length of time between feedings
  Availability of potable water, stove, refrigerator
  Formula preparation, milk storage, cleaning techniques
  Caregiver ability, willingness to prepare formula, handle utensils
  Prevalence of formula switching

- Type of feeding schedule (on demand, structured)
- Use of vitamin and mineral supplements (include iron and fluoride)
- Intake of additional fluids (plain or sweetened water, juice)
- Use of bottle propping; bottle during nap, bedtime
- Introduction of cow's milk, cereal, vegetables, fruit, meat, finger foods, table foods; use of additional salt, sugar, artificial sweeteners, honey, corn syrup
- Presence of food intolerances, allergic reactions; describe
- Evidence of underfeeding or overfeeding, vomiting, diarrhea, constipation, colic

Child
- Caregiver attitudes toward food and eating, child's appetite, weight; interactions during mealtime
- Amount of money spent on food, use of food assistance programs; primary shopper
- Child's age, feeding style (cup, spoon, assisted, unassisted)
- Food likes, dislikes
- Food diary to ascertain actual consumption; note all foods, beverages offered and consumed for 3 to 7 consecutive days; include all sources of nutrients as recommended in food guide pyramid, timing and regularity of meals and snacks, method of food preparation, ethnic/cultural/religious practices; note foods not included in diet, unusual intake (dirt, corn starch, paint chips)
- Use of vitamin and mineral supplements, including iron and fluoride
- Presence of food intolerances or allergies, resulting diet modifications
- Evidence of feeding/eating problems: physical disability, dental problems, toddler safety and assertion issues, obesity
- Family history of food/lifestyle-related illness: atherosclerosis, hypertension, cardiovascular disease, diabetes

CLINICAL EVALUATION
Clinical profile of well-nourished child
- Alert, responsive child; infant with vigorous cry
- Growth pattern within accepted parameters

- Clear, bright eyes
- Smooth, elastic skin
- Lustrous hair, not easily plucked
- Smooth, moist, pink mucous membranes

Anthropometric assessment
- Serial measurements of height/length, weight
- Head circumference of children 2 years of age or younger
- Skinfold thickness of children 5 years of age or older

Biochemical assessment
- Complete blood count, including hemoglobin and hematocrit, cholesterol, albumin, nitrogen, creatinine, amino acid screen
- Complete urinalysis

 Endocrine System Assessment

INSPECTION
- Vital signs, including blood pressure
- Height and weight: crown-to-pubis, pubis-to-heel length; serial measurements, deviations from expected growth trend
- Stature: relationship to family norm, skeletal proportions, noting especially shortness, fat distribution
- Increased head circumference, delayed fontanel closure
- Facial characteristics, structure, defects, symmetry, proportion, overgrowth, deviation in head-to-skull proportions, plethora, infantile features or signs of aging, moon facies, bulging eyes and wide-eyed, staring expression
- Dentition: delayed, atypical pattern, malocclusion, enlarged jaw, tongue thickening, breath odor
- Skin: pigmentation changes, yellow discoloration, decreased turgor, edema, dryness, oiliness, coarseness, ecchymosis, reddened abdominal striae
- Hair: sparsity or abnormal distribution, texture; nail texture, configuration
- Intolerance to room temperature or changes
- Sexual maturity: delayed, ambiguous, precocious

- Weakness, trembling, sweating
- Irritability, restlessness, emotional lability, apathy, crying and relief by water feedings, depression
- Twitching, poor coordination, carpopedal spasms, altered level of consciousness

PALPATION

- Fontanel closure
- Abdominal pain, acute or diffuse
- Muscle wasting, paresthesia of extremities
- Chvostek's sign and Trousseau's sign: positive in tetany
- Thyroid enlargement, symmetry, nodularity, mobility, tenderness, hoarseness (normally not easily examined)

Hematologic System Assessment

INSPECTION

- Vital signs: pyrexia, tachycardia
- General appearance: nutritional status, hydration
- Height, weight, delayed growth, delayed or absent puberty
- Stature, congenital anomalies, facial deformities
- Weakness, irritability, fatigue, activity, intolerances
- Skin color: pallor or jaundice, scleral icterus
- Condition of gums, tongue
- Nail texture and shape: especially thin, brittle, or spoon-shaped
- Inappropriate bleeding after minor trauma; spontaneous bleeding, ecchymosis, petechiae, epistaxis

PALPATION

- Size and span of liver and spleen
- Neck, axillary and inguinal lymph nodes for size (enlargement), tenderness, consistency, mobility, nodularity (generally not palpable)
- Joints for pain, heat, edema, limitation of motion

Musculoskeletal System Assessment

INSPECTION

- General appearance: symmetry, posture, position, contour, alignment, structural relationships; compare left and right; front and back
- Gross deformities, unusual posturing or positioning
- Ability to perform age-dependent activities: sit, stoop, stand, rise from supine to standing position, walk, run
- Gait, stride, balance, coordination, speed, endurance
- General mobility, spontaneity of movement, awkward/involuntary movement, lack of or self-limitation of movement, stiffness
- Tremors, spasms, fasciculations, weakness, paralysis
- Spinal curvature, generally C-shaped in infant, progressing to double-S configuration by 18 months of age; absence of masses
- Presence of scoliosis, kyphosis
- Spinal integrity, defects
- Presence on back of pitting or dimpling, hairy patches, altered pigmentation
- Extremities: size, proportion, symmetry
- Digits: number, configuration, deformities
- Active range of motion of all joints, degree of motion

PALPATION

- Muscles for development, mass, symmetry, strength, tone
- Passive range of motion of all joints, degree of deviation
- Joint edema, tenderness, redness, warmth, crepitus, clicking, masses
- Extremities for length, circumference
- Distances between knees and malleoli for genu varum, genu valgum
- Ortolani and Barlow maneuvers for signs of hip dislocations
- Trendelenberg test for signs of hip disease

Renal Urinary Systems Assessment

INSPECTION

- Vital signs: note blood pressure elevation, fever, tachycardia, tachypnea
- Weight trends: failure to gain, weight loss, failure to thrive, growth retardation
- Poor eating, vomiting, diarrhea
- Characteristics of urine (generally yellow, clear, and odorless), strength and direction of urinary stream
- Change in established elimination pattern, incontinence, enuresis
- Presence of oliguria, polyuria, polydipsia, hematuria; pain on urination
- Congenital anomalies and defects: nonrenal multisystem defects, genitourinary defects; abdominal tone
- Presence of genitourinary lesions, rashes, discharge, trauma, scarring
- Skin color: pallor, mottling, jaundice
- Dehydration: dry skin and mucous membranes, poor tissue turgor, sunken fontanels
- Edema: around eyes, face, hands, legs, feet, sacrum; presence of pitting, ascites
- Fatigue, malaise, lethargy, irritability, muscle weakness, cramps or carpopedal spasms, seizures, coma

PALPATION

- Normal kidney may be felt; note palpability, enlargement
- Abdominal, back, flank pain
- Abdominal tone

 Integumentary System Assessment

INSPECTION

- Skin color: note pigmentation, discoloration, redness, pallor, mottling, cyanosis, jaundice, bronzing; vascular lesions,

petechiae; concurrent assessment of lips, tongue, buccal mucosa, sclera, conjunctiva, nails
- Vascularity, vascular lesions, petechiae, ecchymosis, bleeding
- General temperature, local redness, sunburn
- Dryness, oiliness, edema, diaphoresis, urticaria, peeling, scaling, crusting
- Integrity: note developmental defects, ulcers, fissures, excoriation, erosion, infection, incisions, burns, bites, needle marks, scars
- Cleanliness, odor, exudate, infestation
- Rashes, exudates, vesicles, bullae
- Acne, pustules, cellulitis
- Lesions: note size, shape, pattern, distribution
- Nails: note color, contour, integrity, angle, cleanliness, infection; presence of spooning, clubbing
- Hair quantity, texture, distribution, luster, elasticity, brittleness, oiliness/dryness, color, pubertal changes, cleanliness, lice infestation
- Any transient, temporary, permanent changes

PALPATION

- Triceps skinfold thickness measurement
- Skin temperature, texture
- Skin turgor, atrophy, wrinkling, tenting
- Lesion palpability, firmness, mobility
- Nail texture and adherence to nail plate

 Eye, Ear, Nose, and Throat Assessment

INSPECTION

- General appearance, craniofacial anomalies, use of corrective lenses or hearing aid, responses to visual or auditory stimuli, equilibrium, speech characteristics and difficulty with phonation, ease of sucking/feeding and swallowing, evidence of facial paralysis or trauma, irritability
- Ease of respirations, mouth or nose breather, effect of crying on respiration, hoarseness, cough

- Frequent blinking, squinting, photophobia, nystagmus; rubbing or pulling at ears
- Symmetry and congruity of brows, lids, eyes, nose, ears
- Placement and alignment of eyes, symmetry, spacing, protrusion or retraction, movement
- Lid symmetry, position, ability to completely close, palpebral slant and epicanthal folds, edema, ptosis, masses, condition of eyelashes and direction of hair growth
- Lacrimal puncta: moisture or dryness of eyes, erythema, edema, itching, pain
- Conjunctival and scleral color; vascularity; markings and color of iris
- Cornea: symmetry of reflected light, opacity, ulceration, abrasions, foreign bodies, scarring
- Pupil size, shape, direct and consensual reactivity, movement (PERRLA, *p*upils *e*qual, *r*ound, *r*eact to *l*ight and *a*ccomodation, is the accepted acronym for the normal pupillary finding)
- Visual acuity, peripheral vision, extraocular motility, color acumen; visualization of red light reflex
- External ear: note size, symmetry, deformities, thermal injury, trauma
- Top of pinna, alignment with lateral corner of eye
- Ear canal: note color, discharge, edema, odor, foreign bodies, pain
- Tympanic membrane: note color, integrity, cone of light and bony landmarks, tension, thickness, vascularity
- Hearing acuity
- Nasal patency; nose shape, symmetry, deformities, lesions; septal alignment, integrity; presence of discharge, bleeding, flaring, lesions, foreign bodies, trauma
- Olfactory acuity
- Lips: note color, crying, cracking, ulceration, edema, induration, lesion
- Buccal integrity; architecture for color, texture, moisture, edema, exudate, bleeding; tongue mobility, deviation; gag reflex, taste discernment
- Color and condition of gums; number, distribution, condition of teeth; alignment of jaw; mouth odor

PALPATION

- Nose for structure, deformities, fractures
- Frontal and maxillary sinuses for tenderness
- Temporomandibular joint for crepitus, pain
- Auricles for masses, pain
- Weber and Rinne tests for testing of air and bone conduction in hearing

 ## Psychologic Assessment

The psychosocial development of the child is based on a dynamic and complex interaction of internal (psychic) and external (environmental) factors. Biologic influences are integral, as are growth, development, and maturation. Table 1 outlines prominent conceptual models of childhood development. It is important to note that no single model encompasses all aspects of social, behavioral, emotional, and cognitive development.

 ## Bonding Assessment

PARENTAL HISTORY

- Upbringing, attitudes
- Family relationships, experiences
- Ethnic/cultural practices
- Social/economic status
- Support systems
- Communication skills
- Caregiving abilities
- Emotional/physical health
- Number of past pregnancies and experiences
- Expectations from child
- Influences of pregnancy on personal goals, career aspirations

Table 1　Conceptual Models of Childhood Development

Stage	Infancy	Toddler	Early Childhood (Preschool)	Middle Childhood (School-age)	Adolescent
Age (Years)	0-1	1-3	3-6	6-12	12-18
Significant Other	Mother or mother substitute	Parents or parental substitutes	Extended family	Neighborhood, school, community	Peers, leadership models
Crisis Stage (Erikson)	Trust vs. mistrust	Autonomy vs. shame and doubt	Initiative vs. guilt	Industry vs. inferiority	Intimacy vs. isolation
Psychosexual Stage (Freud)	Oral/sensory Oral activities greatest source of pleasure Id orientation	Anal/muscular Focus on anal sphincter control Persistent id orientation; beginning ego development	Phallic/Oedipal/locomotion Focus on sexual differences and similarities; sexual complexes and anxiety Emerging superego	Latent Focus on expanded skill development; sexual dormancy	Genital Focus on sexuality and relationships
Intellectual Stage (Piaget)	Sensorimotor (approximately 0-2 years)	Preoperational (approximately 2-4 years)	Preoperational (approximately 4-7 years)	Concrete operational (approximately 7-11 years)	Formal operational

Reflexive experiences with progression to response modification, intentional activity, manipulation of environment Information through trial and error, assimilation	Egocentric, concrete thought Use of symbols Singularity of focus Transductive reasoning	Perceptual intuitive stage Invariance of physical properties Prelogical reasoning	Experientially based problem solving Generalization from concrete logical operations Objective thought Inductive reasoning	Abstract thought, reasoning Systematic problem solving
Moral Development Stage (Kohlberg)	Preconventional Punishment and obedience orientation Morality based on consequences of activity	Preconventional Naive, hedonistic orientation Morality based on satisfaction of needs	Conventional "Good boy, good girl" orientation Law and order orientation Based on approval of others, compliance with authority figures	Postconventional Social contract orientation Based on greater good, altruism

Continued.

Table 1   *Conceptual Models of Childhood Development – cont'd*

Stage	Infancy	Toddler	Early Childhood (Preschool)	Middle Childhood (School-age)	Adolescent
Developmental Tasks	Reflexive activity; sensorimotor exploration; emotional and physical dependence on mother; pleasure principle; developing basis for trust and self image	Beginning of pleasure postponement; self-assertion; skill testing; learning to walk, talk, self-feed, control elimination; identification of gender; awareness of	Increased family interactions; cooperative play with peers; increased motor activity; increased vocabulary; beginning to read, count; interest in physical world; use of fa...	Increased cognitive growth: read, write, calculate; increased motor coordination, physical skills; increased socialization; same sex peer/play groups; development of	Establishment of individuality, personality; marked peer influences; emotional independence from family; sexual maturation; preparation or selection of ca-

	sex stereotypes	... iors	self and social groups; sex role identity	
Response to Illness/ Hospitalization	Physiologic irritation; crying Stranger anxiety, delayed bonding	Separation anxiety, escalating from crying to withdrawal to detachment Fear of procedures Increased dependency on caregiver Regressive behaviors	Separation anxiety Refusal to eat; sleep disruption Magical thinking Guilt associated with perceived past bad behavior	Anger, irritability, loneliness, boredom associated with physical restrictions, inactivity Guilt associated with impact of illness on family	Anger, boredom, and frustration associated with dependency and physical restrictions Possible greater dependence on caregiver, isolation

PRENATAL BONDING
- Pleasure derived from fetal movements, development
- Name selection
- Nesting behaviors (preparing home for infant's arrival)

INFLUENCING FACTORS
- Length/severity of labor, type of delivery
- Condition of mother and infant at birth
- Opportunity to greet, touch, handle newborn

BONDING BEHAVIORS
- Claiming processes: identification of infant's physical characteristics with other family members, awareness of infant's uniqueness as an individual, incorporation of individual into family structure; parental comparison of infant with average child
- Eye contact: degree of satisfaction derived from and amount of time spent gazing and exploring; lack/avoidance of eye contact and substitute behaviors
- Touch: performance of typical postdelivery inventory, including fingertip exploration of head, hands, feet; caressing of trunk, enfolding in arms; amount/type of body contacts; ease in handling infant; body part(s) focused on or avoided
- Communication: welcoming responses, use of infant's name; amount of face-to-face contact; displays of affection such as smiling, stroking; time spent talking to infant, tone of voice; use of slow, repetitive, rhythmic speech; mimicry of infant's expressions; slowed exaggeration of own expressions
- Caretaking: readiness and ability to protect, care for, nurture infant; speed, reliability, consistency of responses to infant's cues; amount of time spent with infant; facility with aspects of physical care; disdain or reluctance to bathe, diaper infant
- Consoling: immediacy of response to infant's cry, fussiness, irritability; measures used to console such as holding, rocking, crooning

CUES TO IMPAIRED PARENTING
- Marked delay in naming infant
- Disinterest

- Refusal to see or care for infant
- Unrealistic concerns/expectations about infant
- Blaming infant for circumstances surrounding birth
- Name calling
- Unsafe handling

CUES TO IMPAIRED INFANT ATTACHMENT

- Altered social responsiveness such as decreased smiling, vocalizing, playfulness; absence of exclusive primary emotional relationship, dislike of being held; passivity, fearfulness
- Altered affect such as inability to express feelings, lack of exuberance
- Delayed progression through developmental tasks in absence of physiologic dysfunction

 # Growth and Developmental Assessment

All assessments should be documented, preferably on standardized graphs or forms. Typical measurements taken during a well-child examination include the following:

Length/height (Tables 2 and 3), height velocity
Weight (see Tables 2 and 3), somatotype
Patency and condition of fontanels (in infant)
Head circumference (Fig. 1), chest circumference
Hearing and vision screenings
Dentition (Fig. 2)
General nutritional status
Muscle mass, body fat
Sexual maturity
Developmental maturation of gross motor, language, fine motor/adaptive, personal/social skills (see Denver II on inside back cover)

Table 2   *Height and Weight Measurements for Boys*

	Height by Percentiles						Weight by Percentiles					
	5		50		95		5		50		95	
Age*	cm	in	cm	in	cm	in	kg	lb	kg	lb	kg	lb
Birth	46.4	18¼	50.5	20	54.4	21½	2.54	5½	3.27	7¼	4.15	9¼
3 mo	56.7	22¼	61.1	24	65.4	25¾	4.43	9¾	5.98	13¼	7.37	16¼
6 mo	63.4	25	67.8	26¾	72.3	28½	6.20	13¾	7.85	17¼	9.46	20¾
9 mo	68.0	26¾	72.3	28½	77.1	30¼	7.52	16½	9.18	20¼	10.93	24
1	71.7	28¼	76.1	30	81.2	32	8.43	18½	10.15	22½	11.99	26½
1½	77.5	30½	82.4	32½	88.1	34¾	9.59	21¼	11.47	25¼	13.44	29½
2†	82.5	32½	86.8	34¼	94.4	37¼	10.49	23¼	12.34	27¼	15.50	34¼
2½†	85.4	33½	90.4	35½	97.8	38½	11.27	24¾	13.52	29¾	16.61	36½
3	89.0	35	94.9	37¼	102.0	40¼	12.05	26½	14.62	32¼	17.77	39¼
3½	92.5	36½	99.1	39	106.1	41¾	12.84	28¼	15.68	34½	18.98	41¾
4	95.8	37¾	102.9	40½	109.9	43¼	13.64	30	16.69	36¾	20.27	44¾
4½	98.9	39	106.6	42	113.5	44¾	14.45	31¾	17.69	39	21.63	47¾
5	102.0	40¼	109.9	43¼	117.0	46	15.27	33¾	18.67	41¼	23.09	51
6	107.7	42½	116.1	45¾	123.5	48½	16.93	37¼	20.69	45½	26.34	58
7	113.0	44½	121.7	48	129.7	51	18.64	41	22.85	50¼	30.12	66½

8	118.1	46½	127.0	50	135.7	53½	20.40	45	25.30	55¾	34.51	76
9	122.9	48½	132.2	52	141.8	55¾	22.25	49	28.13	62	39.58	87¼
10	127.7	50¼	137.5	54¼	148.1	58¼	24.33	53¾	31.44	69¼	45.27	99¾
11	132.6	52¼	143.3	56½	154.9	61	26.80	59	35.30	77¾	51.47	113½
12	137.6	54¼	149.7	59	162.3	64	29.85	65¾	39.78	87¾	58.09	128
13	142.9	56¼	156.5	61½	169.8	66¾	33.64	74¼	44.95	99	65.02	143¼
14	148.8	58½	163.1	64¼	176.7	69½	38.22	84¼	50.77	112	72.13	159
15	155.2	61	169.0	66½	181.9	71½	43.11	95	56.71	125	79.12	174½
16	161.1	63½	173.5	68¼	185.4	73	47.74	105¼	62.10	137	85.62	188¾
17	164.9	65	176.2	69¼	187.3	73¾	51.50	113½	66.31	146¼	91.31	201¼
18	165.7	65¼	176.8	69½	187.6	73¾	53.97	119	68.88	151¾	95.76	211

Modified from National Center for Health Statistics (NCHS), Health Resources Administration, Department of Health, Education and Welfare, Hyattsville, Md. Conversion of metric data to approximate inches and pounds by Ross Laboratories.

*Years, unless otherwise indicated.

†Height data include some recumbent length measurements, which make values slightly higher than if all measurements had been of stature (standing height).

Table 3   *Height and Weight Measurements for Girls*

Age*	Height by Percentiles						Weight by Percentiles					
	5		50		95		5		50		95	
	cm	in	cm	in	cm	in	kg	lb	kg	lb	kg	lb
Birth	45.4	17¾	49.9	19¾	52.9	20¾	2.36	5¼	3.23	7	3.81	8½
3 mo	55.4	21¾	59.5	23½	63.4	25	4.18	9¼	5.4	12	6.74	14¾
6 mo	61.8	24¼	65.9	26	70.2	27¾	5.79	12¾	7.21	16	8.73	19¼
9 mo	66.1	26	70.4	27¾	75.0	29½	7.0	15½	8.56	18¾	10.17	22½
1	69.8	27½	74.3	29¼	79.1	31¼	7.84	17¼	9.53	21	11.24	24¾
1½	76.0	30	80.8	31¾	86.1	34	8.92	19¾	10.82	23¾	12.76	28¼
2†	81.6	32¼	86.8	34¼	93.6	36¾	9.95	22	11.8	26	14.15	31¼
2½†	84.6	33¼	90.0	35½	96.6	38	10.8	23¾	13.03	28¾	15.76	34¾
3	88.3	34¾	94.1	37	100.6	39½	11.61	25½	14.1	31	17.22	38
3½	91.7	36	97.9	38½	104.5	41¼	12.37	27¼	15.07	33¼	18.59	41
4	95.0	37½	101.6	40	108.3	42¾	13.11	29	15.96	35¼	19.91	44
4½	98.1	38½	105.0	41¼	112.0	44	13.83	30½	16.81	37	21.24	46¾
5	101.1	39¾	108.4	42¾	115.6	45½	14.55	32	17.66	39	22.62	49¾
6	106.6	42	114.6	45	122.7	48¼	16.05	35½	19.52	43	25.75	56¾
7	111.8	44	120.6	47½	129.5	51	17.71	39	21.84	48¼	29.68	65½

8	116.9	46	126.4	49¾	136.2	53½	19.62	43¼	24.84	54¾	34.71	76½
9	122.1	48	132.2	52	142.9	56¼	21.82	48	28.46	62¾	40.64	89½
10	127.5	50¼	138.3	54½	149.5	58¾	24.36	53¾	32.55	71¾	47.17	104
11	133.5	52½	144.8	57	156.2	61½	27.24	60	36.95	81½	54.0	119
12	139.8	55	151.5	59¾	162.7	64	30.52	67¼	41.53	91½	60.81	134
13	145.2	57¼	157.1	61¾	168.1	66¼	34.14	75¼	46.1	101¾	67.3	148¼
14	148.7	58½	160.4	63¼	171.3	67½	37.76	83¼	50.28	110¾	73.08	161
15	150.5	59¼	161.8	63¾	172.8	68	40.99	90¼	53.68	118¼	77.78	171½
16	151.6	59¾	162.4	64	173.3	68¼	43.41	95¾	55.89	123¼	80.99	178½
17	152.7	60	163.1	64¼	173.5	68¼	44.74	98¾	56.69	125	82.46	181¾
18	153.6	60½	163.7	64½	173.6	68¼	45.26	99¾	56.62	124¾	82.47	181¾

Modified from National Center for Health Statistics (NCHS), Health Resources Administration, Department of Health, Education and Welfare, Hyattsville, Md. Conversion of metric data to approximate inches and pounds by Ross Laboratories.

*Years, unless otherwise indicated.

†Height data include some recumbent length measurements, which make values slightly higher than if all measurements had been of stature (standing height).

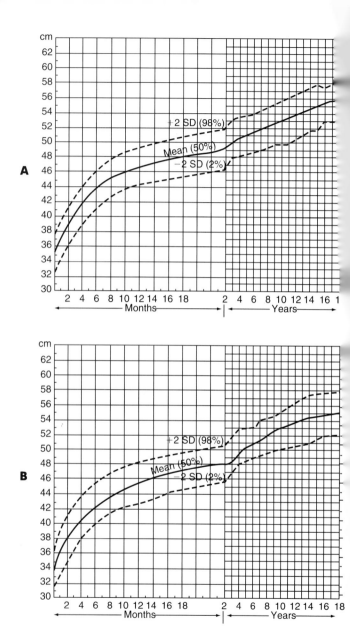

Fig. 1 A, Head circumference chart for boys. B, Head circumference chart for girls. (From Nellhaus G: Composite international and interracial graphs, *Petiatrics* 41:106, 1968.)

Environmental Assessment

GENERAL

- Type of home: private, apartment, condominium, multiple dwelling, trailer, shelter; number of rooms
- Number of floors, steps; accessibility of stairs, elevators; presence of fire escape, functioning fire extinguisher; fire escape plan
- Number of families/occupants; adequacy of sleeping arrangements, toilet facilities, bathing facilities
- Availability of potable, running water, electricity, heating/cooling systems, laundry facilities; use of refrigerator, stove
- General cleanliness of house, environment
- Safe space for medical equipment/supplies
- Presence of environmental hazards: chipped paint, insects/rodents, poor sanitation/faulty waste disposal, pollution
- Type of home security: locks/bars on windows, doors; electronic surveillance; security guards
- Structural modifications: ramp access to home, widened doorways, power failure alarm systems
- Use of secure screens; window safety guards; gaurds around heaters, radiators, fireplaces; smoke, heat, carbon monoxide detectors; electric outlet caps; garage door openers safety features
- Evidence of proper lighting, clear and dry pathways, secured rugs
- Nearest telephone: posted numbers of emergency service, poison control center, nearest hospital or health care facility, location of major intersection
- Presence of pets, amount of handling, immunization status
- Proximity to street; availability of a secure, fenced play area; locked, fenced pool area
- Caregiver knowledge of safety adaptations based on child's developmental stage, locale, season; knowledge of cardiopulmonary resuscitation, first aid
- Caregiver's protective and nurturing responses to child, coping abilities
- Caregiver modeling of safety behaviors

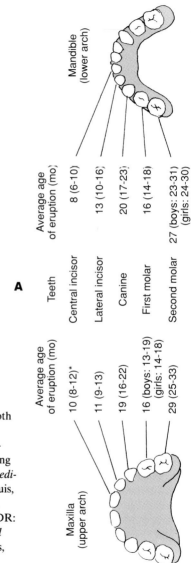

Average age of eruption (mo)	Teeth	Average age of eruption (mo)
10 (8-12)*	Central incisor	8 (6-10)
11 (9-13)	Lateral incisor	13 (10-16)
19 (16-22)	Canine	20 (17-23)
16 (boys: 13-19) (girls: 14-18)	First molar	16 (14-18)
29 (25-33)	Second molar	27 (boys: 23-31) (girls: 24-30)

Maxilla (upper arch)

Mandible (lower arch)

A

Fig. 2 Sequence of tooth eruption and shedding. **A,** Primary teeth. **B,** Secondary teeth. (From Wong DL: *Clinical manual of pediatric nursing,* ed 4, St Louis, 1996, Mosby [Data from MacDonald RE, Avery DR: *Dentistry for the child and adolescent,* ed 6, St Louis, 1994, Mosby].)

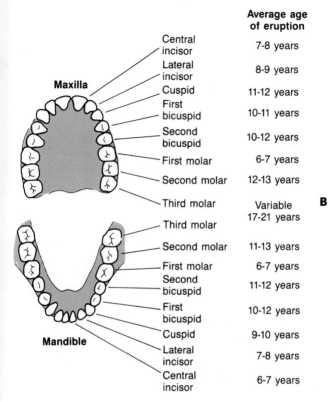

Fig. 2—cont'd

SPECIFIC

Preventing burns

- Keep matches and lighters out of reach of children
- Keep all hot objects or open flames away from children
- Disconnect smaller appliances when not in use
- Do not use gas stove or oven for heating
- Do not overload electric system; replace frayed or broken electric cords or wires
- Keep crib or bed away from radiators or heaters
- Use flame retardant/resistant clothing, bedding, toys
- Set water heater temperature to 120° F (49° C) or below

- Do not hold child when cooking, handling, consuming hot foods or liquids
- Turn pot handles toward back of stove; use back burners
- Avoid tablecloths with hanging edges
- Keep kitchen entry closed or gated
- Secure garage doors

Preventing choking, aspiration, suffocation, strangulation
- Use cribs conforming to federal guidelines with snug-fitting mattress; hang mobiles, toys out of child's reach; do not use soft bedding or fluffy bed clothes; position baby during sleep on back or side; use bunk beds that conform to government guidelines
- Position crib or bed away from other furniture, windows, draperies; tie drapery or blind cords high, cut short, use blind cord safety tassels
- Do not use accordion-style gates; secure playpens in up-right position when in use
- Securely close or lock doors or hinged objects of all kinds as appropriate (e.g., appliances, toys)
- Keep plastic bags away from children; discard after tying in knots
- Do not tie anything, including pacifiers, around infant's/child's neck
- Place monitor cords under clothing
- Remove loose, small, breakable parts from clothing and toys; firmly secure or remove drawstring in clothing; keep all small objects away from children
- Restrict finger foods to soft, noncylindric variety; do not allow running or playing when eating
- Never leave child unattended when bathing or playing in/near water
- Empty pails, pet's deep water bowls, wading pools when not in use
- Empty tub and sink when not in use; keep toilet lid down, bathroom door closed
- Establish emergency backup plan with power and telephone companies, emergency medical service, equipment provider in case of power failure (for child on ventilator, with oxygen pump or monitors); have extra fuses, batteries available

Preventing poisoning
- Store all toxic substances out of child's reach
- Keep all medicines out of reach, in original containers, in childproof containers; use only as directed
- Keep a 30-ml (1-ounce) bottle of syrup of ipecac on hand; check expiration date regularly

Preventing injury
- Keep crib sides up; do not leave child unattended when crib sides are down/changing table is in use
- Use approved car restraints; use appropriate restraints in high chairs, walkers, shopping carts; do not leave child unattended
- Do not use wheeled toys/walkers near stairs/driveways
- Keep all sharp objects out of child's reach
- Keep firearms unloaded; keep weapons, ammunition locked up and out of child's reach
- Use protective helmet, appropriate padding when cycling, skating
- Keep car doors locked; never leave child alone in car under any circumstances
- Teach road, traffic safety
- Enroll teenagers in driver's education course

 Family Assessment

ASSESSMENT FACTORS
- Composition: names, dates of birth, ages, relationships
- Configuration: nuclear, extended, blended/reconstituted, single parent, homosexual, communal, migrant, homeless
- Developmental stage: marriage; families with infants, pre-schoolers, school-age children, adolescents; launching centers, middle-age and aging families, termination
- Occupation: type of employment, principal wage earner, job security, adequacy of income, benefits, alternate source of income and services, expenditures, obligations, expectations
- Education: current status, highest educational level attained, aspirations

- Interactions

  Roles, functions, relationships, hierarchies
  Responsibilities, rules
  Communication styles, channels
  Emotional climate; cohesiveness, affection
  Boundary definition, flexibility
  Decision making, problem solving, behavior control
  Social networks, support groups
  Opportunities for personal growth
  Community involvement/interactions: religious, legal,
      educational, social services, governmental

- Coping

  Perception of stressors
  Emotional history, coping strategies
  Adaptation to life transitions
  Adaptation to crises, acute illness
  Resources, support systems

CULTURAL ASSESSMENT

- Ethnicity, culture, religion, race
- Country of origin, length of time in country, group identi-
  fied with
- Customs, values, beliefs, mores
- Role of family, children, elderly; impact of gender
- Primary language, ability to speak/write English
- Spatial, temporal perceptions
- Food preferences, traditions, subscriptions, restrictions
- Information processing
- Emotional expressiveness
- Physiologic determinants, susceptibility, predisposition to
  health problems
- Health practices, beliefs

 Financial Assessment

FAMILY RESOURCES AND REQUIREMENTS

- Income: salary, primary, and auxiliary wage earners, income fluctuations, benefits, allotments, retirement funds,

public assistance; impact of illness on employment and finances, family stability; ability to manage and prioritize finances
- Expenditures: percentage of income spent on housing, food, utilities, insurance, education, transportation, clothing, health care, recreation, loans, credit cards, savings/investments, gifts/donations
- Extraordinary health care expenses: insurance deductibles/copayments; recurrent hospital, outpatient, pharmacy bills; services of health care professionals, emergency services, transportation to health care facilities; home repair/remodeling to accomodate needs of child; rented/purchased medical equipment, supplies; increased utility bills related to use of specialized equipment; medications; prescribed feeding formulas or diet
- Home health care services: skilled nursing, medical social work, physical therapy, speech therapy, respiratory therapy, occupational therapy, pharmacy and infusion therapy, nursing assistant/home health aide service, counseling; respite care

FUNDING FOR HOME HEALTH SERVICES

- Private health insurance: extent of home health care may be limited by terms and conditions of specific policy, exclusion of preexisting conditions, covered or limited services, ceilings on benefits, stop-loss provisions; reimbursements for home health services may be offered by some insurers if home health costs are lower than in-hospital costs (individual case management)
- Managed care groups: health maintenance organizations (HMOs), preferred provider organizations (PPOs), competitive medical plans—greater emphasis on health promotion and disease prevention; provision of home health services may be limited
- Department of Defense: benefits to dependents of active duty, retired military personnel through Civilian Health and Medical Program of the Uniformed Services. Tricare, a restructuring of military health care system, is currently being phased in, with full implementation planned for 1997. Dependents of active duty, retired military personnel will be eligible for selected health care plans.

All military hospitals, clinics will be combined. Regional military health care centers will provide care with contracting civilian providers

- Children with Special Health Care Needs (Title V): services for children with chronic health problems
- Medicaid, its waivers and amendments, Comprehensive Care Program for children less than 21 years of age: based on income, disability criteria; covered, reimbursable services are defined by federal and state regulations — criteria include homebound client status, medical necessity, financial need; eligibility, benefits vary widely among states
- Health Savings Accounts: alternative to HMOs and PPOs, whereby health care consumer puts aside, tax-free, a proportion of income in anticipation of extraordinary health care costs; permits consumer to shop for best and most affordable provider
- Other: state and local departments of health, social services, education; disease oriented national associations, voluntary agencies, community and religious organizations, private foundations

Note: Most funding is limited and insufficient to meet the individual's need for ongoing or long-term care. Personal resources are quickly depleted. No single source of funds exists. Funding is a complex, time-consuming, and frequently frustrating maneuver. It requires a health care professional to assess, initiate, and coordinate services.

Care Plans

Maternal care

 Postpartum Period

The postpartum period, the puerperium, begins after the third stage of labor (i.e., placental separation and expulsion) and lasts approximately 6 weeks after delivery. It is characterized by a gradual reversal of the anatomic and physiologic adaptations of pregnancy. The involutional process and its attending psychologic and emotional components have been designated the fourth trimester. The most common complications include hemorrhage, infection, and thromboembolic disease. Hospital discharge of a woman who has a low-risk pregnancy and vaginally delivers a full-term, healthy infant occurs approximately 24 hours after delivery. Women who have delivered full-term, healthy infants by cesarean section are discharged approximately 48 hours after delivery. In the absence of problems, generally, only one or two postpartum home visits are made: one visit 24 hours after discharge and possibly a second visit 1 week later; alternatively, there may be one home visit with telephone follow-up, depending on the client's health care plan. Follow-up health care is provided in outpatient settings and physicians' offices.

Home care is primarily concerned with assessment of the puerpera to monitor involutional status, identification, and resolution of existing or potential problems of the puerpera, the newborn, or the mother's and newborn's environment and with teaching maternal self-care and infant care. Home care provides physical care and emotional and educational support and facilitates family-infant attachments.

Nursing diagnosis

Risk for injury
Related factors: involution of uterus and of placental site;

multisystem changes predominantly in genitourinary, endocrine, renal, cardiovascular systems; lactation; relaxation of pelvic musculature, abdominal wall

Defining characteristics: contracted uterus decreasing in size, early diuresis, lochial secretions, breast engorgement, secretion of colostrum

OUTCOMES

Short-term
Prevention of injury evidenced by pattern of normal involution (i.e., firm, contracted uterus descending midline into true pelvis) (1 to 2 weeks), lochial secretions progressing from rubra to serosa to alba, secretion of colostrum, breast engorgement, resolution (expected within 4 to 15 days, individual times vary)

Long-term
Maintenance of optimal health, without injury, evidenced by uncomplicated puerperium, return of menses in non-breastfeeding mother, establishment of lactation in breastfeeding mother (approximately 72 hours) (expected in 2 to 6 weeks, individual times vary)

NURSING INTERVENTIONS/INSTRUCTIONS

1. Assess general well-being and perception of health. Instruct client on anticipated postpartum course, including those signs and symptoms that require contacting physician for immediate intervention. Cluster information so it is most meaningful to client (each visit).
2. Perform complete physical assessment, including fundal height and consistency (each visit).
3. Assess and query regarding lochial secretions. Instruct on anticipated course of secretory activity and on perineal care (each visit).
4. Assess for perineal pain; check perineum for increased erythema, tenseness, ecchymosis, bulging, and type of discharge. Instruct client on pain relief measures (each visit).
5. If client has had a cesarean section, assess incision for erythema, ecchymosis, edema, approximation of wound edges, discharge, infection, and status of sutures or clips.

Instruct client on wound care and on returning, as applicable, to health care for suture removal (per physician's directive, this may be done in home by nurse) (each visit).

6. Take vital signs. Demonstrate and instruct client on temperature taking. Instruct client on signs and symptoms of common infection sites (i.e., cesarean section incision, episiotomy, lacerations, genitourinary system, breast). Report deviations from normal to physician (each visit).

7. Assess renal function, including recent bladder intubation. Instruct client in expected diuresis of early postpartum period (each visit).

8. Assess breasts. Note tenderness, nodularity, engorgement, discomfort, and colostrum secretion. Instruct client on pain relief measures and management of milk production (each visit).

9. Review client history of thromboembolic disease and prolonged immobility. Assess for bilateral calf size, temperature, color, tenderness, pulses, paresthesias, shortness of breath, and chest pain. Notify physician of existing problem (each visit).

CAREGIVER/CHILD AND FAMILY INTERVENTIONS

1. Correctly identifies course of lochial flow (i.e., from rubra, serosa, alba). Reports excessive clots or bright red bleeding to physician.

2. Takes 20-minute sitz bath with water temperature of 100° to 110° F (37.8° to 43.3° C) daily after bowel evacuation and as needed. Applies topical anesthetic spray to perineum afterward. Tenses gluteal muscles before sitting. Takes acetaminophen or nonsteroidal anti-inflammatory drug for pain, as ordered by physician. Reports severe or increasing pain.

3. Keeps abdominal operative site clean and dry. Showers as desired and gently dries site. Immediately reports discharge, increased redness, or swelling. Returns to physician for suture removal, per directive, and schedules follow-up postpartum visits.

4. Demonstrates correct temperature taking and reports increased temperature, constitutional symptoms, and signs and symptoms of infection.

5. Reports urgency, frequency, or dysuria (hematuria not included because it may be difficult to differentiate between hematuria and urine contaminated with lochial secretions). Performs perineal care after elimination, wipes from front to back, and uses fresh pad.
6. Nonlactating client controls breast discomfort by wearing well-fitted bra at all times, applying ice packs to engorged breasts, avoiding breast stimulation, and taking prescribed analgesics (commonly codeine with aspirin or acetaminophen every 4 hours).
7. Lactating client controls breast discomfort by wearing well-fitted bra at all times, taking warm showers, massaging breasts, taking acetaminophen every 4 hours as needed, and putting infant to breast every 2 to 3 hours.

Nursing diagnosis

Knowledge deficit
Related factors: early hospital discharge, lack of readiness to learn, inadequate/insufficient prenatal instruction, lack of experience, absence of role model, energies focused on infant care and family concerns, lack of help/support
Defining characteristics: expresses concerns about self-care

OUTCOMES
Short-term
Adequate knowledge evidenced by puerpera's ability to identify learning strengths/deficits and to identify measures to facilitate return to desired health status (expected in 1 week)

Long-term
Adequate knowledge evidenced by resumption of life-enhancing, satisfying activities (expected in 6 weeks)

NURSING INTERVENTIONS/INSTRUCTIONS
1. Assess client's readiness to learn, learning style, ethnic or cultural background, coping mechanisms, family support systems, and participation (each visit).

2. Assess complaints and nonverbal cues of fatigue. Note sleep, rest, and activity patterns. Instruct client on normalcy of fatigue response, scheduling of activities, and inclusion of family members for assistance and support (each visit).
3. Assess for predelivery and current bowel function. Instruct client on bowel regimen, including diet, hydration, and toilet habits (each visit).
4. Assess prepregnant, ideal, and current weights and client's expectation of loss. Instruct client on dietary needs, depending on breastfeeding status (each visit).
5. Assess level of activity and exercise/activity tolerance, immediate plans for employment or education, range of activities permitted, and degree of family participation in household chores and child care (each visit).
6. Assess family planning. If home visit is made after first or second postpartum week, query when (not if) sexual relations were resumed. Instruct client on resumption of menses, need for family planning, and importance of postpartum examination (each visit).

CAREGIVER/CHILD AND FAMILY INTERVENTIONS

1. Recognizes it may take weeks to regain previous energy level. Paces activities; takes rest periods during day when infant sleeps. Enlists support and participation of child's father, siblings, and significant others in home management and child care.
2. Verbalizes regimen to facilitate bowel evacuation: well-balanced diet high in fiber, adequate hydration, exercise, and time to toilet. Uses stool softeners as prescribed. Relieves hemorrhoidal pain by taking warm sitz baths after evacuation and as needed and by applying witch hazel compresses, corticosteroid suppositories, or anesthetic creams.
3. Nonlactating client resumes a regular diet. Lactating client modifies diet to include an additional 600 calories, 20 g of which are protein, and calcium; drinks to quench thirst, not excessively. Well-balanced weight-loss programs may be initiated. Takes vitamin and mineral supplements as recommended. Sees nutritionist for long-term diet maintenance.

4. With physician's approval, performs abdominal exercises as soon as tolerated, (any time after vaginal delivery and after soreness has disappeared with cesarean sections). Performs perineal strengthening Kegel exercises. Resumes full activities such as bathing, climbing stairs, cleaning, driving, using internal body cues to stop and rest. Resumes employment, preferably no earlier than 6 weeks after delivery.
5. Schedules postpartum physician or clinic visit. Identifies family planning method selected.

Nursing diagnosis

Parental role conflict
Related factors: stress of pregnancy and delivery; young maternal age; parity; marital status; strained relationship; interrupted employment, career, or school
Defining characteristics: expresses ambiguity or confusion over parental role; expresses concerns or feelings of inadequacy regarding child care; inability, unwillingness to modify lifestyle; reluctance to participate in child care

OUTCOMES
Short-term
Adequate parenting evidenced by increasing frequency of attachment behaviors and participation in child care (expected in 1 to 3 weeks)

Long-term
Role acceptance evidenced by verbalization of feelings of adequacy and demonstration of nurturing behaviors (expected in 1 to 2 months)

NURSING INTERVENTIONS/INSTRUCTIONS
1. Identify primary caregiver and assess support systems (see "Family Assessment," p. 41). Assess maternal-infant attachment, father's presence and involvement with the family unit, and role of siblings and extended family, especially grandparents. Refer to parenting classes or counseling as indicated (each visit).

2. Assess maternal perceptions of infant's health. Solicit and answer questions. Provide written information on child care (first visit).

3. Assess home and safety environments (see "Environmental Assessment," p. 37). Observe infant being bathed and diapered; base teaching on observed need; have caregiver give return demonstration (each visit).

4. Assess sleeping infant, noting position, color, respirations, and sleep-activity state. Inform caregiver of findings; focus on normalcy of findings. Instruct on infant positioning (each visit).

5. Perform complete physical examination of infant. Inform caregiver of infant behavior, responses, and findings. Reinforce positive aspects of infant's physical and emotional health. Report deviations from normal to physician (each visit).

6. Assess feeding regimen and technique of bottle-fed infant. Observe infant being fed. Instruct client on formula preparation and storage, bottle cleaning methods, and feeding techniques, as needed (first visit).

7. Observe feeding session of breast-fed infant. Note infant hunger cues, suck/swallow reflexes and coordination, infant latching, duration and times of suckling, infant satiety, and diaper wetness. Instruct mother on relaxation, breastfeeding techniques, positioning, infant cues of satiety; reassure and encourage. Provide written and illustrated directions and information on La Leche League. Concurrently, observe for condition of breasts and nipple soreness. Instruct on care of breasts (first visit).

8. Assess infant's umbilical stump for color, odor, drainage, and degree of healing. Instruct on cord care (first visit).

9. In circumcised infant, assess area for erythema, edema, and discharge. Instruct on circumcision care (first visit).

10. Instruct on conditions that warrant immediate intervention, how to activate Emergency Medical Service (EMS), and importance of immunizations and well-baby care (each visit).

11. Provide list of community resources (health clinics; women, infants, and children [WIC] programs; and breast pump rental services) (first visit).

CAREGIVER/CHILD AND FAMILY INTERVENTIONS

1. Demonstrates attachment behaviors (calls infant by given name or diminutive, gazes at, cuddles, strokes, hugs, and talks to infant).
2. Includes infant's father, siblings, and other significant family members in infant care, either as active participants or as observers.
3. Verbalizes expectations. Compares infant with siblings and children of comparable age.
4. Seeks out information on child care. Attends parenting classes with significant other.
5. Recognizes range of infant sleep-activity patterns, respirations, color, responses, and behavior.
6. Changes and bathes infant using appropriate technique and safety controls, maintains a safe environment for infant.
7. For bottle-fed infant, caregiver prepares formula following package instructions. Identifies hunger cues and feeds infant 2 to 4 ounces of formula on demand (approximately every 3 to 4 hours). Holds infant during feeding; does not prop bottle. Does not add cereal to formula. Positions infant in crib on side (preferably the right) after feeding.
8. For breast-fed infant, caregiver suckles newborn on demand, beginning with several minutes at each breast, increasing to 10 minutes or more. Recognizes it takes 72 to 96 hours for milk production to be established (shorter in multiparas) but that infant's nutritional needs are being met. Does not supplement breastfeedings with water or formula. Uses pacifiers only after consultation. Consults with lactation specialist or La Leche League for questions and support.
9. Identifies infant health and progress: feeds well, has lusty cry, sleeps well between feedings, wets 6 to 8 diapers a day, stools at least once a day, gains weight, develops routine.

10. Cares for breasts by avoiding excess suckling, does not go more than 5 hours between feedings, removes breast secretions by washing with plain water; expresses small amount of milk, lets breasts air dry, and does not use plastic bra liners.

11. Cleans umbilical stump with alcohol. Diapers infant below stump level. Does not use moist or airtight covers.

12. Diapers newly circumcised infant to prevent pressure on area. Keeps petrolatum gauze in place, if ordered. Reports increased swelling, bleeding, and difficulty in urination.

13. Identifies conditions that warrant health care follow-up: marked change in activity pattern, respiratory distress, marked pallor, jaundice, cyanosis, fever, refusal to feed, unrelieved constipation or diarrhea, and rash.

14. Verbalizes knowledge of EMS activation.

15. Returns to health care facility for diagnostic screenings, immunizations, and ongoing well-baby visits.

16. Demonstrates increasing competence with handling feeding, diapering, and bathing infant.

17. Demonstrates enjoyment of infant. Takes time for self and schedules satisfying activities separate from home and child care.

SAMPLE DOCUMENTATION INCLUSIONS

1. Specific assessment
   Mother: Assess vital signs, fundal height and consistency, lochial flow, condition of episiotomy or abdominal operative site, condition of breasts, establishment or suppression of lactation; extent of attachment; and environmental hazards.
   Infant: Assess vital signs, weight, skin color, level of alertness, cry and consolability, feeding and elimination patterns, hydration, condition of umbilical stump, and circumsised area.

2. Specific care/teaching
   Maternal care: Teach care of perineum, operative site, and breasts; health maintenance activities and follow-up visits.
   Infant care: Teach feeding, bathing, diapering, circumcision and cord care, safety, when to seek assistance, ap-

pointments for screening, well-baby visits and immunizations, correct temperature taking.
3. General
   Note responses to care and teaching, follow up on problems found.
4. See "Documentation and Family Home Record Keeping" in Appendix for required documentation components for all home care visits.

Pulmonary system

Apnea

Pathologic apnea in the infant is the cessation of respirations and/or respiratory movement for 20 seconds or longer that is associated with color change (cyanosis), change in pulse rate (bradycardia of <100 beats per minute), decreased peripheral blood flow (pallor), hypotonia (limpness), or change in level of consciousness. Although the cause of apnea is unknown, it is considered a life-threatening event and symptomatic of premature birth (25% of infants who weigh less than 2500 g, and 80% of those who weigh less than 1000 g experience apnea), upper airway obstruction and hypoxia, cardiac disorders, gastroesophageal reflux, hypoglycemia, seizure activity, or serious infection. Types of apnea are central, obstructive, and mixed (50%), involving the absence of thoracic muscle movement that changes respiratory effort and air flow, movement of muscles without air exchange, or a combination. The episodes generally begin at 1 to 2 days of age and are unlikely to occur if not apparent during the first 7 days. Apnea that continues without restoration of breathing activity can result in respiratory arrest and death.

Home care is primarily concerned with recognition and management of apneic episodes by cardiorespiratory monitoring, drug therapy, and provision of various levels of interventions as needed to restore breathing. An additional consideration includes parental and family stressors created by caring for the infant with apnea.

Nursing diagnosis

Ineffective breathing pattern
Related factors: tracheobronchial obstruction, infant apneic
    episodes, premature status

Defining characteristics: apnea lasting 20 seconds, choking, cyanosis, bradycardia, hypotonia, unresponsive to tactile stimulation, apnea monitor alarm sound

OUTCOMES

Short-term
Restoration of cardiorespiratory rate and rhythm evidenced by proper application of apnea monitor and leads and correct response with rapid interventions for each event (expected immediately)

Long-term
Cardiorespiratory rate and rhythm maintained evidenced by use of monitor and successful interventions to restore breathing, compliance with medication regimen (expected ongoing)

NURSING INTERVENTIONS/INSTRUCTIONS

1. Ensure that caregiver is trained in infant cardiopulmonary resuscitation before hospital discharge. Collaborate with caregiver to develop a protocol to activate Emergency Medical Service (EMS) (first visit, reinforce on subsequent visits).

2. Assess caregiver's knowledge and understanding of apneic episodes and instruct on determination of false alarms, observations of signs and symptoms associated with an event, possible causes, and interventions based on specific type of episode (first visit, review second visit).

3. Assess respiration and pulse rates, respiratory pattern, skin color (circumoral cyanosis), any changes associated with feeding, sleep, environmental temperature, humidity, bowel elimination, and abdominal distention and discuss findings with caregivers (each visit).

4. Instruct on taking apical pulse and assessment of respirations and allow for demonstration by caregiver (first visit, reinforce second visit).

5. Instruct and provide detailed information for correct placement and application of electrodes/belt, for leads to belt to skin, to reposition every 2 to 3 days or if loose to preserve skin integrity, to thread wires under cloth-

ing, to avoid use of skin lotions at electrode sites, and on general skin care (first visit, reinforce as needed).

6. Instruct and provide detailed information about type and use of monitor, settings per physician's order (usually preprogrammed at 20 seconds for apnea and 80 beats per minute for heart rate), lead connection to electrodes/belt, alarms and meanings, basic troubleshooting activities according to manufacturer's directions, and connection to electricity or batteries, placing monitor on flat surface away from other children (first visit, reinstruct every visit).

7. Do not use cellular phone in home. Instruct on safety measures involved in use of monitor and to report problems immediately (first visit).

8. Instruct and provide detailed information about interventions in response to alarm and symptoms first by observing skin color and chest movement and then by placing ear to infant's nose for 10 seconds to hear breathing. If breathing and color are good, note on record; but if skin color changes and infant is not breathing, rub back, wait 10 seconds, and if breathing does not resume, stimulate bottom of feet by slapping. If breathing still has not resumed, activate EMS and begin cardiopulmonary resuscitation (CPR). If breathing does resume at any point, observe for 10 seconds and reset alarms (first visit, review each visit).

9. Supply flow sheet and instruct on false alarms, recording apnea patterns, associated symptoms, and actions taken. Review record for comments of concern (each visit).

10. Assess accuracy of monitor, number, duration, cause, and type of alarms and symptoms noted and caregiver response to each type of alarm. Collaborate with caregiver when reviewing record of episodes and actions taken (each visit).

11. Instruct on and observe administration of physician-ordered respiratory stimulant (caffeine or theophylline) with feedings to include correct dose measurement, frequency, and side effects (gastrointestinal, cardiac, and central nervous systems). Inform of need for laboratory testing for theophylline level (first visit, reinstruct as needed).

12. Inform of criteria for future weaning from and discontinuation of monitor and assist caregiver to recognize improvement and stability in infant's condition (any visit as applicable).

CAREGIVER/CHILD AND FAMILY INTERVENTIONS

1. Maintains apnea monitor on infant, especially during sleep or if out of eyesight, but may remove during waking and play time or during feeding, if possible.

2. Administers medications as ordered and notes and reports adverse reactions to physician (increased heart rate, poor feeding, and irritability).

3. Properly applies electrodes attached to belt and changes every 2 to 3 days, peels off of skin carefully, washes sites with mild soap and warm water, pats skin dry, prepares new electrodes by attaching monitor leads, peels cover off back, and attaches to skin.

4. Avoids use of lotions and electrode exposure to water during bathing and reports any skin redness or irritation at electrode sites.

5. Observes frequency, duration, and symptoms such as decreased or absent pulse and respirations, cyanosis, limpness, choking, or gagging associated with each episode; records episode on flow sheet; and calls physician, if necessary or as ordered.

6. Responds to monitor alarm indicating apneic event by observing chest for respiratory movement, providing gentle to vigorous tactile or voice stimulation for milder episode, and, if no response, activating EMS, performing mouth-to-mouth resuscitation, and CPR for severe episode, if necessary.

7. Follows manufacturer's manual to check monitor several times a day; reviews trouble-shooting actions to take for false, lead, or battery alarms; avoids electric interference from household appliances and use of cellular phones in home; and calls supplier with any questions regarding monitor (24-hour availability for assistance).

8. Notifies local electric company and emergency services of home monitoring, has emergency numbers near telephone, unplugs monitor and removes leads to electrodes when not in use.

9. Maintains emergency plan information and telephone numbers in strategic place for immediate access and uses if needed.

Nursing diagnosis

Altered health maintenance/fear (parental)
Related factors: ineffective family coping, potentially life-threatening situation (death of infant)
Defining characteristics: reported lack of support system and feelings of inadequacy, apprehension, anxiety, tension, fatigue, altered parenting, poor bonding, history of apnea or sudden infant death syndrome in family

OUTCOMES

Short-term
Family members acknowledge fears and demonstrate ability to plan and care for infant/child evidenced by family members recognizing need for monitor with reduction of anxiety and feelings of inadequacy; integration of information about family needs, parenting, and support in daily care of infant/child; signing of informed consent, if required (expected within 1 to 2 weeks)

Long-term
Family coping and adaptation are evidenced by development of family responsibility for optimal support and participation in care and maintenance of infant's/child's well-being and family relationships, acceptance of extensive psychosocial support (expected within 1 to 2 months or length of time monitor is used)

NURSING INTERVENTIONS/INSTRUCTIONS

1. Assess educational level of caregiver and information provided on discharge from hospital to provide consistent instruction. Identify deficits and reinforce health plan to reduce confusion and frustration (first visit).

2. Meet and collaborate with family members to assess anxiety, feelings about monitor, knowledge about monitor management, effect on caregiver's daily routines, and planning of care (see "Family Assessment," p. 41, for guidelines) (first visit, repeat as needed).

3. Reinforce information to promote family understanding of disorder and care needs and review and document monitor functions of alarms, electrode placement, and trouble-shooting activities (each visit).

4. Discuss and allow family to express feelings of guilt, anxiety, and depression. Promote communication among members to verbalize feelings and expectations with each other (first and any other visit).

5. Collaborate with family members to develop new patterns of responsibilities and provide sensitivity and positive reinforcement for attempts and changes as they occur (each visit).

6. Suggest that caregiver write down questions and assist in maintaining a log of daily changes, events, and items to discuss at next visit (first visit, review on subsequent visits as needed).

7. Explore possible instruction on infant CPR and monitoring to grandparents or other possible caregivers to provide respite for family members (child crisis center that provides nursing care at no cost). Impress on family importance of leaving infant with someone trained in CPR (any visit).

8. Instruct on methods to develop appropriate coping skills and to meet family's medical and other needs (emotional, financial, food, supplies, and equipment) by referral to social or counseling services and support groups (first visit, reinforce as needed).

CAREGIVER/CHILD AND FAMILY INTERVENTIONS

1. Displays and verbalizes decreasing anxiety and anger and provides a supportive, cooperative family environment with recognition of seriousness of child's needs and focuses on maintaining infant's health.

2. Develops trust in home care personnel, progressively accepts their presence within family group, and collaborates in developing and modifying daily care.

3. Prioritizes and provides effective care and treatment within daily family routines.
4. Develops coping skills to deal with feelings of constant responsibility for infant's survival, which can be overwhelming. Seeks and accepts family support.
5. Recognizes and assumes role changes within family and maintains integrity. Includes siblings in family planning for health maintenance of infant.
6. Develops self-assurance and coping mechanisms that have positive effect within family.
7. Identifies problem areas and obtains community or professional assistance or services as needed.
8. Understands ongoing medical evaluation of need for continuing monitoring and long-term follow-up plan.

SAMPLE DOCUMENTATION INCLUSIONS

1. Specific assessment
   Assess cardiorespiratory rate, skin color, hypotonia, skin integrity, unresponsiveness, correct use and response to monitor, knowledge and adaptive capacity of caregiver and family, and need for referral to professional services.
2. Specific care/teaching
   Teach correct administration of medications, pulse and respirations, application and care of monitor, skin care, appropriate actions/responses to alarms, troubleshooting and safety hazards during monitoring, and infant CPR.
3. General
   Note responses and involvement in care and teaching, changes in plan, adaptation to care, and family successes and problems in maintaining relationships.
4. See "Documentation and Family Home Record Keeping" in Appendix for general required documentation components for all home care visits.

 Assisted Ventilation

Assisted ventilation, or *artificial* or *mechanical ventilation,* is a method of applying positive or negative pressure to support inflation of the lungs. It can provide temporary or permanent assistance to take over the action of the diaphragm and chest wall muscles. Negative pressure devices are applied to the outside of the chest wall to create negative pressure in the lungs and initiate inspiration in those with neuromuscular conditions, obstructive (bronchitis), and restrictive (poliomyelitis) diseases. Positive pressure ventilators increase airway pressure above atmospheric pressure to inflate the lungs and improve gas exchange by better distribution of gases within the lungs and reinflation of collapsed areas of the lungs. They can be invasive (with an artificial airway such as a tracheostomy tube) or noninvasive (with a facial or nasal mask). These are used in infants with prematurity, tracheomalacia, bronchopulmonary dysplasia, and central control breathing disturbances, as well as in children with neuromuscular and musculoskeletal disorders. These are the most common types of ventilators used in the home, and they are small, portable, and easily moved within the environment. The type of ventilator selected depends on the medical diagnosis and is based on regulating the cycle (pressure, volume, and time cycled) before discharge from the hospital, requirements each day, needed oxygen concentration, and resources to acquire, maintain, and repair the equipment. Supplemental oxygen may also be required for children receiving assisted ventilation.

Home care is primarily concerned with management of the ventilator-dependent child and the various levels of interventions needed to maintain, monitor, and troubleshoot the ventilator. Of additional importance is the ability of the family to become trained and participate in the total care of the ventilator-dependent child. For tracheostomy care associated with mechanical ventilation, combine the information in this plan with the tracheostomy care plan.

Nursing diagnosis

Ineffective breathing pattern/airway clearance/gas exchange
Related factors: decreased energy and fatigue; tracheobronchial obstruction versus a pneumothorax; altered oxygen supply; loss of lung function, inflammatory/infectious process; decreased lung expansion

Defining characteristics: dyspnea, tachypnea, use of accessory
   muscles (retractions), nasal flaring, grunting, cyanosis
   (dusky color), tachycardia, irritability, diaphoresis,
   elevated temperature, restlessness, abnormal breath
   sounds (crackles/rhonchi), inability to clear increased
   thick secretions, hypoxia, hypercapnia, elevated peak in-
   spiratory pressure on ventilator, or ventilator dyssyn-
   chrony

OUTCOMES

Short-term
Optimal functioning ventilator and airway patency with adequate ventilation (caregiver response to alarms) and
oxygenation (determined by pulse oximetry) established and
evidenced by clearance of loosened secretions by cough or
suction; maintenance of skin and mucous membrane color
based on racial baseline parameters with no hypoxia; breath
sounds clear and equal bilaterally, no infection; adequate
rest, sleep, relaxation; comfortable breathing pattern
(expected within 2 days and ongoing)

Long-term
Respiratory baseline measures and gas exchange maintained
with ventilator, absence of signs of respiratory distress with
clear breath sounds, progressive withdrawal of oxygen or
ventilation support when appropriate, management of safe
home-assisted ventilation demonstrated by caregivers
(expected within 1 month)

NURSING INTERVENTIONS/INSTRUCTIONS

1. Explain importance of and ensure that caregiver has
   been trained in CPR before hospital discharge. Collaborate with caregiver to develop protocol to activate
   EMS (first visit, reinforce).
2. Assess caregiver knowledge and understanding of disease etiology, status and need for assisted ventilation,
   ability to adapt and manage ventilator and care of child
   (first and second visits).
3. Assess and instruct caregiver to assess and monitor respiratory status for distress, chest expansion for symmetry, counting respiratory rate with ventilator cycle,
   and child's respiratory efforts that include absence

or presence of effort, depth, and normal rate and
rhythm to determine effectiveness of assisted ventilation
and if settings need changing. Include color of skin,
oral mucous membranes, and nailbeds for hypoxia; abnormal breath sounds on auscultation; presence and
characteristics of secretions in assessment (see "Pulmonary System Assessment," p. 10, for guidelines) (every visit).

4. Provide information and instruction using language that
   is easily understood and provide written instructions
   and care plan (first visit, reinforce regularly).

5. Assess caregiver's baseline knowledge. Demonstrate
   procedure for encouraging coughing, postural drainage
   of lung segments using gravity to assist in clearing
   airway and how to monitor with use of stethoscope
   (first and second visits).

6. Instruct on symptoms of respiratory distress, including
   sudden dyspnea, increased respiratory rate (>24
   breaths per minute), rapid pulse (>100 beats per
   minute), circumoral or nail bed cyanosis, wheezing, nasal flaring, steps to correct (i.e., clearing airway and
   orthopneic position), and taking child to emergency department, or calling EMS if condition does not improve (first visit).

7. Instruct child on how to become synchronous with ventilator. Inform caregiver to stay with child and provide
   emotional support when anxious (first and second
   visits).

8. Assess and instruct to assess all ventilator connections,
   settings, alarms, and function daily. Monitor for effects
   of changes in ventilatory settings (every visit).

9. Instruct caregiver on cleaning and changing circuits,
   machine, suctioning equipment and supplies, and resuscitation bag (first visit, reinstruct as needed).

10. Collaborate with caregiver to review potential nonmedi-
    cal problem-solving or troubleshooting of equipment
    malfunction, ventilator management of settings, alarms,
    and cleaning outlined in manufacturer's guidelines; and
    corrective actions to take (first visit, review as needed).

11. Administer and instruct caregiver to provide supple-
    mental humidified oxygen with ventilator via system

based on ordered pressure input and flow rate requirements of ventilator and on portability and availability of oxygen system (assist as needed) (first and second visits).

12. Instruct on safety measures in use of oxygen (first visit).

13. Instruct caregiver to humidify inspired air by cascade, jet nebulizer, or humidifier to prevent drying of secretions and loss of body fluids and heat (first visit).

14. Instruct on removing secretions by suctioning if child is dyspneic or gurgling, using resuscitation bag to preoxygenate child between each suctioning effort (see "Tracheostomy," p. 114) (first visit, as needed).

15. Instruct on and observe medication administration ordered in conjunction with ventilation therapy (first visit, as needed).

16. Demonstrate elevation of head of bed and positions of optimal comfort for sleeping and resting that allow for diaphragmatic movement and chest expansion (first visit).

17. Review and collaborate with caregiver about equipment needed for times away from home (portable suction, oxygen tank, spare tracheostomy tubes, artificial nose to replace cascade, fully charged ventilator, and others if needed) (any visit).

18. Assist caregiver in organizing environment for immediate access to supplies and equipment and ease of care (first visit).

19. Assess response to ventilatory assistance and report untoward responses to physician (each visit).

20. Inform caregiver and family of availability of American Lung Association and local support groups for information and services (first visit).

CAREGIVER/CHILD AND FAMILY INTERVENTIONS

1. Becomes CPR certified before child's discharge from hospital, obtains training in emergency procedures associated with ventilator, and places list of emergency activities and telephone numbers in strategic place for easy access.

2. Locates resources and acquires special equipment and supplies (e.g., oxygen source and backup tank with

gauge, ventilator and accessories, suctioning equipment and supplies, and extra tracheostomy tubes).

3. Verbalizes understanding and rationale for physical care, airway management, treatments and procedures, and need for constant monitoring.

4. Makes list of questions to ask for each home care visit.

5. Completes training or classes in all aspects of care before independent care of child receiving assisted ventilation.

6. Assesses respirations for rate and effort compared with ventilator effectiveness, child's color during suctioning, and signs of respiratory distress or deterioration to report.

7. Complies with ordered medication regimen.

8. Complies with treatments, monitoring schedules, and equipment care and cleaning.

9. Demonstrates maintenance of ventilator function using ventilator checklist and uses manufacturer's guidelines for troubleshooting equipment problems.

10. Correctly administers humidified oxygen (continuous or intermittent) and uses resuscitation bag when needed, provides adequate humidification to airway by cascade or artificial nose when ventilated via tracheostomy tube.

11. Follows safety precautions during oxygen use, including posting sign stating "oxygen in use, no sparks, no open flames, no oil or grease, no smoking" and maintains a standby oxygen source.

12. Performs chest physiotherapy by gravity and use of pillows and positioning, without fatigue to child (frequency and time depend on need for airway clearance) and encourages coughing or removes secretions by suctioning, if needed.

13. Positions child, with use of foam rubber wedge or pillows, to elevate head for sleep and rest and reports change in mentation or orientation following naps or changes in sleep patterns caused by hypercapnia.

14. Develops trust in home care providers (nurse, respiratory therapist, and nursing assistant) and confidence in own competence in managing total care.

15. Notifies local electric company and emergency services of having child on ventilator, maintains emergency plan

information, and has emergency numbers near telephone for immediate access.
16. Uses emergency services when life-threatening changes
occur and cannot be resolved.

Nursing diagnosis

Impaired physical mobility
Related factors: decreased strength and endurance, intolerance to activity and limited movement with ventilator
use, anxiety
Defining characteristics: inability to purposefully move
within physical environment; imposed restriction of
movement, including mechanical apparatus; limited
range of motion

OUTCOMES

Short-term
Progressive mobility, independently/with assistance, with/
without ventilator, evidenced by positioning of comfort,
range of motion maintained, use of assistive aids (expected
within 1 week)

Long-term
Optimal independent movement, use of extremities within
level of endurance while attached to ventilator, evidenced
by absence of muscle atrophy, contractures, participation in self-care and play as able (expected within 3
weeks)

NURSING INTERVENTIONS/INSTRUCTIONS

1. Assess energy level, physical restrictions while attached
to ventilator, neuromuscular or musculoskeletal impairments, and ability to participate in movement and play
activities appropriate to age (first visit).
2. Assess availability of portable ventilator and wheelchair
to support ventilator and to enhance movement within
environment. Instruct on use of devices to operate on
chair (first and second visits).
3. Assess for response to activity such as respiratory
changes or distress (each visit).

4. Perform range-of-motion exercises and instruct caregiver to perform these daily (first visit, reinforce).

5. Instruct to use position changes as needed to perform self-care or to engage in play activities (first visit).

6. Obtain order for physical therapy referral or reinforce teaching by therapist for exercises and mobility while receiving assisted ventilation and for occupational and speech therapy, if appropriate.

CAREGIVER/CHILD AND FAMILY INTERVENTIONS

1. Schedules and assists or participates in daily activities for periods of time as tolerated.

2. Avoids extremes in activity while allowing for as much independence as possible.

3. Discontinues activity if fatigue or respiratory distress results.

4. Follows recommendations of physical therapist to maintain mobility, muscle tone, and range of motion.

5. Uses resource to acquire wheelchair with mount for ventilator, if appropriate.

Nursing diagnosis

Caregiver role strain

Related factors: amount of caregiving tasks, duration of caregiving required, unpredictable illness course or instability in care receiver's health, discharge of child with significant home care needs

Defining characteristics: worry about child's health; having enough time, energy to provide care needed; feeling of loss because child never met caregiver's expectations; conflict in family about issues of providing care, 24-hour care, and supervision of child

OUTCOMES

Short-term

Identification of role strain evidenced by verbalization of stress or nervousness, worry, interference with other important roles in life, loss of independence, need for assistance and support (expected within 1 week)

Long-term
Resolution of role strain by provision of continued, progressive, safe care without compromising caregiver's physical and emotional needs (expected within 1 month)

NURSING INTERVENTIONS/INSTRUCTIONS

1. Assess extent of needs of child and ability and feeling of adequacy of caregiver to perform role and care, feelings of caregiver about demands and complexity (exhaustion and resentment) of care, and feelings of being alone and having no pride in caregiving activities (first visit).
2. Assess relationship between caregiver and family and stressors placed on relationships, breakdown in family relationships, role confusion, or competing demands from family and care responsibilities (ongoing).
3. Assist caregiver to monitor continued ability to perform care and treatments, day-to-day needs that must be changed or learned, changes in strains or stressors, maintenance of routines, and need for additional resources or assistance (each visit).
4. Provide time for caregiver and family to discuss frustrations, anxiety, fear, and fatigue; praise attempts and accomplishments in coping and providing care (each visit).
5. Help locate sitter or nursing student and instruct in CPR and care of child to give relief from constant attendance and care by primary caregiver (any visit).
6. Encourage sharing of caregiver roles and responsibilities among family members, friends, and extended family to provide relief to immediate family (any visit).
7. Listen to family feelings, concerns, expectations, and preferences for caregiving. Answer all questions (each visit).
8. Support caregiver's need for relief services and counseling referral, if necessary (any visit).

CAREGIVER/CHILD AND FAMILY INTERVENTIONS

1. Prepares for emotional changes associated with caregiving during discharge planning and teaching.
2. Develops ability to cope with caregiver role and incorporates flexibility into day-to-day functioning.
3. Explores and uses community resources (e.g., United

Way) to provide physical and psychologic assistance and relief from role strain (respite care).
4. Maintains own health and well-being in caregiver role and as much independence and privacy as possible. Becomes involved in outside activities.
5. Maintains diary for ventilation settings, vital signs, respiratory status, and other concerns to share with family members, physician, or home care nurse.
6. Develops new coping skills and strategies for role changes by family members needed to support or participate in care of child.
7. Preserves family relationships and minimizes stressors by sharing feelings, fears, and concerns with one another.
8. Progressively adapts to and accepts ventilatory care by caregiver and family members.
9. Participates in outside support groups; refers to clergy or counseling as needed.

SAMPLE DOCUMENTATION INCLUSIONS

1. Specific assessment
   Assess respiratory status; airway patency and secretions; oxygenation; hypoxia; ventilator function/dysfunction; ventilator settings and monitoring; strength and endurance; level of anxiety; caregiver ability; coping ability and adaptive capacity of child, caregiver, and family; tracheostomy characteristics; and needs from tracheostomy plan.
2. Specific care/teaching
   Teach administration of medications, oxygen, and care of equipment; operation of ventilator and monitoring of connections, settings, and alarms; troubleshooting, cleaning, and changing circuitry; rest and mobility needs; chest physiotherapy; infection prevention; humidification of air flow and environment; removal of secretions by coughing or suctioning; synchronous breathing with ventilator; use of resuscitation bag; and exercising of extremities.
3. General
   Note response to care and teaching, plan modification, changes in health status, adaptation to care associated with ventilator, need for professional referrals, interven-

tions to prevent caregiver strain and to promote family health, and documentation summary.
4. See "Documentation and Family Home Record Keeping" in Appendix for general required documentation components for all home care visits.

 ## Bronchial Asthma

Bronchial asthma, an airway reactive disease responsive to stimuli that cause narrowing of the bronchi and bronchioles, is a common respiratory condition in children. Extrinsic asthma, the type found in children, is characterized by allergic responses, usually to something inhaled (antibody-antigen reaction) that causes smooth muscle bronchospasm, edema of the mucous membrane of the bronchi, and accumulation of tenacious secretions. These responses can be precipitated by specific allergens, climate changes, or excessive exercise or activity. Intrinsic asthma is characterized by responses to emotional upset or respiratory infection. Bronchial asthma is not as common as bronchiolitis in children younger than 2 years old.

Home care is primarily concerned with the education of the child and family about the disease and its management: control and relief of asthma symptoms, prevention or correction of acute episodes with a medication regimen, allergen control and reduction in precipitating factors, and promotion of a normal lifestyle for the child.

Nursing diagnosis

Anxiety/fear (child and parent)
Related factors: change in health status, environment (hospitalization); threatening situation of bronchospasms; respiratory obstruction; irreversible asthmatic attack
Defining characteristics: difficult breathing, apprehension, restlessness, facial tension, feeling of fear regarding ex-

acerbation of asthmatic episode, fear of suffocation, increased respiration rate with wheezing

OUTCOMES

Short-term
Minimal anxiety associated with chance of asthma attack evidenced by caregiver and child understanding and accepting disorder; fewer trips to emergency room; ability to remain calm, take measures to correct or manage attack (expected within 1 to 2 weeks)

Long-term
Fear, anxiety at manageable level evidenced by effective use of coping mechanisms; ongoing support, adaptation to chronic nature of disease with lifestyle as free of fear or anxiety as possible (expected within 1 month)

NURSING INTERVENTIONS/INSTRUCTIONS

1. Assess emotional and mental status of caregiver and child and ability to adapt to long-term care and supervision (see "Psychologic Assessment," p. 25, for guidelines) (first visit, as needed).
2. Provide information about disease in easily understandable language. Inform of treatments and progress (each visit).
3. Maintain a calm, quiet environment during assessment and teaching (each visit).
4. Provide opportunity for caregiver and child to verbalize fears and concerns. Encourage acceptance of disease and changes needed to minimize attacks (each visit).
5. Suggest that caregiver stay with child during anxious times and provide calmness and support, especially during asthma attack (first visit).
6. Assist caregiver to reduce feelings of guilt and blaming self for child's condition (each visit).
7. Inform of long-term effects of diagnosis. Refer to parent support group, if available, and national agencies such as Asthma and Allergy Foundation of America (any visit).

CAREGIVER/CHILD AND FAMILY INTERVENTIONS

1. Recognizes anxiety associated with chronic condition, chance of attack, and onset of acute symptoms of attack.

2. Maintains calm, supportive environment and controls situation during episode by remaining with and reassuring child during attack. Administers appropriate treatment before or at onset of attack.
3. Child uses familiar relaxation techniques, diversion, and interventions such as remaining quiet, breathing control exercises, medication, and quiet play activities to avoid episode.
4. Uses appropriate coping mechanisms and support resources as needed.

Nursing Diagnosis

Ineffective airway clearance/breathing pattern
Related factors: decreased energy and fatigue, tracheobronchial obstruction, airway reaction to allergens
Defining characteristics: dyspnea, prolonged expirations, tachypnea, audible wheezing; intercostal, substernal, and suprasternal retractions; air hunger, nasal flaring, cyanosis of lips and nailbeds; abnormal breath sounds (wheezing, rhonchi), hyperresonance on percussion, dry cough, clammy skin, increased and tenacious mucus, hypoxia, hypercapnia, chest x-ray film and pulmonary function tests revealing pulmonary changes; results of skin testing for allergens; noncompliance with treatment regimen

OUTCOMES
Short-term
Optimal breathing pattern, airway patency with adequate ventilation established evidenced by respiratory rate, ease, depth maintained at baseline levels with audible wheezing absent; control of symptoms, relief of airway obstruction by medications; maintenance of skin, mucous membrane color based on racial baseline parameters; environmental measures to prevent asthmatic episodes implemented; breath sounds clear, equal bilaterally (expected within 2 to 4 days and ongoing)

Long-term
Respiratory baseline levels maintained within disease parameters with progressive reduction in asthmatic attacks

with effective treatment regimen, improvement in long-term prognosis, reduction in hospitalizations by prevention of acute asthmatic attacks, optimal management of total home, environmental respiratory care demonstrated by caregivers and child (age-dependent) (expected within 1 month)

NURSING INTERVENTIONS/INSTRUCTIONS

1. Assess caregiver knowledge and understanding of disease and status (incidence and severity of attacks), including distress, signs, and symptoms caused by condition and reason for them, and ability to adapt to long-term therapy (first visit).

2. Provide information based on knowledge deficit assessed about disease, signs and symptoms to note, and what actions to take. Use easily understandable language or provide written instructions (first visit, review as needed).

3. Assess trends in respiratory status, including rate, depth, and ease or effort; chest expansion; retractions and nasal flaring; color of skin, oral mucous membranes, and nailbeds; abnormal breath sounds on auscultation; presence and characteristics of secretions; and frequency and severity of attacks (see "Pulmonary System Assessment," p. 10, for guidelines) (each visit).

4. Collaborate with caregiver and child to assess factors that trigger asthmatic attacks that include substances in home (odors from perfumes, general household fumes, cooking odors, tobacco smoke, house dust, or fireplaces), contact with allergens (pollens, weeds, plants, or feathers), or other factors (cold air, smog, pets, or mites in mattresses) (first visit and reassess as needed).

5. Instruct on positioning child during asthma attack to achieve optimal comfort and chest expansion for ventilation in either semi-Fowler's or high-Fowler's position or leaning child forward on a pillow (first visit).

6. Instruct child to increase fluid intake to help expectorate mucus (first visit).

7. Instruct on administration of ordered liquid form of bronchodilator, antiasthmatic medications, and steroid therapy (in feedings or by dropper in young children); assess expiration date and need for refill for bronchodilator inhaler, use aerosol therapy with small volume nebulizer or hand-held measured dose inhaler, vital signs before and after use of bronchodilator drugs, and response for medication effectiveness and side effects (first visit and until instruction given for all medications).

8. Instruct caregiver and child of actions to take for an impending attack (controlled breathing, breathing exercises, medication administration, and rest) (first and second visits).

9. Instruct on administration of subcutaneous injection of adrenergic medication in acute attacks and frequency allowed for temporary relief of bronchospasms (first visit, reinforce second visit).

10. Instruct on side effects or toxicity of bronchodilator medication, including nausea, vomiting, abdominal discomfort or pain, and restlessness and to discontinue drug and report to physician immediately (first visit).

11. Assess for and report ineffective responses to medications that lead to increased respiratory rate with dyspnea, continued coughing, cyanosis, and fatigue to physician (any visit).

12. Instruct on effective breathing exercises and coughing. Note changes in sputum color/consistency. Initiate referral to physiotherapy, if ordered (first and second visits).

13. Instruct on use of peak flow meter and abdominal diaphragmatic breathing; use games such as blowing ping pong balls and bubbles to teach (first and second visits).

14. Instruct caregiver in procedure to activate EMS if child does not respond to treatment (first visit).

15. Inform caregiver and family of availability of American Lung Association, and local support groups for information and services (first visit).

CAREGIVER/CHILD AND FAMILY INTERVENTIONS

1. Locates resource to acquire special equipment and supplies (small-volume nebulizer, tubing, medication con-

tainers, and standby oxygen equipment, if ordered).

2. Assesses respirations for rate and ease, use of accessory muscles, and pulse for rate and rhythm; determines care for day based on changes; and modifies plans for treatment if deviations from baseline values are noted.

3. Safely administers medications in correct form, frequency, and route and detects adverse reactions and inability of medications to control bronchospasms or clear secretions from airway and reports this to physician.

4. Avoids delay in starting asthma medications, starts oral or inhalant medications at first sign of coughing or itching and before exercises, checks expiration date, and replaces medications before they run out.

5. Avoids administration of any over-the-counter medications to treat attack.

6. Offers clear fluids, popsicles, and frozen juices every 2 hours to liquify mucus; offers warm fluids to sip if wheezing; and uses humidifier in child's bedroom.

7. Avoids exposure to outside and home pollutants such as sprays, fumes, cooking odors, feather pillows or comforters, smog, tobacco smoke, pet hair, weeds, pollens, plants/allergens; changes filters from heating and air conditioning units; washes and dusts child's room; forbids smoking in child's environment; and cleans equipment correctly.

8. Avoids strenuous exercise, especially running in cold weather (takes oral medication 90 minutes before and inhalant 10 minutes before exercise); preferred exercise is swimming because it does not involve rapid breathing; jogging, soccer, and playing a wind instrument promote lung development.

9. Informs school nurse and teacher of condition and what signs and symptoms to note; child takes inhaler to school to use as needed and avoids physical education on days when mild attacks occur.

10. Reports severe wheezing and if wheezing is not improved after a second dose of medication; if child is unable to speak, has bluish or dusky lips, has chest pain, vomits medication, or has yellowish color to nasal discharge or mucus, reports to physician or calls EMS.

11. Writes questions or concerns for discussion during next
    nurse visit or physician appointment.

Nursing diagnosis

Activity intolerance/sleep pattern disturbance
Related factors: generalized weakness, fatigue, presence of
    respiratory disorder
Defining characteristics: exertional discomfort/dyspnea,
    change in activity level, insomnia, coughing at night, fre-
    quent shortness of breath, restlessness, anxiety, inabil-
    ity to lie down for sleep

OUTCOMES
Short-term
Optimal energy conservation with ability to perform normal daily activities for age evidenced by normal respiratory status, reduced dyspnea during activity, adequate
sleep, quiet rest pattern established (expected within 3 to
4 days)

Long-term
Progressive increase or maintenance in play and other activities within baseline respiratory and energy parameters
demonstrated (expected ongoing)

NURSING INTERVENTIONS/INSTRUCTIONS
1. Assess energy level and deficit in activity level; changes
   in respiratory status during activity; and ability and interest in participating in favorite play activities, school,
   and self-care appropriate to age (each visit).
2. Inform caregiver and child of relationship between pulmonary condition and inability/interference in performing activities and possible consequences of activity and
   effect of breathing difficulty on ability to rest and sleep,
   resulting in fatigue (first visit).
3. Inform of alternate methods of performing activities and
   conserving energy (first and second visits).
4. Assist to plan changes in types and timing of activities such as quiet play when necessary, depending

on response to activity and age of child (each visit).

5. Advise to administer bronchodilators before activities and to plan to include rest periods following activities (first visit).
6. Instruct to increase activity as tolerated within child's physical/psychologic capabilities and to decrease activity with signs and symptoms of fatigue or respiratory distress (each visit).
7. Demonstrate elevation of head of bed and positions of optimal comfort for sleeping and resting that allow for ease in breathing (first visit).
8. Collaborate with caregiver to modify environment to accommodate exercises and play activities and to create quiet, stress-free surroundings to promote sleep. Use nonallergenic pillows and mattress cover (first and second visits).

CAREGIVER/CHILD AND FAMILY INTERVENTIONS

1. Participates in planned activities appropriate for age and development.
2. Schedules activities in daily routine for periods of time as tolerated. Organizes and balances activities around rest and sleep times.
3. Performs activities when bronchodilator medication is at optimal level.
4. Avoids extremes in activities that cause fatigue and substitutes with less strenuous activities.
5. Identifies signs and symptoms that require adjustment in type of activities. Discontinues activity if needed.
6. Monitors and documents in daily log child's progress toward achieving optimal activity and rest levels, if realistic and helpful in determining interventions that are successful.
7. Allows the child to select and include favorite activities and play.
8. Provides quiet, safe environment conducive to promoting activities within identified restrictions.
9. Positions child, with use of foam rubber wedge or pillows, to elevate head for sleep and rest.

Nursing diagnosis

Ineffective family coping: compromised/individual coping (child)

Related factors: prolonged disease that exhausts supportive capacity of significant people, frequent hospitalizations, family disorganization and role changes

Defining characteristics: significant person's expression of inability to cope and feelings of fear, anxiety, guilt, anger; inadequate understanding of chronic illness and long-term care by family; inability of child to cope or ask for help; chronic fatigue and anxiety of child

OUTCOMES

Short-term

Family members demonstrate ability to plan and care for child evidenced by provision of a normal environment, decreased anxiety and feelings of inadequacy, and integration of information about family needs into care and support of child (expected within 1 to 2 weeks)

Long-term

Family coping and adaptation evidenced by optimal support and participation in care and maintenance of family relationships (expected within 1 to 2 months)

NURSING INTERVENTIONS/INSTRUCTIONS

1. Meet and collaborate with family members to assess stressors, coping mechanisms, and planning of care (first visit, repeat as needed).
2. Reinforce information to promote family understanding of illness and care needs (each visit).
3. Discuss and allow family to express feelings of guilt, anxiety, and depression. Promote communication among members to verbalize feelings and expectations with each other (any visit).
4. Instruct on methods to develop appropriate coping skills and to meet family's medical and other needs (emotional, financial, food, respite, supplies, and equipment)

by referral to social or counseling services (first visit, as needed).

CAREGIVER/CHILD AND FAMILY INTERVENTIONS

1. Displays decreasing anxiety and anger and provides a supportive family environment.
2. Develops trust in home care personnel and collaborates in developing and modifying daily care.
3. Provides care and treatments effectively. Supports child during stressful times or when feeling most vulnerable and unable to participate in daily life routines with family or friends.
4. Avoids overprotection or rejection of child by caregiver or family members.
5. Recognizes and assumes role changes and maintains family integrity.
6. Develops coping mechanisms that have positive effect within family.
7. Identifies problem areas and obtains community, professional, or social service assistance as needed.

SAMPLE DOCUMENTATION INCLUSIONS

1. Specific assessment
   Assess respiratory rate, ease, lung sounds, and deviations; onset of new problems; changes in sputum characteristics; effectiveness of medication regimen and pulmonary physiotherapy; exacerbation of symptoms; nutritional and hydration status; environmental hazards/factors that can trigger attack; and adaptive capacity of family.
2. Specific care/teaching
   Teach correct administration of medications via oral, parenteral, and inhalation routes; rest and activity needs and precautions; energy conservation; postural drainage and chest percussion; coughing and deep breathing exercises; prevention and treatment of attacks; disease course, expectations, and skills to enhance coping; infection and stress prevention; and humidified oxygen administration, if appropriate.
3. General
   Note responses to care and teaching, goal achievement, changes in plan, progression or regression of health

status, adaptation to long-term care, need for medical follow-up and professional referrals, and test and procedure results.
4. See "Documentation and Family Home Record Keeping" in Appendix for general required documentation components for all home care visits.

 ## *Bronchopulmonary Dysplasia*

Bronchopulmonary dysplasia (BPD) is a chronic condition of the lungs, resulting from injury to the airways and alveoli. It most commonly develops in the premature infant after treatment for idiopathic respiratory distress syndrome (IRDS), also known as hyaline membrane disease. BPD is associated with endotracheal intubation, high positive pressure mechanical ventilation, and high concentrations of oxygen administered for long periods of time (more than 28 days) to treat IRDS and disorders such as congenital heart defects and meconium aspiration. The disease involves four stages based on the time that the change occurred (from 0 to 30 days) and what type of alveolar and bronchial damage and repair occurs. The process begins with IRDS, progresses to obstruction and ventilatory difficulty, then develops to dysplasia and increased mucus production with reduced ciliary activity that prevents clearing from the lungs, and finally to chronic hypoxemia, emphysema, and fibrosis. Recovery can be complete by 2 to 3 years of age, but symptoms can persist from 5 to 7 years of age or longer and pulmonary x-ray results remain abnormal for many years.

Home care is primarily concerned with lung growth and adequate oxygenation, with the maintenance of airway patency and adequate exchange of gases by administration of medications, optimal nutrition for growth and healing, supplemental oxygen, and prevention of respiratory infections. The long-term nature of the disease requires additional home nursing assistance and instruction on equipment monitoring, oxygen and chest therapy, growth and development needs of the child, and adaptation needs of the family. If the child is techology-dependent, see the assisted ventilation and tracheostomy care plans for nursing and caregiver interventions.

Nursing diagnosis

Ineffective breathing pattern/gas exchange
Related factors: decreased energy and fatigue, tracheobronchial obstruction, alveolar-capillary membrane changes
Defining characteristics: dyspnea, tachypnea, use of accessory muscles (retractions), nasal flaring, cyanosis (dusky color), irritability, abnormal breath sounds (possible wheezing, crackles), inability to clear mucus, hypoxia, hypercapnia, chest x-ray film revealing pulmonary changes

OUTCOMES
Short-term
Optimal breathing pattern and airway patency with adequate ventilation and oxygenation established and evidenced by respiratory rate, ease, and depth maintained at normal levels; maintenance of skin and mucous membrane color based on racial baseline parameters; reduced dyspneic episodes; mobilization and removal of mucus; breath sounds clear and equal bilaterally; adequate rest and sleep (expected within 2 days)

Long-term
Respiratory baseline values maintained within disease parameters with progressive withdrawal of oxygen or ventilation support, management of home respiratory care with continued humidified oxygen supply to the tissues demonstrated by caregivers and child (expected within 1 month)

NURSING INTERVENTIONS/INSTRUCTIONS
1. Ensure that caregiver has been trained in cardiopulmonary resuscitation (CPR) before hospital discharge. Col-

laborate with caregiver to develop an emergency protocol. Place picture above bed with CPR steps to follow
(first visit, reinforce).

2. Assess caregiver knowledge and understanding of disease, including signs and symptoms caused by condition
and reason for them and ability to adapt to long-term
therapy (first visit).

3. Provide information based on assessment about disease,
signs, symptoms to note, and what actions to take. Use
easily understandable language or provide written instructions (first visit, review as needed).

4. Assess trends in respiratory status, including rate,
depth, and ease or effort; chest expansion; retractions and nasal flaring; color of skin, oral mucous membranes, and nailbeds; abnormal breath sounds on
auscultation; and presence and characteristics of secretions (see "Pulmonary System Assessment," p. 10, for
guidelines) (every visit).

5. Instruct on taking pulse and assessment of respirations
and establish baseline values. Collaborate with caregiver
to plan care based on respiratory status (first visit, reinstruct on plan changes as needed).

6. Assess apnea monitor function, readings, and false
alarms. Instruct in use if ordered for infant (see "Apnea," p. 57) (first and follow-up visits).

7. Instruct caregiver to provide supplemental oxygen at
dose and method prescribed (usually nasal cannula)
with adjustments made, in collaboration with physician,
at times when needed such as during feeding, crying,
dyspnea, or postural drainage (first and second visits).

8. Instruct on safety measures in use of oxygen (first visit).

9. Monitor oxygen saturation by oximetry with a portable
unit during rest and activity, with and without supplemental oxygen. Assess for restlessness and agitation
or mentation changes that occur with hypoxemia (first
and every second visit as needed).

10. Demonstrate and allow for return demonstration in administration of bronchodilator and aerosol therapy to
remove mucus and advise to perform before postural
drainage (first visit, reinstruct based on need).

11. Instruct caregiver to humidify inspired air by cool vaporizer in room to prevent dry mucosa (first visit).

12. Assess caregiver's knowledge. Demonstrate procedures for encouraging coughing and postural drainage of lung segments using gravity and chest percussion (first visit).

13. Instruct caregiver to perform postural drainage procedures while positioning the infant on lap or bed (first visit, reinstruct as needed).

14. Instruct on suction of secretions if unable to remove by coughing or postural drainage. If tracheostomy is present, instruct to suction via tube and perform tube and site care (see p. 114) to maintain patency (first visit, subsequent visits as needed).

15. Instruct on administration of ordered liquid form of bronchodilator medicine, steroid therapy (usually in feedings), and inhalation of bronchodilator medicine by small volume nebulizer or hand-held measured dose inhaler. Assess and instruct caregiver to assess response for medication effectiveness and side effects (first visit, until instruction given for all medications).

16. Demonstrate elevation of head of bed and positions of optimal comfort for sleeping and resting that allow for ease in breathing and chest expansion (first visit).

17. Assess vital signs. Collaborate with caregiver to note and record presence of edema or water retention (irritability, poor feeding, labored breathing, or skin color change), signs and symptoms of heart failure (see p. 10) or pulmonary hypertension, or other complications that can occur (each visit).

18. Assess response to interventions and report untoward responses to physician (each visit).

19. Inform caregiver and family of availability of American Lung Association and local support groups for information and services (first visit).

CAREGIVER/CHILD AND FAMILY INTERVENTIONS

1. Becomes CPR certified. Places list of emergency activities and telephone numbers in strategic place for easy access.

2. Locates resource to acquire special equipment and supplies (oxygen concentrator and back-up tank with gauge, tubing, small volume nebulizer, tubing, and medication containers).

3. Assesses respirations for rate and ease, use of accessory muscles, pulse for rate and rhythm. Determines care for day based on changes. Modifies plans for treatment if deviations from baseline values are noted.

4. Correctly applies and monitors cardiopulmonary status with an apnea monitor, if appropriate.

5. Correctly administers humidified oxygen (continuous or intermittent) using correct size nasal prongs and increases oxygen when cyanosis, crying, or dyspnea persists or during feedings or postural drainage. Decreases oxygen level as soon as respiratory assessment baseline values are achieved; notifies physician if oxygen level cannot be decreased.

6. Follows safety precautions in oxygen use, including posting a sign stating, "oxygen in use, no sparks, no open flames, no oil or grease, no smoking." Maintains a standby oxygen source if not administered continuously.

7. Administers medications safely in correct form and frequency. Detects adverse reactions and inability of medications to control dyspnea or clear secretions from airway and reports to physician.

8. Stores medications safely and avoids administration of any medications not prescribed.

9. Performs chest physiotherapy by gravity and use of pillows and positioning without causing fatigue to infant. Percusses only over rib areas. Frequency and time limit depend on need for mucus removal; removes mucus by suctioning, if needed.

10. Performs postural drainage for child before, 2 hours after meals, or in morning and before bedtime. Encourages coughing during and after procedure and spitting mucus into tissue.

11. Positions child, with use of foam rubber wedge or pillows, to elevate head for sleep and rest.

12. Identifies any deterioration in respiratory status and reports to physician.

13. Takes child for monthly or periodic chest x-ray examination as prescribed to monitor disease stage and assess lung damage; complies with flu immunization appointments.

Nursing diagnosis

Fluid volume excess
Related factors: compromised regulatory mechanism
Defining characteristics: edema, weight gain, intake greater than output, abnormal breath sounds (crackles)

OUTCOMES
Short-term
Reduction in fluid volume excess evidenced by respiratory status within baseline parameters, intake and output (I&O) ratio within baseline parameters, decreasing edema and weight gain with effective diuretic therapy and adequate hydration (expected within 2 to 3 days)

Long-term
I&O balance maintained with stable respiratory function and optimal weight maintenance (fluid related) (expected within 2 weeks)

NURSING INTERVENTIONS/INSTRUCTIONS
1. Assess for respiratory distress with tachypnea, dyspnea, retractions, crackles on auscultation, increased oxygen needs, associated edema, and reduced urine output (each visit).
2. Assess and instruct caregiver to assess I&O every 2 to 8 hours, depending on status. Instruct in measurement of fluid intake with or without restrictions and estimation of output (first and second visits).
3. Instruct on amount of fluids allowed and frequency of administration. Administer gastrostomy feeding of ordered low fluid volume if fluid amounts are restricted (see "Altered Nutrition," nursing diagnosis) (first and second visits).

4. Assess and instruct on taking and recording weight daily or more frequently if ordered with same scale and child wearing same clothing (every visit).
5. Instruct on administration of diuretic regimen with or without a potassium supplement as ordered and instruct caregiver to assess responses to expect such as weight loss and improved breathing; include dose, route, frequency, and side effects (first and second visits with reinstruction as needed).
6. Instruct to observe and report edema, respiratory changes, skin color changes, irritability, and poor feeding or tolerance of feedings to home health care nurse (each visit).

CAREGIVER/CHILD AND FAMILY INTERVENTIONS

1. Assesses for respiratory changes and need for additional oxygen.
2. Monitors intake by amount of feedings and output by estimating number of diapers used or weighing diapers every 8 hours or daily based on fluid excess.
3. Weighs daily or more frequently based on persistent signs and symptoms of fluid retention.
4. Maintains fluid restrictions within prescribed limits over 24-hour period.
5. Correctly administers diuretic and potassium in feedings as ordered and assesses for side effects, primarily dehydration.
6. Reports adverse responses or reactions to physician.

Nursing diagnosis

Risk for infection

Related factors: inadequate primary defenses (stasis of secretions), chronic disease (lung damage), insufficient knowledge of caregiver to avoid exposure of child to pathogens

Defining characteristics: inability to mobilize and cough up secretions, change in color of sputum to yellow or green, temperature instability, hyperirritability, vomiting, diarrhea

OUTCOMES

Short-term
Early detection of signs and symptoms of infection
and respiratory infection prevented evidenced by optimal respiratory parameters and airway patency maintained; afebrile status; and secretions that are colorless,
thin, and easily removed (expected with daily assessment)

Long-term
Adaptation to lifestyle that promotes clean, safe environment and actions to minimize risk for respiratory infections demonstrated (expected ongoing)

NURSING INTERVENTIONS/INSTRUCTIONS

1. Assess home and living conditions (see "Environmental
   Assessment," p. 37, for guidelines) (first visit, follow-up
   for additional modifications on second visit).
2. Assess for changes in respiratory rate, depth, and ease
   and for diminished breath sounds on auscultation (each
   visit).
3. Assess temperature for increases/decreases from baseline norm, increased viscosity, change in color/odor of
   pulmonary secretions, skin color changes, irritability,
   and changes in feeding or elimination pattern (each
   visit).
4. Instruct on changes in respiratory pattern, sputum, and
   behavior to note and report to physician (first visit).
5. Instruct on taking axillary temperature (oral for child)
   (first visit).
6. Instruct on administration of oral liquid antibiotic
   and antipyretic medication in proper form, usually
   in feedings or by dropper, depending on child's
   age and responses to expect (first visit, reinforce).
7. Instruct on precautions such as washing hands, avoiding contact with those having an upper respiratory
   infection, and importance of adequate nutritional intake and rest to prevent infection (first visit, ongoing).
8. If ordered, obtain sputum specimen, when possible, for
   culture (any visit).

CAREGIVER/CHILD AND FAMILY INTERVENTIONS

1. Takes oral or axillary temperature if sputum changes color or respirations change.
2. Observes for changes in respiratory status and in sputum amount, color, odor, or consistency and presence of productive or nonproductive cough. Reports changes to physician.
3. Administers antibiotic therapy correctly until all medication is taken.
4. Avoids possible exposure of child to family members or others with suspected upper respiratory infections. Wears face mask, if appropriate.
5. Performs proper handwashing frequently, especially before and after caring for child. Uses clean or sterile technique as appropriate during care and procedures.
6. Cleanses oxygen cannula every 8 hours with hot soapy water. Washes humidifier and refills daily with sterile water. Washes filter on concentrator weekly.
7. Maintains an environment free from respiratory contaminants, humidified, and well-ventilated.
8. Properly disposes of all articles and supplies used in giving care or performing procedures according to universal precautions.

Nursing diagnosis

Altered nutrition: less than body requirements/ineffective infant feeding pattern

Related factors: inability to ingest enough nutrients because of biologic factor of increased caloric need resulting from work of breathing, fluid restrictions, esophageal reflux, feeding aversion

Defining characteristics: inadequate food intake (prematurity, inability to suck/swallow while breathing) and poor weight gain, low–birth-weight status, increased energy expenditure related to work of breathing

OUTCOMES

Short-term

Adequate nutritional intake by gastrostomy, nasogastric tube, or oral feedings with minimal effort evidenced by

weight gain (not attributed to fluid retention), daily intake
by child of planned meals (expected within 1 week)

Long-term
Nutritional status for optimal growth, development, and
healing demonstrated by adequate feedings and weight
maintenance or weight gains at recommended level for age
and normal nutritional needs/pattern and activities that
facilitate successful feeding behaviors performed by caregiver (expected within 1 to 3 months)

NURSING INTERVENTIONS/INSTRUCTIONS

1. Assess nutritional requirement for age and weight,
   including needed caloric intake, weight deviation
   from standard for age, food and fluid preferences for
   child, and times of meals or feedings (see "Gastrointestinal System Assessment," p. 16, for guidelines) (first visit).
2. Demonstrate and instruct on administration of formula feedings of 24 to 28 calories to infant via gastrostomy, or adding a hyperosmolar nutritional
   supplement of high glucose or triglyceride oil if ordered to reduce volume when fluid is restricted (see
   "Alternative Feeding Management," p. 205) (first and
   second visits).
3. Instruct on formula preparation and storage, provide
   written instructions to follow, or obtain home referral
   of nutritionist for instructions (first visit, reinstruct
   as needed).
4. Check gastrostomy/nasogastric tube patency and placement. Change tube and instruct in daily gastrostomy
   site and tube care (each visit).
5. Collaborate with caregiver to plan, prepare, and offer
   small feedings or meals of preferred foods of appropriate consistency to child to meet additional caloric
   needs at as normal feeding times as possible (first and
   second visits).
6. Suggest allowing rest periods and avoiding rushing
   during meals. Place infant or child in position of
   comfort by holding infant upright and child in sitting
   position at table within easy reach of food and with

appropriate amounts of food and properly sized utensils (first visit).

7. Suggest providing quiet, relaxing environment and remaining with child during meals. Increase oxygen during meals and assist to eat if weak or lacks energy to feed self (first visit).
8. Instruct to weigh child every 3 to 7 days to assess for gains or losses with allowances for possible fluid retention (first visit).
9. Support participation of caregiver and family in care regimen (each visit).
10. Initiate social services referral for assistance in obtaining food and other supplies for respiratory care (any appropriate visit).

CAREGIVER/CHILD AND FAMILY INTERVENTIONS

1. Provides ordered caloric intake via gastrostomy tube to increase or maintain weight.
2. Follows instructions for mixing and refrigerating formula correctly and preparing for administration of gastrostomy feedings.
3. Positions infant and feeds at appropriate times. Increases oxygen if respirations change during feeding.
4. Provides pacifier to infant for nonnutritive sucking if fed via gastrostomy.
5. Checks gastrostomy tube patency by instillation of 10 to 30 ml of water after feeding or medication administration.
6. Prepares nutritional foods and fluids of proper consistency and texture (e.g., finger foods and other appealing selections for child) and offers at appropriate times and frequency.
7. Feeds or assists to ingest meals, if needed, to conserve energy and paces feedings according to breathing pattern.
8. Promotes pleasant environment for child to enhance intake.
9. Measures weight using same scale, with the child wearing same clothing, and at same time on specified days. Compares changes with I&O ratio to determine if gains or losses are related to fluid imbalance.

Nursing diagnosis

Risk for impaired skin integrity
Related factors: external factors of pressure and irritation at tube sites (gastrostomy, nares)
Defining characteristics: tissue damage or disruption of skin or mucous membranes

OUTCOMES
Short-term
Skin and mucous membranes protected from irritation and minimal tube pressure to susceptible tissue sites evidenced by clean, dry, intact areas free of redness or other color changes and predisposition to breakdown (expected within 1 to 2 days)

Long-term
Intact skin and mucous membranes free from infection, discomfort, breakdown; gastrostomy and nasal cannula site maintained (expected within 1 week)

NURSING INTERVENTIONS/INSTRUCTIONS

1. Assess gastrostomy tube site for redness, drainage, edema, rash or irritation, tension or movement of tube, use of tape or dressing to secure tubing, and nares mucosa for dryness, cleanness, redness, crusting, lesions, or breaks caused by oxygen nasal cannula (each visit).
2. Instruct to apply petrolatum at gastrostomy tube site and to use diaper to cover site and prevent tube movement (first visit).
3. Suggest using only small amount of tape to secure tube or to place tape on gauze square and then tape to skin (first visit).
4. Instruct on care of gastrostomy site to maintain clean, dry skin and in application of bandage or diaper to prevent tube manipulation (first visit, reinforce on second visit).
5. Apply water-soluble lubricant to nares during oxygen therapy and instruct on procedure using soft-tipped

applicator. Change cannula tape site daily or as needed (first visit).

6. Apply and instruct on application of ointment or creams (antimicrobial or corticosteroid) to tube site, if ordered, for rashes or breaks in skin at gastrostomy site (first and second visits).

7. Instruct caregiver to report any irritation or soreness at tube areas to physician immediately (first visit).

CAREGIVER/CHILD AND FAMILY INTERVENTIONS

1. Assesses perigastrostomy skin site and nares mucosa daily. Gently washes and pats dry, avoiding excess movement or tension of tubes on tissues.

2. Applies petrolatum or ordered ointments at gastrostomy site, uses gauze dressing around tube, if needed, and tapes sparingly or secures in place with diaper.

3. Applies water-soluble ointment to nares as needed and pads facial tissue under cannula tubing to prevent irritation.

4. Reports any reddened areas, drainage, swelling, or breaks in skin at tube sites.

Nursing diagnosis

Altered growth and development
Related factors: environmental and stimulation deficiencies, effects of chronic illness, inadequate parental caregiving, prescribed dependence, nutritional deficit

Defining characteristics: delay or difficulty in performing skills (motor, social, expressive) typical of age group, altered physical growth, inability of child to perform self-care or self-control activities appropriate for age

OUTCOMES
Short-term
Growth and development behavior and activities evidenced by absence of deficits, delays, or regression of functioning; performance of age-appropriate growth and development within limits imposed by illness (expected within 6 to 12 weeks)

Long-term
Progressive age-appropriate steady growth and development advances and achievement of normal physical, emotional, and social parameters (expected ongoing)

NURSING INTERVENTIONS/INSTRUCTIONS

1. Assess expected growth and developmental level for age and extent of deficits from normal patterns that include fine and gross motor skills, language and social development, psychosocial, interpersonal skills, and cognitive development (see "Growth and Developmental Assessment," p. 31, for guidelines) (every visit).
2. Assess caregiver, family, and environment for stressful events and ability to provide love and care, adequate stimulation, and play activities (each visit).
3. Assess for caregiver overprotection or negligence (each visit).
4. Instruct on normal growth and development patterns for child's age and possible lag in development caused by chronic illness (first visit).
5. Assist caregiver and family to develop goals and participate in care to achieve optimal development (ongoing).
6. Instruct to monitor child activity tolerance and collaborate to develop a plan based on this information to provide visual, auditory, and tactile stimulation; gross motor skills for infant; time with child for talking or play activities; and self-care activities (ongoing).
7. Provide encouragement and support for efforts made by child and caregivers (each visit).
8. Provide early referral to professional resources to assist child in specific areas of need such as speech or physical therapist, special education teacher, psychosocial counselor, and social worker (any visit).

CAREGIVER/CHILD AND FAMILY INTERVENTIONS

1. Complies with provision of age-related activities to enhance stimulation, independence, and developmental progression (cognitive, psychomotor, and psychosocial).
2. Sets realistic goals for growth and development achievement.
3. Maintains consistent caregiver and schedule of care and activities.

4. Provides an organized and consistent program of daily activities that includes mobiles, music, toys, books, and other age-related objects.
5. Provides time for talking and playing with other children and family members.
6. Holds, rocks, and cuddles child to provide touch and loving care.
7. Provides opportunity to participate in age-related self-care activities, including dressing, bathing, eating, and toileting with adaptations as needed.
8. Attends parenting classes for child stimulation, growth and development milestones, and age-related discipline and expectations.
9. Identifies and uses specialized services to assist with growth/developmental lags.

Nursing diagnosis

Ineffective family coping: compromised
Related factors: prolonged disease that exhausts supportive capacity of significant people, frequent hospitalizations, family disorganization and role changes
Defining characteristics: significant person's expression of inability to cope and feelings of fear, anxiety, guilt, anger, inadequate understanding of chronic illness, and long-term care by family

OUTCOMES
Short-term
Family members demonstrate ability to plan and care for child evidenced by provision of normal environment, decreased anxiety and feelings of inadequacy, and integration of information about family needs into care and support of child (expected within 1 to 2 weeks)

Long-term
Family coping and adaptation evidenced by optimal support and participation in care and maintenance of family relationships (expected within 1 to 2 months)

NURSING INTERVENTIONS/INSTRUCTIONS

1. Meet and collaborate with family members to assess stressors, coping mechanisms, and planning of care (first visit, repeat as needed).
2. Reinforce information to promote family understanding of illness and care needs (each visit).
3. Discuss and allow family to express feelings of guilt, anxiety, and depression and promote communication among members to verbalize feelings and expectations with each other (any visit).
4. Instruct on methods to develop appropriate coping skills and to meet family's medical and other needs (e.g., emotional, financial, food, respite, supplies, and equipment) by referral to social or counseling services (first visit, each visit as needed).

CAREGIVER/CHILD AND FAMILY INTERVENTIONS

1. Displays decreasing anxiety and anger and provides a supportive family environment.
2. Develops trust in home care personnel and collaborates in developing and modifying daily care.
3. Provides care and treatments effectively.
4. Recognizes and assumes role changes and maintains family integrity.
5. Develops coping mechanisms that have positive effect within family.
6. Identifies problem areas and obtains community or professional assistance or services as needed.

SAMPLE DOCUMENTATION INCLUSIONS

1. Specific assessment
   Assess respiratory rate, ease, sputum characteristics, vital signs, weight, I&O, skin integrity, growth and development status, environmental hazards, and adaptive capacity of family.
2. Specific care/teaching
   Teach correct administration of medications, antimicrobial therapy, gastrostomy feedings, postural drainage, oropharyngeal suctioning, skin and site care, and universal precautions, administration and care of oxygen, oximetry, preparation, and care.

3. General
   Note responses to care and teaching, changes in plan, progression or regression of health status, and adaptation to long-term care.
4. See "Documentation and Family Home Record Keeping" in Appendix for general required documentation components for all home care visits.

 Cystic Fibrosis

Cystic fibrosis (CF) is an autosomal, recessive, multisystem life-threatening genetic disease of children affecting the exocrine glands. CF is characterized by increased viscosity of mucous gland secretions. This causes obstruction as mucus accumulates and dilates small passages in organs, primarily in the pancreas and lungs. The sweat glands lose the ability to conserve salt, resulting in an increase in sodium and chloride in sweat and saliva (electrolyte deficit). Pancreatic function is affected by loss of the ability to secrete enzymes (trypsin, lipase, and amylase), affecting fat and protein digestion and absorption with the obstruction of pancreatic ducts by thick secretions that prevent the flow of enzymes into the duodenum. This leads to malnutrition and malabsorption, and intestinal function is affected by obstructive mucus, leading to fecal impaction, intussusception, and rectal prolapse. Liver function is affected by obstruction of ducts, causing cirrhosis and digestive problems. Pulmonary function is affected by impaired ciliary action and bronchial obstruction, leading to infection (pneumonia and bronchitis) and chronic hypoxemia. The presence of the disease is confirmed by 6 months of age and varies in severity.

Home care is primarily concerned with pulmonary function, prevention of pulmonary infection, and nutritional support. The long-term nature of the disease requires additional home nursing assistance and instruction on the growth and development needs of the child and adaptation needs of the caregiver and family.

Nursing diagnosis

Ineffective airway clearance/gas exchange
Related factors: decreased energy, fatigue, tracheobronchial obstruction (thick mucus), altered oxygen supply
Defining characteristics: dyspnea; tachypnea; cyanosis; abnormal breath sounds (wheezing, crackles); inability to move secretions; dry, nonproductive cough; hypoxia; hypercapnia; barrel chest; hemoptysis; chest x-ray film revealing pulmonary changes (hyperinflation, eventual lung fibrosis)

OUTCOMES

Short-term
Stable breathing pattern, airway patency with effective ventilation established, evidenced by respiratory rate, ease, and depth maintained without distress; normal color of skin, mucous membranes; expectoration of mucus; breath sounds clear, equal bilaterally (expected within 2 to 4 days, ongoing)

Long-term
Management of home respiratory care evidenced by respiratory baselines maintained within disease parameters; effective treatments, medication regimen demonstrated; pulmonary complications, infections prevented (expected within 1 month)

NURSING INTERVENTIONS/INSTRUCTIONS

1. Assess caregiver knowledge; proper understanding of disease and status, including pulmonary signs, symptoms caused by condition and reason for them; ability to adapt to lifetime therapy (first visit).
2. Assess trends in respiratory status, including rate, depth, ease, or effort; dyspnea; wheezing; thick, tenacious secretions; cough (dry, nonproductive, paroxysmal); color of skin, oral mucous membranes, and nailbeds; finger clubbing; and abnormal breath sounds, (see "Pulmonary System Assessment," p. 10, for guidelines) (every visit).

3. Provide information based on assessment and instruct on signs, symptoms to note, and actions to take. Use language that is easily understood or provide written instructions (first visit, review as needed).

4. Instruct on assessment of respirations, establish baselines, and collaborate with caregiver to plan care based on respiratory status (first visit, reinstruct on plan changes as needed).

5. Demonstrate and instruct on bronchodilator aerosol therapy to remove mucus. Advise to perform before postural drainage (first visit, reinstruct as needed).

6. Instruct on administration of liquid form of bronchodilators, expectorants (usually in feedings), and inhalation of bronchodilator by small volume nebulizer or handheld measured dose inhaler. Assess response for medication effectiveness and side effects (first visit, until instruction given for all medications).

7. Assess caregiver's baseline knowledge, demonstrate procedure for encouraging coughing, and teach child to cough and expectorate into tissue (first visit).

8. Instruct caregiver and child or reinforce instruction given by physiotherapist on postural drainage of lung segments using gravity and chest percussion with portable automatic percussor or hands cupping or clapping, with frequency depending on severity of condition (first visit, reinforce second visit).

9. Instruct caregiver and child on breathing exercises by participating in games and play activities (first visit, second visit if needed).

10. Instruct on methods to provide humidified environment and increased fluid intake if allowed (first visit).

11. Demonstrate elevation of head of bed; high-Fowler's position and sitting positions for optimal comfort during rest that allow for ease in breathing, chest expansion, and conservation of energy (first visit).

12. Suggest loose, nonrestrictive clothing and linens (first visit).

13. Secure referral for respiratory physical therapist to teach and perform chest physiotherapy and breathing exercises if treatments are ineffective, if unable to remove mucus (any visit).

14. Assess response to interventions. Report untoward responses to physician (each visit).
15. Inform caregiver and family of availability of services provided by American Lung Association and Cystic Fibrosis Foundation and local support groups for information (first visit).

CAREGIVER/CHILD AND FAMILY INTERVENTIONS

1. Locates resource to acquire special equipment/supplies (small volume nebulizer, tubing, medication containers, humidified oxygen, and suction equipment, if appropriate). Collaborates with social services to secure financial assistance, if needed.
2. Assesses respirations for rate, ease, and ability to remove secretions. Modifies plans for treatment if deviation from baseline is noted.
3. Administers ordered medications safely via correct form, method, route, and frequency. Detects adverse reactions, inability of medications to ease respirations, or clear secretions from airway and reports to physician. Avoids use of cough suppressants.
4. Allows independence of child in self-administration of medications based on age and abilities.
5. Maintains environment with optimal humidity, temperature, and ventilation.
6. Performs chest physiotherapy by gravity, use of pillows, and positioning without fatigue to child and percusses only over rib areas (frequency and time limit dependent on need for mucus removal). Performs deep breathing exercises daily as part of therapy.
7. Performs postural drainage and percussion for child before or 2 hours after meals, in morning, before bedtime, or as frequently as every 4 hours, if needed; uses battery-operated percussor, if available.
8. Encourages and remains with child if coughing is severe during and after procedure and reminds child to expectorate mucus into tissue instead of swallowing secretions.
9. Provides oral care following physiotherapy for mouth odors and comfort.
10. Participates in play and games such as blowing bubbles,

ping-pong balls (incentive spirometry), pinwheels; hanging on trapeze by knees; performing somersaults; standing on head; and other nonstressful activities to encourage breathing exercises and effective postural drainage.
11. Identifies any deterioration in respiratory status or blood in sputum (common in older children) and reports to physician.

Nursing diagnosis

Risk for infection
Related factors: inadequate primary defenses (stasis of secretions), chronic disease (lung damage), insufficient knowledge of caregiver to avoid exposure of child to pathogens
Defining characteristics: inability to cough up secretions, change in color of sputum to yellow or green, temperature instability, chills, hyperirritability, respiratory distress, frequent hospitalizations for infections

OUTCOMES
Short-term
Early detection and interventions for signs, symptoms of respiratory infection evidenced by optimal respiratory parameters, airway patency maintained; afebrile status; secretions that are slightly yellow, colorless, loosened, expectorated (expected with daily assessment)

Long-term
Adaptation to lifestyle that promotes clean, safe environment; actions to prevent, minimize risk for pulmonary infections demonstrated by infection-free respiratory system; avoidance of hospitalizations (expected ongoing)

NURSING INTERVENTIONS/INSTRUCTIONS
1. Assess home and living conditions (see "Environmental Assessment," p. 37, for guidelines) (first visit, follow-up for additional modifications on second visit).

2. Assess for changes in respiratory rate, depth, and ease and diminished breath sounds (each visit).

3. Assess body temperature, increased viscosity, change in color/odor of pulmonary secretions, skin color changes, irritability, and changes in feeding or elimination pattern (each visit).

4. Instruct on changes in respiratory pattern, sputum, behavior to note. Report to physician (first visit).

5. Instruct on taking rectal (oral for child) temperature (first visit).

6. Instruct on importance of continuing chest physiotherapy and deep breathing to remove secretions (first visit, as needed).

7. Instruct on administration of ordered prophylaxis or therapy with oral liquid antibiotic and antipyretic medications in proper form, usually in feedings by dropper or in tablet form depending on child's age (first visit, reinforce on subsequent visits).

8. Inform and support need for hospitalization to treat infection with intravenous (IV) antibiotic therapy (any visit as appropriate).

9. Instruct on intermittent administration of IV antibiotic therapy in home via venous access device (peripheral or central venous catheter) if caregiver is willing and able to perform procedure (see "Medication Administration and Teaching Guidelines," pp. 450-463) (each visit during length of therapy).

10. Monitor vital signs, equipment effectiveness, diagnostic studies as available, supplies on hand, adverse reactions to antimicrobial medications (e.g., diarrhea and sore mouth), and IV insertion site (each visit).

11. Instruct on precautions to prevent infection such as washing hands and avoiding contact with people who have respiratory infection and on importance of adequate nutritional intake and rest (ongoing).

12. Obtain sputum specimen if possible for culture; obtain blood specimen, if ordered (any visit).

CAREGIVER/CHILD AND FAMILY INTERVENTIONS

1. Observes for changes in respiratory status; changes in sputum amount, color, odor, and consistency; decreased

appetite; and irritability indicating infection. Reports changes to physician.

2. Takes oral or axillary temperature if sputum color or respirations change.

3. Administers oral antibiotic therapy correctly until all medication is taken or ongoing administration for prophylactic therapy.

4. Administers intermittent antibiotic therapy over 24 hours via venous access device (heparin lock for short-term, central venous catheter for long-term), including aseptic technique, drug preparation, flushing of device, site care, disposal of syringes and needles according to universal precautions. Uses infusion pump if appropriate.

5. Has knowledge of, notes, and reports side effects of antibiotic therapy to physician because high doses are usually administered.

6. Continues daily postural drainage and chest percussion.

7. Avoids possible exposure of child to family members or others with respiratory infections. Wears face mask if appropriate.

8. Performs proper handwashing frequently, especially before caring for child. Uses clean or sterile technique as appropriate during care and procedures.

9. Maintains environment that is clean, free from respiratory contaminants, humidified, and well ventilated. Avoids extremes in environmental temperature.

10. Properly disposes of all articles/supplies used in giving care or performing procedures according to universal precautions.

11. Ensures physician follow-up visits and yearly immunization for influenza.

Nursing diagnosis

Altered nutrition: less than body requirements
Related factors: inability to ingest enough nutrients because of anorexia, refusal of meals; inability to digest, absorb nutrients because of lack of pancreatic enzymes
Defining characteristics: inadequate food intake; weight loss

(malnutrition); failure to thrive; irritability during feedings/meals; coughing; dyspnea resulting in emesis; poor skin turgor; bulky, foul-smelling feces; steatorrhea (fat); azotorrhea (protein); thin extremities; abdominal pain; cramping; distention; prolapse of rectum

OUTCOMES

Short-term
Improved appetite with adequate nutritional, increased fluid intake; functional bowel elimination evidenced by soft-formed feces; weight gain or minimal loss; daily intake by child of planned balanced meals, feedings (expected within 1 week)

Long-term
Nutritional status for optimal growth, development, prevention of malnutrition demonstrated by nutritionally balanced food; satisfactory weight gains at recommended level for age; normal nutritional needs/pattern, bowel elimination characteristics, activities that facilitate successful feeding (expected within 1 to 3 months)

NURSING INTERVENTIONS/INSTRUCTIONS

1. Assess nutritional requirement for age and weight; needed caloric intake; weight deviation from standard for age; appetite and child's food and fluid preferences; times of meals/feedings (see "Gastrointestinal System Assessment and Nutritional Assessment," pp. 16 and 17, for guidelines) (first visit).
2. Assess bowel elimination pattern; feces characteristics for looseness, light color, foul smell, frothiness, and frequency; and abdominal discomfort (each visit).
3. Instruct and collaborate with caregiver on planning and administration of a high-calorie, high-protein, moderate-carbohydrate dietary intake with possible fat inclusions to increase calories, and increased salt intake, especially in hot weather (first and second visits).
4. Instruct to avoid giving respiratory treatments after meals because this can cause coughing and vomiting (first visit).
5. Instruct on administration of pancreatic enzymes mixed

with cool food during middle of meal and with snacks, fat-soluble vitamins (A, D, E, and K), iron supplement, as ordered (first visit, until instruction for all medications has been given).

6. Collaborate with caregiver to offer small feedings or meals of preferred foods of appropriate consistency and supplemental liquid protein to meet additional caloric needs as near routine feeding times as possible (first and second visits).
7. Observe feedings and note irritability, breathing difficulty, or coughing. Assist and suggest calm environment during meals and feedings and actions to take to minimize frustrations (allow rest periods, avoid rushing during meals, place infant in position of comfort by holding infant upright, and place child in sitting position at table within easy reach of food with appropriate amounts of preferred foods and properly sized utensils) (any visit).
8. Instruct on importance of increasing fluids, if allowed, especially in summer (first visit).
9. Demonstrate and instruct caregiver to weigh child every 3 to 7 days or daily, using same scale at same time of day (infant more frequently) to assess for change (first visit).
10. Support participation and presence of caregiver and family at mealtime (each visit).
11. Administer nutritional intake by nasogastric tube, gastrostomy, or total parenteral nutrition as ordered (see "Alternative Feeding Management," p. 205) (any visit).
12. Initiate social services referral for assistance in obtaining food, nutritionist for diet planning if needed (first or appropriate visit).

CAREGIVER/CHILD AND FAMILY INTERVENTIONS

1. Plans and provides menus of diet that contain caloric, protein, carbohydrate, and fat intake with supplements (Pediasure) as needed.
2. Prepares nutritional foods and fluids of proper consistency and texture and finger foods, snacks, and other appealing selections for child. Offers food at appropriate times and frequency in appropriate amounts.

3. Feeds or assists to ingest meals, if needed, to conserve energy. Paces feedings according to appetite, breathing pattern, and coughing.
4. Promotes pleasant environment for child that can enhance intake. Integrates meal times into family routine.
5. Monitors bowel elimination, failure to pass feces, and abdominal distention. Modifies enzyme administration based on physician's orders.
6. Changes soiled diapers frequently as needed.
7. Obtains daily weight using same scale, with child wearing same clothing, at same time on specified days. Records and compares changes.
8. Complies with collection of feces for laboratory measurement of fat and enzyme content and sweat test for chloride concentration, as ordered.

Nursing diagnosis

Risk for activity intolerance
Related factors: generalized weakness; presence of respiratory disorder, imbalance between oxygen supply and demand
Defining characteristics: exertional dyspnea, verbalization of fatigue, inability to play, perform self-care activities

OUTCOMES
Short-term
Optimal endurance, ability to perform normal daily activities evidenced by normal respiratory status, dyspnea absent during activity (expected within 1 week)

Long-term
Progressive increase in play, other activities demonstrated within baseline respiratory, energy parameters (expected ongoing)

NURSING INTERVENTIONS/INSTRUCTIONS
1. Assess energy level, deficits in activity level, changes in respiratory status during activity, and ability and interest in participating in favorite play activities and self-care appropriate to age (every visit).

2. Inform caregiver and child of relationship between disease and inability or interference in performing activities and possible consequences of activity (first visit).
3. Inform of alternate methods of performing activities while conserving energy (first and second visits).
4. Assist to plan changes in types and timing of activities such as quiet play, depending on response to activity and age of child (each visit).
5. Advise to administer bronchodilators before activities and plan to include rest periods following activities (first visit).
6. Instruct to increase activity as tolerated within child's physical and psychologic capabilities and on signs and symptoms of fatigue or respiratory distress (each visit).
7. Assist to modify environment to accommodate exercises and play activities. Encourage caregiver to participate in activities (first and second visits).
8. Encourage school attendance. Inform family to advise school nurse and teacher of child's limitations. Encourage feedback to ensure understanding (any visit).

CAREGIVER/CHILD AND FAMILY INTERVENTIONS

1. Participates in planned activities within limitations. Attends school appropriate for age and development.
2. Schedules activities into daily routine as tolerated.
3. Performs activities when bronchodilator is at optimal therapeutic level.
4. Avoids extremes in activities that cause fatigue and substitutes less strenuous ones.
5. Identifies signs and symptoms that require adjustment in type of activities and discontinues activity if needed.
6. Monitors and documents progress toward achieving optimal daily activity and adverse responses to activity.
7. Allows child to select and include favorite activities and play.
8. Provides quiet, safe environment conducive to promoting activities within identified limitations.

Nursing diagnosis

Altered growth and development
Related factors: environmental, stimulation deficiencies; ef-

fects of chronic illness; inadequate parental caregiving; prescribed dependence; nutritional deficit

Defining characteristics: delay, difficulty in performing skills (motor, social, expressive) typical of age group; altered physical growth from effect of disease on ingestion, digestion, absorption of nutrients; inability of child to perform self-care, self-control activities appropriate for age; anxiety; anger; depression

OUTCOMES

Short-term
Expected growth, development, activities for age evidenced by minimal deficits, delays, regression of functioning; performance of age-appropriate growth, development skills within limits imposed by illness (expected within 6 to 12 weeks)

Long-term
Progressive age-appropriate growth, development advances, achievement of normal physical, emotional, social parameters (expected ongoing with respect to age)

NURSING INTERVENTIONS/INSTRUCTIONS

1. Assess expected growth, developmental level for age; extent of deficits from normal patterns that include fine and gross motor skills, language, social development, psychosocial and interpersonal skills, and cognitive development (see "Growth and Developmental Assessment," p. 31, for guidelines) (every visit).
2. Assess caregiver, family, and environment for stressful events and ability to provide love, caring, adequate stimulation, and play activities (each visit).
3. Assess for caregiver overprotection or negligence of child (each visit).
4. Instruct on normal growth and development patterns for child's age and possible lag in development, maturation, and physical changes caused by chronic illness (first visit).
5. Assist caregiver and family to develop goals and participate in care plan to achieve optimal development potential (first visit, ongoing).
6. Instruct to monitor child activity tolerance. Collaborate

to develop plan based on this information to provide visual, auditory, and tactile stimulation; gross motor skills for infant; time with child for talking, play activities, and self-care activities (first visit, ongoing).

7. Provide encouragement and support for efforts made by child and caregivers (each visit).

8. Provide early referral to professional resources such as speech or physical therapist, special education teacher, psychosocial counselor, or social worker to assist child in specific areas of need (any visit).

CAREGIVER/CHILD AND FAMILY INTERVENTIONS

1. Complies with provision of age-related activities to enhance stimulation, independence, developmental progression (cognitive, psychomotor, and psychosocial).

2. Sets realistic goals for growth and developmental achievement.

3. Maintains consistent caregiver and schedule of care/activities.

4. Implements consistent encouragement and appropriate discipline.

5. Provides organized, consistent program of daily activities that include mobiles, music, toys, books, swimming, painting, sandbox, other age-related articles, and school attendance for school-age child.

6. Provides time for talking and playing with other children and family members. Invites friends to visit and play. Involves in age-appropriate social and sex role activities.

7. Holds, rocks, and cuddles child to provide touch and loving care.

8. Provides opportunity to participate and promotes independence in age-related self-care activities, including dressing, bathing, eating, and toileting with adaptations as needed.

9. Attends parenting classes for child stimulation, growth/development milestones, age-related discipline, and expectations.

10. Identifies and uses specialized services to assist with growth/developmental lags.

Nursing diagnosis

Ineffective family coping: compromised

Related factors: prolonged disease that exhausts supportive capacity of significant people; frequent hospitalizations; family disorganization, role changes

Defining characteristics: significant person's expression of inability to cope; feelings of fear, anxiety, guilt, anger; inadequate understanding of chronic illness, long-term care by family; physical changes noted in child (cachexia, barrel chest, cyanosis)

OUTCOMES

Short-term

Family members demonstrate ability to plan, care for child evidenced by provision of normal environment, decreased anxiety, feelings of inadequacy; integration of information about family needs into care, support of child (expected within 1 to 2 weeks)

Long-term

Family coping; adaptation evidenced by optimal support, participation in care; maintenance of family relationships, marriage; demonstrates positive feelings, acceptance of child's body image; self-esteem changes; ability to provide support to child, explain the condition and treatments (expected within 1 to 2 months)

NURSING INTERVENTIONS/INSTRUCTIONS

1. Meet and collaborate with family members to assess stressors, coping mechanisms, planning of care (first visit, repeat as needed).
2. Assess understanding of condition and prescribed treatments. Reinforce information to promote family understanding of illness and care needs (each visit).
3. Discuss and allow family to express feelings of guilt, anxiety, and depression. Promote communication among members to verbalize feelings, expectations, and need for family counseling (any visit).

4. Instruct on methods to develop appropriate coping skills and to meet family's needs (medical, emotional, financial, food, respite, supplies, and equipment) by referral to social or counseling services (first visit, as needed).
5. Encourage and support all efforts to participate in care of child by family members. Assist to modify family activities according to daily needs of child (each visit).
6. Allow for and support anticipatory grieving as appropriate as disease progresses (any visit).
7. Inform of resources that provide genetic counseling. Encourage interactions with other CF families to obtain information and support (any visit).

CAREGIVER/CHILD AND FAMILY INTERVENTIONS

1. Displays decreasing anxiety and anger. Provides supportive family environment.
2. Develops trust in home care personnel. Collaborates in developing and modifying daily care.
3. Provides care and treatments effectively. Modifies family activities to meet needs of child.
4. Recognizes and assumes role changes. Maintains family integrity.
5. Develops coping mechanisms that have positive effect within family.
6. Identifies problem areas and obtains community or professional assistance and other services as needed.

SAMPLE DOCUMENTATION INCLUSIONS

1. Specific assessment
   Assess respiratory rate, ease, sputum characteristics, vital signs, nutritional intake, weight, bowel elimination, characteristics, I&O, family hygiene practices, growth, development status, effectiveness of medication regimen, pulmonary physiotherapy, exacerbation of symptoms, failure to thrive, environmental hazards, adaptive capacity of family, and pertinent diagnostic findings.
2. Specific care/teaching
   Teach correct administration of medications via oral, parenteral, inhalation routes; administration, care of oxygen; dietary regimen; alternate feeding methods if appropriate; rest; activity needs; postural drainage;

chest percussion; coughing; deep breathing exercises; universal precautions; disease implications; skills to enhance coping, growth, development program; infection control; and early interventions.

3. General
Note responses to care, teaching, goal achievement, changes in plan, progression, regression of health status, adaptation to long-term care, need for professional referrals.

4. See "Documentation and Family Home Record Keeping" in Appendix for general required documentation components for all home care visits.

 Tracheostomy

A tracheostomy is a surgically created opening in the skin of the neck into the trachea (between the second and fourth tracheal cartilage rings) to allow for passage of air. A tracheostomy is performed when upper airway obstruction is present (infections, edema, congenital conditions), in cases of underlying pulmonary disease, following lung or cardiac surgery, or in conditions that require long-term assisted ventilation. Usually pediatric tracheostomy tubes are made of soft plastic or Silastic material that is pliable to fit into the trachea without an inner cannula; in instances where metal tubes are used, an inner cannula is present. The tracheostomy can be cared for in the home by a caregiver who is instructed in and capable of performing the complex procedures and providing the child's safe, total care.

Home care is primarily concerned with assessment and instruction on the management of the tracheostomy with preservation of respiratory status and prevention of skin, tube, or infection complications. Additional attention is provided to support the adaptive capacities and participation of the family in the tracheostomy care. For the child who requires a tracheostomy associated with mechanical ventilation, see the assisted ventilation care plan.

Nursing diagnosis

Anxiety/fear (child and parental)
Related factors: change in health status, presence of tracheostomy, threat of death, threatening situations (tube obstruction, accidental dislodgement)
Defining characteristics: difficult breathing, fear of suffocation, apprehension, restlessness, facial tension, inability to speak, fear of responsibility of providing tracheostomy care

OUTCOMES
Short-term
Progressive reduction in anxiety, fear associated with care of tracheostomy evidenced by caregiver becoming acquainted with and verbalizing increased ability to remain calm and participate in care measures as needed (expected within 1 to 2 weeks)

Long-term
Fear, anxiety at manageable level evidenced by effective, ongoing support, care required for tracheostomy (expected within 1 month)

NURSING INTERVENTIONS/INSTRUCTIONS
1. Assess emotional/mental status of caregiver and child and their ability to adapt to presence of tracheostomy, anxiety, fear, and concerns about care of child (see "Psychologic Assessment," p. 25, for guidelines) (any visit as needed).
2. Provide information about reasons for tracheostomy. Inform of treatments and procedures involved in home management and how child's safety and comfort will be facilitated in easily understandable language (first and second visits).
3. Maintain calm, quiet environment. Comfort child who is fearful when unable to produce sounds or cry. Inform that voice will return when tube is removed, if temporary; support caregiver that is upset by child's fear (each visit).

4. Provide opportunity for caregiver and child to express fears and concerns. Encourage modes of communication to replace lack of vocal sounds (each visit).
5. Suggest that caregiver stay with child during anxious times (first visit).
6. Assist caregiver to reduce feelings of apprehension, anxiety, fear about child's condition (each visit).
7. Provide link of communication between family and health professional referrals for information and problem solving (any visit as needed).
8. Refer to support group, community agency, respite care, or psychologic counseling as appropriate (any visit).

CAREGIVER/CHILD AND FAMILY INTERVENTIONS

1. Recognizes anxiety associated with care of tracheostomy, unknown possibility of tube obstruction, or other complications.
2. Verbalizes anxiety, frustration, fatigue, and stress related to management of tracheostomy.
3. Maintains calm, supportive environment; controls stimuli; reassures child; and reinforces positive effects of tracheostomy.
4. Child uses distraction techniques such as remaining quiet and at rest, quiet music, and age-appropriate quiet play activities.
5. Uses appropriate coping mechanisms and support resources if needed.

Nursing diagnosis

Ineffective airway clearance/risk for aspiration

Related factors: decreased energy, fatigue; tracheobronchial obstruction (thick mucus); presence of tracheostomy tube; impaired swallowing; vomiting

Defining characteristics: dyspnea; tachypnea; cyanosis; abnormal breath sounds (rhonchi, crackles); retractions; nasal flaring; inability to move increased, thick secretions; increased nonproductive cough

OUTCOMES

Short-term
Stable breathing pattern, airway patency with effective ventilation via tracheostomy established evidenced by respiratory rate, ease, depth maintained via tracheostomy without
distress; removal of mucus; obstruction of airway prevented;
tube dislodgement prevented; breath sounds clear, equal
bilaterally (expected within 2 days, ongoing)

Long-term
Management of home respiratory care evidenced by respiratory baselines maintained; absence of respiratory distress,
injury associated with tracheostomy; complete, effective tracheostomy care demonstrated (expected within 1 month)

NURSING INTERVENTIONS/INSTRUCTIONS

1. Ensure that caregiver is trained in CPR via tracheostomy before hospital discharge. Collaborate with caregiver to develop protocol to activate EMS (first visit, reinforce on subsequent visits).
2. Assess caregiver's knowledge and understanding of reason for tracheostomy, pulmonary status, need for airway
   patency, and risk for airway obstruction (first visit).
3. Assess trends in respiratory status, including rate,
   depth, ease, and effort; dyspnea; tachypnea; retractions;
   thickness and color of secretions; cough (increased,
   nonproductive); color of skin, oral mucous membranes,
   and nailbeds; abnormal breath sounds (see "Pulmonary System Assessment," p. 10, for guidelines) (every
   visit).
4. Provide instruction on pulmonary assessment, signs, and
   symptoms to note. Collaborate with caregiver to plan
   daily care based on respiratory status. Use language
   that is easily understood or provide written instructions
   (first visit, reinstruct on plan changes as needed).
5. Instruct to assess for possible tube dislodgement, decan-
   nulation, and measures to take to secure tube, adjust
   ties, and replace tracheostomy tube. Assist to devise
   emergency kit containing extra tube, clean ties, suction
   tube, lubricant, and scissors to keep nearby (first and
   second visits).

6. Administer and instruct caregiver to provide supplemental oxygen to tracheostomy tube via air compressor at dose and method prescribed with adjustments made in collaboration with physician when needed. Advise to have portable oxygen unit and resuscitation bag available (first and second visits).

7. Instruct on safety in use of oxygen. Post sign that oxygen is in use (first visit).

8. Instruct caregiver to humidify inspired air by cool vaporizer in room. Provide fluids hourly to prevent dry mucosa and thick mucus (first visit).

9. Instruct on suction of secretions using clean technique if unable to remove by coughing, via tube at correct amount of pressure, correct number of thrusts for appropriate amount of time, preoxygenation before and during suctioning (first visit, subsequent visits based on auscultation or sounds of gurgling).

10. Change and clean inner tracheostomy tube and ties several times a day if needed, depending on secretions. Instruct caregiver to perform procedure for tube removal, cleansing, disinfecting, and reinserting to remove mucus accumulation and to maintain airway patency (first visit, subsequent visits as needed).

11. Instruct on inflation of cuff if receiving assisted ventilation or IPPB treatment, and deflation when child is off ventilator and during food ingestion regardless of feeding method (first and second visits).

12. Demonstrate procedure for encouraging coughing for older child and allow return demonstration (first and second visits).

13. Instruct to offer small amounts of food that are easy to swallow, to place child in upright position during meals to prevent aspiration, and to use infant seat for infant feeding. Encourage fluids unless restricted (first visit).

14. Demonstrate elevation of head of bed, positions of optimal comfort for sleeping/resting that allow for ease in breathing, chest expansion, and aspiration prevention (first visit).

15. Suggest wearing loose, nonrestrictive clothing near neck (first visit).

16. Assess response to interventions. Report any deviations from established norm to physician (each visit).
17. Inform caregiver and family of availability of services provided by American Lung Association and local support groups for information and services (first visit).

CAREGIVER/CHILD AND FAMILY INTERVENTIONS

1. Becomes CPR certified and performs CPR, if necessary, on child with tracheostomy tube in place. Places list of emergency activities and telephone numbers in strategic place for easy access.
2. Locates resource to acquire special equipment and supplies (oxygen, suctioning, extra tracheostomy tube, ties, dressings). Collaborates with social services to secure financial assistance if needed.
3. Assesses respirations for rate, ease, and ability to remove secretions. Modifies plans for treatment if deviation from baseline is noted.
4. Suctions tracheostomy at correct pressure (< 100 mm Hg for infant, < 120 mm Hg for child), for correct length of time as frequently as needed using clean technique, and with preoxygenation to remove thick mucus or mucus that is difficult to cough up, or if respiratory status changes resulting from airway obstruction caused by mucus accumulation. Instills drops of normal saline in tracheostomy (0.5 ml for infant, 1 to 2 ml for young child, and 2 to 3 ml for older child) if mucus is thick.
5. Ensures availability of portable suction apparatus with back-up batteries, portable oxygen tank, and resuscitation bag on hand.
6. Correctly administers humidified oxygen when needed (continuous, intermittent).
7. Follows safety precautions in oxygen use, including posting sign stating, "oxygen in use, no sparks, no open flames, no oil or grease, and no smoking"; maintains standby oxygen source if not administered continuously.
8. Provides optimal humidity by cool room vaporizer, environmental temperature, ventilation at comfortable level, and environment free from respiratory contaminants

(smoke, food crumbs, cleaning, hair sprays, dust, powders, hair from animals) that can irritate trachea.

9. Provides oral care for mouth dryness, odors, and comfort.
10. Provides tracheostomy tube care (usually 2 hours after meals to prevent vomiting and aspiration). Removes ties and tube, cleanses with soapy water and pipe cleaners, rinses with water, reinserts, secures in place with clean ties, and inflates/deflates cuff as appropriate if receiving assisted ventilation.
11. Avoids tub baths and activities near water without supervision.
12. Cleanses reusable suction catheter with soap and water and stores in clean plastic bags. Cleanses then sterilizes tracheostomy tube with germicidal solution.
13. Identifies any deterioration in respiratory status and reports to physician.

Nursing diagnosis

Risk for infection

Related factors: inadequate primary defenses (stasis of secretions), invasive procedure (tracheostomy), insufficient knowledge of caregiver to avoid exposure of child to pathogens

Defining characterstics: ineffective cough to remove secretions, change in odor/color of secretions from tracheostomy to yellow or green, increased secretions, fever, irritability

OUTCOMES

Short-term
Early detection of signs, symptoms of respiratory infection; use of clean technique to perform procedures evidenced by optimal respiratory parameters; airway patency with colorless, odorless secretions removed; afebrile status (expected with daily assessment)

Long-term
Adaptation to lifestyle that promotes clean, safe environment; preventive measures performed to minimize

risk for pulmonary infections demonstrated by patent, infection-free respiratory system (expected ongoing)

NURSING INTERVENTIONS/INSTRUCTIONS

1. Assess home and living conditions (see "Environmental Assessment," p. 37, for guidelines) (first visit, follow-up for additional modifications on second visit).
2. Assess for changes in respiratory rate, depth, and ease and diminished breath sounds and changes in oxygen saturation (each visit).
3. Assess temperature for deviations from norm, increased viscosity or change in color/odor of secretions from tracheostomy, irritability, and changes in feeding/elimination pattern, all of which indicate pulmonary infection (each visit).
4. Instruct about possible changes in respiratory pattern, sputum, and behavior to note, if child has cold and becomes restless or pale. Report to physician (first visit).
5. Instruct on taking axillary (oral for child) temperature (first visit).
6. Instruct on handwashing and importance before and after care of child.
7. Instruct on use of clean technique during tracheostomy suctioning procedure, cleansing tube, and changing dressing (first visit, review).
8. Instruct on administration of medications, and responses to expect with oral liquid antibiotic and antipyretic (first visit, reinforce).
9. Instruct on precautions to prevent infection, such as washing hands and avoiding contact with people who have respiratory infection, and importance of adequate nutritional intake and rest (first visit, ongoing).
10. Obtain sputum specimen when possible for culture, if ordered (any visit).

CAREGIVER/CHILD AND FAMILY INTERVENTIONS

1. Observes for difficulty in breathing; yellow or green color, foul odor, increased amount of sputum from tube; any blood from tube; pallor, decreased appetite, irritability. Reports changes to physician.
2. Suctions tracheostomy using clean technique at correct suction pressure and for correct length of time if child

appears restless, has difficulty breathing with whistling
sound heard, has difficulty sucking/eating, or if mucus is
copious or thick to prevent stasis.
3. Takes temperature if sputum color or respirations
change. Reports elevations above 100.4° F or level specified by physician.
4. Administers oral antibiotic therapy correctly until all
medication is taken. Notes and reports side effects.
5. Maintains personal hygiene. Avoids use of contaminated articles when performing care and possible exposure of child to family members or others with suspected respiratory infections. Wears face mask if
appropriate.
6. Performs proper handwashing (washes to count of 10),
especially before caring for child. Uses clean technique
during care and procedures. Washes and stores supplies appropriately.
7. Properly disposes of all articles and supplies according to
universal precautions.

Nursing diagnosis

Impaired skin or tissue integrity
Related factors: external factor of irritants (secretions), mechanical pressure of tracheostomy tube
Defining characteristics: moisture caused by secretions; irritation, excoriation, tissue damage around tube insertion
site; redness, accumulation of crusting at site

OUTCOMES

Short-term
Skin at tracheostomy site is dry, intact evidenced by absence of redness, irritation, bleeding, pressure resulting
from tube movement during care (expected within 1 to 2
days)

Long-term
Optimal skin integrity maintained evidenced by absence of
any abnormal color, irritants, breakdown at tracheostomy
tube site (expected within 1 week)

NURSING INTERVENTIONS/INSTRUCTIONS

1. Assess skin and tissue at tube site for signs indicating risk for breakdown such as excessive moisture, irritation, redness, rash, excoriation, and crusting and tube not secured in proper position (see "Integumentary System Assessment," p. 22, for guidelines) (every visit).

2. Demonstrate and instruct on assessing skin at least twice daily and cleansing procedure around tube, softening and removal of dried secretions with half strength hydrogen peroxide, soap, and water; gently rinsing with water, drying thoroughly twice daily with careful attention to avoid manipulation of tube; and allowing return demonstration (first visit, reinstruct second visit if needed).

3. Instruct on application of clean dressing around tube, application of antiseptic or antibiotic ointment if ordered (first visit).

4. Instruct and inform to change tracheostomy ties and pad when needed. Rotate position of knots on ties to avoid pressure areas. Allow to practice procedure under supervision (first and second visits).

5. Inform to increase environmental humidity to prevent dry skin and mucous membranes (first visit).

6. Instruct to report any bleeding, rash, or excoriation at tube site to physician (first visit).

CAREGIVER/CHILD AND FAMILY INTERVENTIONS

1. Assesses skin at tracheostomy site daily. Reports changes or breakdown.

2. Maintains clean, dry, tracheostomy site with tube in secure position.

3. Avoids allowing secretions to accumulate or to dry at tube site by cleansing, redressing, and changing ties and pad if wet, soiled, or loose.

4. Applies ointment or protective skin barrier at site as ordered.

5. Notes fit of tube and if manipulation irritates site. Consults with physician to replace tube if fit is not proper (too tight, too loose).

6. Provides optimal humidity by cool room vaporizer, tracheostomy collar during night, naps to prevent drying, excess moisture to skin.

Nursing diagnosis

Impaired verbal communication
Related factors: tracheostomy
Defining characteristics: inability to speak/cry (vocal sounds),
  unwilling to attempt other methods of communication,
  frustration of child or caregiver

OUTCOMES

Short-term
Alternate modes of communication attempted evidenced by
satisfactory nonverbal interactions among child, caregiver,
family members (expected within 3 to 4 days)

Long-term
Effective methods of communication adopted (expected for
duration of tracheostomy tube placement)

NURSING INTERVENTIONS/INSTRUCTIONS

1. Assess child's and family's willingness to attempt and to
   adapt to different methods of communications; coping
   skills; and presence of frustration, anger, and depression
   (first visit and as needed).
2. Reassure child that voice will return when tube is removed, if appropriate (first visit).
3. Assess for possible downsizing of tracheostomy tube (requiring physician order) to allow air movement around
   tube and vocal sounds to be produced (any visit as
   appropriate).
4. Suggest various modes of communication and devices available to aid in communication (first and second visits).
5. Initiate order for speech pathologist consultant (any
   visit).

CAREGIVER/CHILD AND FAMILY INTERVENTIONS

1. Maintains effective use of age-related alternate modes of
   communication such as computer, magic slate, paper,
   pencil, hand grasps, signs, signals, eye blinking,
   movements, mouth sounds, or picture cards.

2. Supports child's attempts to communicate with peers and family members.
3. Displays patience. Anticipates child's extra needs.
4. Reinforces recommendations and teaching by speech pathologist.

Nursing diagnosis

Ineffective family coping: compromised

Related factors: presence of tracheostomy that exhausts supportive capacity of significant people; family disorganization, role changes

Defining characteristics: significant person's expression of inability to cope; feelings of fear, anxiety, guilt, anger related to tracheostomy, providing care; inadequate understanding, stress causing impatience with child's needs, physical changes (tracheostomy)

OUTCOMES

Short-term
Family members demonstrate ability to plan and care for child evidenced by provision of normal environment, decreased anxiety or feelings of inadequacy, integration of information about family needs into care, support of child (expected within 1 to 2 weeks)

Long-term
Family coping and adaptation evidenced by optimal support, participation in care, maintenance of family relationships, demonstration of positive feelings, acceptance of child's needs within family structure, respite care if needed (expected within 1 to 2 months)

NURSING INTERVENTIONS/INSTRUCTIONS

1. Meet and collaborate with family members to assess stressors, coping mechanisms, and planning of care (first visit, repeat as needed).
2. Reinforce information to promote family understanding of tracheostomy and care needs (each visit).
3. Discuss and allow family to express feelings of guilt,

anxiety, and depression. Promote communication among members to verbalize feelings and expectations with each other (any visit).

4. Instruct on methods to develop appropriate coping skills and to meet family's needs (medical, emotional, financial, food, respite, supplies, and equipment) by referral to social or counseling services (first visit, as needed).

5. Encourage and support all efforts to participate in care of child by family members. Assist to modify family activities according to daily needs of child (each visit).

6. Inform family of resources that provide counseling, social services, and respite care to obtain information and support (any visit).

CAREGIVER/CHILD AND FAMILY INTERVENTIONS

1. Displays decreasing anxiety and anger. Provides supportive family environment.

2. Develops trust in home care personnel. Collaborates in developing/modifying daily care.

3. Provides care and treatments effectively. Modifies family activities to meet needs of child.

4. Recognizes and assumes role changes. Maintains family integrity.

5. Develops coping mechanisms that have positive effect within family.

6. Identifies problem areas. Obtains community or professional assistance or services as needed.

SAMPLE DOCUMENTATION INCLUSIONS

1. Specific assessment
   Assess respiratory rate, ease via tracheostomy; condition of stoma; airway obstruction; mucus characteristics; nutritional/fluid intake; hygiene practices; effectiveness of oxygen, mucus removal regimen; environmental hazards; possible communication modes; anxiety level; and adaptive capacity of family.

2. Specific care/teaching
   Teach correct suctioning, administration/care of oxygen, complete tracheostomy care, outcome of care, caregiver's and family member's care of tracheostomy, respiratory assessment, dietary/fluid regimen, rest, activity needs, care of supplies, universal precautions, skills to enhance

coping, infection prevention, and various communication methods.

3. General
Note responses to care, teaching, goal achievement, changes in plan, progression or regression of health status, adaptation to and provision of physical and emotional needs of child, family, and need for professional referrals.

4. See "Documentation and Family Home Record Keeping" in Appendix for general required documentation components for all home care visits.

 ## Tuberculosis

Tuberculosis (TB) is an infectious disorder of the lungs that has become an increased health hazard in children living in large cities of the United States. TB is caused by *Mycobacterium tuberculosis* and is usually contracted and transmitted by inhalation of air contaminated by droplets containing the organism. The source of TB in children is usually an infected member of the family, a visitor, or an employee of the family. Initially, an inflammatory reaction appears followed by bronchopneumonia. Tissue destruction spreads from the primary site to areas within the lung. Spread via blood vessel erosion can affect distant sites such as bone and lymph nodes.

Home care is primarily concerned with monitoring of respiratory status of the child and instruction of the parents in nutrition, rest, and personal hygiene needs of the child and family. The most important aspect of care involves teaching the administration of and subsequent compliance with the long-term medication regimen.

Nursing diagnosis

Ineffective breathing pattern/risk for activity intolerance
Related factors: decreased energy and fatigue, presence of respiratory problem (inflammatory process)

Defining characteristics: cough with mucus production, pain, or tightness in chest; diminished breath sounds and crackles; dullness on percussion; altered chest expansion on affected side; possible hemoptysis

OUTCOMES

Short-term
Breathing pattern improved, airways patent, initial resolution of signs and symptoms of acute inflammation evidenced by respiratory rate, ease, and depth; breath sounds within normal parameters; limited participation in daily activities (expected within 2 to 3 days)

Long-term
Respiratory baselines and optimal pulmonary function maintained evidenced by complete resolution of inflammatory process, chest x-ray film revealing inactive or arrested disease, management of home respiratory care demonstrated by caregiver and child (expected within 1 month)

NURSING INTERVENTIONS/INSTRUCTIONS

1. Assess trends in respiratory status and associated signs and symptoms of active disease such as fever, anorexia, malaise, weakness, weight loss, and chest pain in child and weakness, anemia, pallor, and weight loss in infants (see "Pulmonary System Assessment," p. 10, for guidelines) (each visit).

2. Instruct on taking respirations, temperature, and weight and asessment of activity tolerance and appetite (first visit).

3. Inform caregiver to maintain bedrest during acute phase to prevent increased respirations, to avoid fatigue, and to reduce metabolic demands. Collaborate with caregiver and child to plan daily activities to conserve energy (first visit).

4. Instruct child on coughing procedure and how to expectorate into tissue instead of swallowing sputum. Suggest oral hygiene for frequent coughing. Collect sputum specimen if ordered and if possible (any visit as needed).

5. Assess and instruct caregiver to assess response to planned interventions, provide diary, instruct on how to

log any untoward pulmonary signs and symptoms (each visit).

6. Monitor results of x-ray studies, tuberculin tests, and sputum analysis as available. Incorporate this information into clinical profile and interventions (any visit).

CAREGIVER/CHILD AND FAMILY INTERVENTIONS

1. Takes temperature and respiratory rate daily or more often as needed. Records in diary.
2. Identifies any deterioration in respiratory status. Reports to physician.
3. Child adapts to restricted activity routine and allows for optimal rest.
4. Complies with x-ray examinations, laboratory, or other testing when requested.

Nursing diagnosis

Ineffective home maintenance management/knowledge deficit (parental)

Related factors: lack of information about disease, treatment of regimen, prevention of reinfection and transmission of disease; insufficient planning, organization, finances, support system

Defining characteristics: expression of need for information about disease, health needs of child, expectations, responsibilities of caregiver; lack of necessary hygienic surroundings; toileting wastes; odors; unwashed clothing, linens; dirty utensils

OUTCOMES

Short-term
Adequate knowledge evidenced by verbalization of causes; progression, transmission, susceptibility, prognosis of disease; medication; nutritional, activity regimens; facilitation of personal/family, environmental cleanliness (expected within 1 to 2 weeks)

Long-term
Adequate knowledge evidenced by ongoing compliance with medication regimen, optimal lifestyle adaptations,

return to normal activities in healthy environment; maintenance of personal cleanliness, surroundings; diagnostic tests, procedures revealing disease in dormant state; periodic TB screening; contact prophylaxis (expected within 2 to 5 months, continued for length of therapy)

NURSING INTERVENTIONS/INSTRUCTIONS

1. Assess education and knowledge of caregiver and family. Identify deficits and strengths and collaborate in planning instruction needed to manage daily care routines (see "Family Assessment," p. 41, for guidelines) (first and second visits).

2. Instruct caregiver on cause, dormancy, and progression of disease. Relate information to plan of care. Clarify misconceptions and importance of cooperation in implementing continuous long-term care. Advise caregiver that most children recover from disease with proper treatment (first visit).

3. Assess home environment; financial status for modifications needed to ensure supportive measures needed to enhance personal hygiene, nutrition, and follow-up care. Consider referral to social services for assistance (see "Family and Financial Assessments," pp. 41-42, for guidelines) (first and second visits).

4. Assess nutritional status, food preferences, caloric requirements, and cultural considerations (see "Gastrointestinal System Assessment and Nutritional Assessment," pp. 16 and 17, for guidelines) (first visit).

5. Collaborate with caregiver in instructions to incorporate assessment data into planning of menus with high protein and vitamin/mineral inclusions (first and second visits).

6. Instruct on administration (names, times, frequency, dosage, side effects, food/drug interactions) of medication protocol, usually of two or more drugs simultaneously, with specific selections based on child's tolerance (given daily 1 to 2 hours before meals for 1 to 2 months, then daily or twice weekly for 9 months) and signs and symptoms of hypersensitivity to drugs. Observe for adverse reactions (first visit, until all medication instruction is completed).

7. Assess for compliance with medication regimen (each visit).

8. Instruct on daily administration of prophylactic drug therapy to children at high risk of exposure to TB (first and second visits).

9. Instruct to avoid exposure to others with respiratory or other infections that can cause reinfection (first visit).

10. Instruct on TB preventive and control measures, including avoidance of contact with infective organism, periodic skin testing for positive reactions, and receiving limited immunity by bacillus Calmette-Guérin (BCG) vaccination from health department (first visit).

11. Instruct and support daily routines of attending school, notifying school nurse, restricting contact sports and excessive activities, and setting aside time for rest (first visit).

12. Inform caregiver and family to avoid overprotecting child or pressuring child to adhere to planned care such as meals or play (any visit).

13. Inform caregiver and family contacts (within last 3 months) to obtain TB skin testing and possible follow-up x-ray scans at local health department (first visit, evaluate for compliance on subsequent visits).

14. Follow-up and report contacts and possible exposure to other persons to prevent further transmission of disease (any visit).

15. Report case to local Health Department for appropriate follow-up (first visit).

CAREGIVER/CHILD AND FAMILY INTERVENTIONS

1. Collaborates with plan of care with reduced anxiety and constructive attitude about disease and its treatment and prognosis.

2. Describes disease process, risk for recurrence, or complications.

3. Manages home environment for child as needed, including comfort, cleanliness, ventilation, temperature, pollutants, or infestations.

4. Maintains optimal dietary, activity, and rest routines.

5. Attends school, if asymptomatic, with physician permission.

6. Secures medication in advance from public health services or home health nurse to facilitate compliance. Administers daily prescribed medication regimen correctly for duration of long-term therapy.
7. Administers medication regimen for family contacts.
8. Reports side effects or hypersensitivities to medications to physician such as rash, urticaria, breathing difficulty, urinary changes, and visual or auditory changes.
9. Carries out measures to prevent infection by handwashing, proper disposal of contaminated articles, covering nose and mouth when coughing/sneezing, and initiating respiratory isolation procedures if necessary.
10. Complies with repeat diagnostic test appointments.
11. Contacts American Lung Association for educational materials.

SAMPLE DOCUMENTATION INCLUSIONS

1. Specific assessment
   Assess respiratory status, nutrition, activity needs, personal hygiene factors, environmental conditions, TB testing, and chest x-ray results.
2. Specific care/teaching
   Teach correct administration of long-term medication therapy, dietary regimen of high caloric and protein content, activity restrictions, environmental and personal hygiene modifications, measures to prevent pulmonary infection/reactivation of disease, screening, immunization, and medication regimen of contacts.
3. General
   Note adaptation and compliance to long-term care, referral to social services, and responses to treatment (resolution of or dormant status of disease).
4. See "Documentation and Family Home Record Keeping" in Appendix for general required documentation components for all home care visits.

Cardiovascular system

 ## Congenital Heart Defects

Congenital heart defects are structural abnormalities of the heart and great vessels that are present at birth. Associated factors include chromosomal defects and maternal diabetes mellitus, systemic lupus erythematosus, phenylketonuria, congenital rubella syndrome, and exposure to environmental teratogens (e.g., ethanol, valproate, hydantoin, phenytoin, and cocaine). There may be many causes, but the specific cause in a given individual is generally unknown. Further, cardiac symptoms may be a manifestation of a variety of noncardiac disorders.

Cardiac defects are characterized as cyanotic or acyanotic. Cyanotic heart defects occur with cardiac lesions and associated pulmonary blood flow obstruction, or with right-to-left shunting of blood, resulting in the mixing of deoxygenated blood with oxygenated blood in the arterial circulation. Examples of cyanotic defects include tetralogy of Fallot, transposition of the great vessels, tricuspid atresia, total anomalous pulmonary venous connection, pulmonary valve atresia, persistent truncus arteriosis, and Ebstein's anomaly. Acyanotic defects occur with left-to-right shunting of blood or with obstruction of the left heart or aorta, resulting in decreased blood flow to the general circulation. Examples of acyanotic defects include ventricular septal defect, atrial septal defect, patent ductus arteriosus (notably with prematurity), coarctation of the aorta, pulmonic stenosis, and aortic stenosis.

Congenital defects vary in severity as well as in type, symptoms, age of onset, and sequelae. Hypoxemia and congestive heart failure are distinctive signs of serious congenital heart defects. Extracardiac defects may also be present. Certain conditions are self-limiting or may resolve with time. Surgical repair may be immediately necessary to sustain life.

Medical management of congenital heart disease may include a drug regimen of cardiotonics, diuretics, vasodilators, iron preparations, antibiotics, and surgical repair of the defect.

Home health care is primarily concerned with maintaining optimal cardiac output, promoting optimal physical growth and psychosocial development, and teaching signs and symptoms of complications. These are accomplished by managing the fear of the caregiver and instructing the caregiver on the skills necessary to optimize pediatric outcome. Skills include proper medication administration, use of energy conservation techniques, effective feeding techniques, recognition and management of distressing symptoms, handling complications and emergencies, helping the child perform health maintenance activities, preparing for tests and surgery, and using community resources.

Nursing diagnosis

Ineffective family coping: compromised
Related factors: situational, maturational crises; mourning loss of healthy child
Defining characteristics: confusion, anger, guilt, loss of control, emotional immobility, overt concerns about child's condition, nonverbal stress behaviors, somatic complaints, underlying fear of sudden death, overprotective parenting, continual focus on prognosis

OUTCOMES
Short-term
Adequate coping evidenced by family's ability to verbalize true feelings, needs; decreased stress behaviors; receptivity to health care teaching (expected in 1 to 4 weeks)

Long-term
Optimal coping evidenced by adaptation, management of child's condition; maintenance/strengthening of family unit (expected within 1 to 3 months)

NURSING INTERVENTIONS/INSTRUCTIONS

1. Ask about and actively listen to caregiver's concerns and fears. Be sensitive to cultural nuances of eye contact, space, and touch (each visit).
2. Encourage expression of feelings. Avoid blame or criticism. Be supportive. Provide factual information and leave written information (lists of community resources and local support groups). Repeat as needed (each visit).
3. Assess caregiver's perception of condition, its cause, treatment, and prognosis and their role in care. Clarify misinformation. Answer questions simply and honestly. Explain defect, draw diagrams when appropriate (each visit).
4. Explore with family meaning of illness to family and their own sources of support and assistance. Emphasize need to meet both family's and child's needs, to incorporate child into family rather than making child central to it, and to treat child as normal as possible. Avoid focusing on child to detriment of mate and siblings (each visit).
5. Query as to coping strengths and past experiences. Affirm positive coping skills. Assist with skill development and problem solving (each visit).
6. Keep caregiver informed of child's progress and strengths based on physical examination. Point out developmental milestones, traits, characteristics, and behaviors unique to child (each visit).
7. Include caregiver in treatment plan. Affirm parenting skills (each visit).
8. Instruct caregiver on recognition of child's needs, self-care, and general health care concerns such as hygiene, discipline, education, and recreation (ongoing).
9. Encourage caregiver to write list of questions for practitioner visits (each visit).
10. Encourage parenting classes/counseling, as appropriate (as needed).
11. Explore sources of alternate or respite care. Provide list of community resources, local support groups (first visit, reinforce as needed).
12. Assist in developing list of contacts for emergency questions or services (e.g., home health nurse, pediatric car-

diologist, Emergency Medical Services [EMS]) (first visit, reinforce as needed).

13. Inform caregiver of community support resources (e.g., American Heart Association, Program for Children with Special Health Care Needs, local support groups). Refer to social worker or Department of Human Services as means to provide financial support or other available resources (first and second visits).

CAREGIVER/CHILD AND FAMILY INTERVENTIONS

1. Establishes rapport with nurse.
2. Verbalizes concerns about child's condition and progress.
3. Maintains/strengthens family unit with positive interaction and communication. Participates in family activities.
4. Participates in treatment plan as well as care of child.
5. Uses home remedies and cultural health care practices with physician's approval.
6. Actively seeks assistance.
7. Takes time for and pleasure in meeting own needs. Identifies and uses respite care.
8. Seeks sources of support.
9. Attends parenting classes and sees counselor as needed.

Nursing diagnosis

Decreased cardiac output
Related factors: structural or functional cardiac defect
Defining characteristics: fatigue; activity/exercise intolerance; dyspnea or cyanosis, especially with feeding, straining, crying; inappropriate diaphoresis; poor feeding; failure to gain weight; weakness; squatting; digital clubbing; anoxic spells; frequent respiratory infections; increased blood pressure

OUTCOMES

Short-term
Adequate cardiac output evidenced by stabilization or decrease in symptoms, caregiver compliance with health care regimen (expected within 1 to 4 weeks)

Long-term
Optimal cardiac output within limitations of condition evidenced by ability to perform age-dependent activities without distress, complications (expected in 4 to 6 weeks)

NURSING INTERVENTIONS/INSTRUCTIONS

1. Assess caregiver's perception of child's health status including general behavior, respiratory patterns, color, feeding and feeding behavior, age-appropriate activity tolerance, urinary output, respiratory infection, and latest developmental tasks (each visit).

2. Perform complete physical assessment. Assess/instruct on oxygen saturation by pulse oximetry per physician's directive and protocol (first visit).

3. Assess circulatory status including rate, rhythm, and volume of apical pulse (1 full minute), peripheral pulses and discrepancies; blood pressure; location of and deviations in heart sounds; respiratory ease, rate, and depth; any evidence of respiratory grunting, nasal flaring, use of accessory muscles; crackles; color of skin, nails, buccal mucosa; unusual posturing; digital clubbing; weight changes; and edema. Give caregiver realistic appraisal of examination and affirm positive findings. Notify physician of deviations from established baselines (each visit).

4. Demonstrate taking apical pulse and respirations of quiet child. Have caregiver return demonstration. Based on performance, repeat and reinforce. Include norms and when to seek assistance. Leave agency telephone number (first and second visits, reinforce as needed).

5. Assess posture of client. Instruct caregiver on positioning maneuvers that may facilitate respiration. Instruct on oxygen administration per physician's order. Include rate of flow; indications for use/increase, comfort, and safety measures; and logistics of ordering equipment/supplies (first and second visits, reinforce as needed).

6. Assess accuracy of medication administration of cardiac glycoside and all drugs being given. Instruct on purpose, dosage, schedule, delivery method, and side effects and their remediation; laboratory monitoring of serum levels; and barriers to compliance (ongoing).

7. Note ambient temperature. Instruct caregiver to avoid extreme temperatures. Refer to community resources that supply fans and heaters (first visit).

CAREGIVER/CHILD AND FAMILY INTERVENTIONS

1. Reports persistent changes (pulse >160 beats per minute [bpm], respirations >60 breaths per minute in infant); changes in breathing pattern or color; decreased feeding or activity tolerance; and unusual weight gain, fever, or infection.
2. Uses pulse oximetry at night, during feedings, and at other designated times. Reports low oxygen saturation to physician.
3. Correctly takes apical pulse for 1 minute before administration of digoxin. Withholds drug if pulse is less than 100 bpm in infants or 70 bpm in children per physician's directive. Pulse-taking procedure may be stopped for less family intrusion and more accurate serum levels.
4. Administers digoxin correctly.

   - Gives at same time each morning; if more than one dose is prescribed per day, gives at regular intervals.
   - Gives 1 hour before or 2 hours after feeding.
   - Gives missed dose only if less than 3 hours have elapsed.
   - Withholds second dose if child vomits; withholds drug completely and contacts physician for persistent vomiting, decreased appetite, or slow/irregular pulse.
   - Enforces general drug and child safety protocols.
   - Returns to laboratory for digoxin serum level tests.

5. Positions child to enhance respiratory function and comfort.

   - Elevates head of bed 45 to 60 degrees or uses several bed pillows (child).
   - Positions infant in prone position in crib or at shoulder in knee-chest position.
   - Child assumes squatting position.

6. Safely administers and maintains supplemental oxygen and does not reduce oxygen flow unless approved by physician.

7. Maintains optimal environment temperature. Avoids sudden thermal changes.

Nursing diagnosis

Activity intolerance
Related factors: imbalance between oxygen supply and metabolic demands
Defining characteristics: increased heart, respiratory rates in response to activity; increased pallor; cyanosis; dyspnea after feeding, activity; irritability; verbal complaints; self-imposed rest

OUTCOMES
Short-term
Satisfactory activity tolerance evidenced by decreased hypoxic responses, minimal increases in baseline vital signs (expected within 1 to 3 weeks)

Long-term
Optimal activity tolerance evidenced by stabilized endurance within limitations of underlying condition (expected within 1 month)

NURSING INTERVENTIONS/INSTRUCTIONS

1. Assess color, respirations, and position of sleeping/resting child (each visit).
2. Identify activities that tire client, self-comforting techniques of child, and comfort measures used by caregiver (each visit).
3. Based on needs assessment, instruct caregiver on measures that decrease oxygen consumption when holding and feeding child. Concurrently instruct another family member to prevent caregiver exhaustion (first and second visits).
4. Instruct caregiver to structure and pace activities so there are rest periods for child and caregiver (each visit).
5. Assist child and caregiver on acceptable play activities (ongoing).
6. Instruct caregiver to allow child to set own pace; to rest

when tired; and to avoid rough play, isometric exercises, and competitive or contact sports (first visit, as needed).

7. Instruct caregiver to consult with physician before extensive travel, travel by plane, or travel to areas of high altitude (as needed).

CAREGIVER/CHILD AND FAMILY INTERVENTIONS

1. Feeds smaller, higher caloric amounts at more frequent intervals with times integrated into child's own sleep-wake pattern. Does not wait for infant to cry before feeding.

2. Feeds infant in upright position, never props bottle, uses soft preemie nipple, and burps frequently.

3. Structures daily activities. Provides rest periods for self and child.

4. Avoids overstimulating environments and activities that tire child. Monitors activity and provides for quiet play. Child stops/rests as needed.

5. Consults with physician before travel or vacation.

Nursing diagnosis

Altered nutrition: less than body requirements
Related factors: inadequate intake of nutrients, energy expenditure of feeding/eating, iron deficient diet
Defining characteristics: fatigue, weakness, disinterest in food, altered respirations during feeding/eating, falls asleep during bottlefeeding or breastfeeding, slow weight gain, frail build, failure to thrive

OUTCOMES
Short-term
Adequate nutrition evidenced by consumption of well-balanced, nutritionally adequate meals, establishment of satisfying feeding/eating schedule, weight gain (expected in 2 to 4 weeks)

Long-term
Optimal nutritional status evidenced by intake of required nutrients to facilitate growth/development within limitations of condition (expected in 1 to 3 months)

NURSING INTERVENTIONS/INSTRUCTIONS

1. Assess caregiver's perception of intake and feeding experience (each visit).
2. Weigh child weekly, note changes, compare with expected trends (see "Growth and Developmental Assessment," p. 31). Notify physician of marked or suspicious changes (each visit).
3. Observe child eating or being fed to assess caregiver's technique and child's intake, response, and energy expenditure. Based on observed need, instruct caregiver on energy conservation measures for child (first and second visits).
4. Take diet history (see "Gastrointestinal System Assessment and Nutritional Assessment," pp. 16 and 17) including food preferences and ethnic/cultural prescriptions or limitations. Assess for use of unsupplemented, iron-poor formula, cow's milk; and iron content of diet. Query concerning use of mineral supplementation (first visit).
5. Instruct caregiver to provide nutritionally adequate meals. Refer to local health department; social service agencys; and women, infants, and children (WIC) program for additional instruction and procurement of food products (first and second visits).
6. Instruct caregiver on administration of prescribed iron preparations (first and second visits).
7. Per physician's directive only, change formula concentration. Instruct caregiver on formula preparation and on possible side effects of less dilute formula (each visit).
8. Instruct on feedings via nasogastric/gastrostomy tube (see "Alternate Feeding Management," p. 205) (first visit).

CAREGIVER/CHILD AND FAMILY INTERVENTIONS

1. Feeds infant small amounts in upright position, burps infant frequently, and uses soft nipple.
2. Uses iron-fortified formula or iron supplementation per physician's directive. Uses community resources for milk and foodstuffs.
3. Per physician's order, offers infant correctly prepared, more concentrated formula. Notifies physician of diarrhea, vomiting, or signs of resulting dehydration.

4. Per physician's order, conserves infant's energy expenditure by feeding through nasogastric/gastrostomy tube.
5. Infant gains up to 1 oz/day; older child gains appropriate to age.
6. Prepares well-balanced, nutritious meals. Includes palatable foods with high iron content (e.g., dried peaches, raisins, farina, beans). Only occasionally allows food with low nutritional value.
7. Correctly calculates liquid iron preparation. Administers iron between meals with vitamin C-fortified juice. Anticipates possible side effects of dark, black stools or tooth staining (temporary).
8. Increases fluid intake and dietary fiber to prevent constipation. Offers prune juice in 1-oz increments to avoid constipation.

Nursing diagnosis

Risk for infection
Related factors: underlying defect, poor nutritional status, associated immunodeficiency syndromes
Defining characteristics: impaired gas exchange, fever, frequent respiratory infections

OUTCOMES

Short-term
Absence of infection evidenced by normal temperature; absence of specific, constitutional symptoms of infection (expected within 1 week)

Long-term
Absence of infection evidenced by optimal functioning within limitations of condition (expected ongoing)

NURSING INTERVENTIONS/INSTRUCTIONS

1. Assess temperature, presence of constitutional symptoms, and overt infection. Notify physician of deviation from norm (each visit).
2. Instruct caregiver on temperature taking; reinforce per return demonstration. Ensure caregiver has thermometer. Instruct to take child's temperature if child feels

hot or is shivering (unrelated to activity or ambient temperature) and to notify physician of elevations (first visit).
3. Instruct caregiver on measures to prevent infection and to maintain health (each visit).

CAREGIVER/CHILD AND FAMILY INTERVENTIONS

1. Washes hands as appropriate.
2. Avoids taking child out in crowds; avoids exposure to infected persons.
3. Provides adequate rest, nutrition, and hygiene.
4. Reports fever, signs of infection, vomiting, and diarrhea to physician.
5. Obtains age-appropriate immunizations.
6. Regularly sees physician for noncardiac care. Regularly sees dentist.
7. Informs caregiver of child's diagnosis before dental care, instrumentation, and surgery. Administers prophylactic antibiotics per physician's order.

Nursing diagnosis

Risk for injury
Related factors: congenital cardiac defect, medical complication of condition, therapies
Defining characteristics: paroxysmal hyperpnea, hypoxic episodes, congestive heart failure (CHF), dehydration with compensatory polycythemia, digitalis toxicity, possible corrective surgery, caregiver inability to recognize or deal with distressing symptoms

OUTCOMES

Short-term
Decreased risk of injury evidenced by compliance with medical regimen; early reporting of adverse symptoms, stabilization, cardiac condition (expected within 1 week)

Long-term
Absence of injury evidenced by optimal cardiovascular functioning within limitations of condition (expected within 1 month)

NURSING INTERVENTIONS/INSTRUCTIONS

1. Assess caregiver's response to illness, readiness to learn, and barriers to compliance (first visit).
2. Include caregiver in care plan. Write clear, explicit directions. Instruct to post directions in accessible, permanent place (e.g., by telephone) (first visit).
3. Instruct primary caregiver and others involved in child's care to obtain training in cardiopulmonary resuscitation (CPR) and to establish emergency protocol (first visit, reinforce).
4. After consultation with physician, prepare child and family for, or arrange for, diagnostic procedures or surgery.

   - Instruct to visit hospital cardiac unit as appropriate and point out hospital garb, visiting hours, and waiting areas.
   - Use doll to demonstrate procedure.
   - Give general explanation of expectations (e.g., frequent taking of vital signs; length of surgery and postoperative course and care) (first visit).

5. Assess for episodes of paroxysmal hyperpnea, hypoxia, or increased cardiac distress. Report deviations from norm to physician. Instruct caregiver on recognition and management of symptoms (each visit).
6. Assess for manifestations of CHF (see "Nursing Care Plan, Congestive Heart Failure," p. 148). Report findings to physician. Instruct caregiver on recognition of symptoms and need to seek medical assistance (each visit).
7. Evaluate compliance with digitalis administration protocol. Review recognition of toxicity and need to seek medical advice (first visit, as needed).
8. Assess fluid and electrolyte status including unusual losses, decreased intake, and digoxin or diuretic therapy. Instruct caregiver on need for adequate hydration, electrolytes, signs of dehydration, and need to report to physician (first and second visits).

CAREGIVER/CHILD AND FAMILY INTERVENTIONS

1. Posts list of protocols and activities in prominent place.
2. Obtains CPR certification.

3. Recognizes persistent increased respirations, restlessness, deep cyanosis, and gasping respirations as signs of distress; intervenes accordingly.

   • Stays calm.
   • Comforts infant/child.
   • Places child in knee-chest position with head and chest elevated.
   • If symptoms do not decrease or escalate, calls EMS.

4. Immediately reports early signs of CHF (increased pulse, especially on rest, with minimal exertion; increased respirations; dyspnea) and later signs and symptoms (wheezing, grunting, hacking cough, orthopnea, cyanosis, nasal flaring, chest retractions, inappropriate profuse sweating [especially of face, head, and neck], decreased output, and increased weight) to physician.

5. Correctly administers digitalis and takes blood for serum levels. Immediately reports vomiting, especially if unrelated to intake, decreased pulse, or bradycardia.

Nursing diagnosis

Altered growth and development

Related factors: effects of chronic illness; environmental, stimulation deficiencies; inadequate parental caregiving; prescribed dependence; nutritional deficit

Defining characteristics: delay, difficulty in performing skills (motor, social) typical of age group; altered physical growth; inability of child to perform self-care or self-control activities appropriate for age

OUTCOMES

Short-term

Appropriate growth/development behavior and activities evidenced by absence of deficits, delays, regression of functioning; performance of age-appropriate growth/development within limits imposed by illness (expected within 6 to 12 weeks)

Long-term
Progressive age-appropriate steady growth/development advances; achievement of normal physical, emotional, social parameters (expected ongoing)

NURSING INTERVENTIONS/INSTRUCTIONS

1. Assess expected growth/developmental level for age and extent of deficits. Include fine and gross motor skills, language/social development, psychosocial development, interpersonal skills, and cognitive development (see "Growth and Developmental Assessment," p. 31, for guidelines) (every visit).
2. Assess caregiver, family, and environment for stressful events and ability to provide love and caring, adequate stimulation, and appropriate play activities (each visit).
3. Assess for caregiver overprotection or negligence (each visit).
4. Instruct on normal growth/development patterns for child's age and possible lag in development caused by illness (first visit).
5. Assist caregiver and family to develop goals and to participate in care to achieve optimal development (ongoing).
6. Instruct caregiver to monitor child activity tolerance. Collaborate to develop plan based on this information to provide visual, auditory, and tactile stimulation; gross motor skills for infant; time with child for talking or play activities; and self-care activities (ongoing).
7. Provide encouragement and support for efforts made by child and caregivers (each visit).
8. Provide early referral to professional resources such as special education teacher, psychosocial counselor, or social worker to assist child in specific areas of need (any visit).

CAREGIVER/CHILD AND FAMILY INTERVENTIONS

1. Complies with provision of age-related activities to enhance stimulation, independence, and developmental progression (cognitive, psychomotor, and psychosocial).
2. Sets realistic goals for growth/developmental achievement.

3. Maintains consistent caregiver and schedule of care/ activities.
4. Provides organized, consistent program of daily activities that include mobiles, music, toys, books, and other learning tools.
5. Provides time for talking and playing with other children and family members.
6. Holds, rocks, and cuddles child to provide touch and loving care.
7. Provides child opportunity to participate in self-care activities including dressing, bathing, eating, and toileting with adaptations as needed.
8. Attends parenting classes for child stimulation, growth/ developmental milestones, age-related discipline and expectations.
9. Identifies and uses specialized services to assist with growth/developmental lags.

SAMPLE DOCUMENTATION INCLUSIONS

1. Specific assessment
   Assess peripheral and apical pulses (rate, volume, rhythm); location of heart sounds; pulse deficit; murmurs; thrills; ease, rate, and depth of respirations; breath sounds; four limb blood pressures; signs of respiratory distress; activity tolerance; weight; color; developmental milestones; and signs of complications (CHF, anoxia, dehydration, or digitalis toxicity).
2. Specific care/teaching
   Teach taking of temperature, pulse, and respirations; reading pulse oximetry measurements; administering oxygen, digitalis, and iron; feeding, holding techniques; diet; activity restrictions; health maintenance activities; symptom recognition, management; emergency protocols; and preparation for surgery.
3. General
   Note responses to care, teaching, changes in plan, and progression/regression of illness status.
4. See "Documentation and Family Home Record Keeping" in Appendix for required documentation components for all home care visits.

Congestive Heart Failure

CHF is a syndrome characterized by the inability of the heart to pump sufficient blood to the systemic circulation to meet metabolic needs or to support growth. Compensatory mechanisms assist in producing more efficient cardiac output. When these mechanisms become ineffective, signs of CHF occur. CHF in children is most frequently associated with congenital heart disease (see "Nursing Care Plan, Congenital Heart Disease," p. 133). Causes of CHF include volume overload (left-to-right shunts or valve incompetence), pressure overload (obstructive lesions such as coarctation of the aorta or aortic stenosis), myocardial abnormalities and depression (tachycardia, heart block, asphyxia, anemia, acidemia, polycythemia, hypoglycemia, hypocalcemia, or hypomagnesemia), and other nonstructural conditions (sepsis, hyperthyroidism, drug toxicity, or some systemic diseases).

Clinical signs of left ventricular or biventricular CHF include restlessness, marked irritability, fatigue or activity intolerance, weak and thready pulse, tachycardia, tachypnea, coughing, wheezing, rales, dyspnea, grunting respirations, orthopnea, inappropriate diaphoresis, cool extremities, intercostal retractions, nasal flaring, poor feeding, inappropriate weight gain (edema), and failure to thrive. Right ventricular failure, rarely seen exclusively, is characterized by hepatomegaly and peripheral edema. Older children also have tenderness or pain at the hepatic site and jugular venous distention.

Age of onset varies and may occur prenatally and be detected at birth or in early infancy, with most congenitally related failure occurring by the first year of life. Symptoms may manifest gradually or rapidly; severity depends on cardiac reserve.

Treatment is directed at controlling CHF. Congenital defects may heal spontaneously or may require surgical correction. Outcome depends on controlling CHF and on treating the underlying condition. Children with cardiomyopathies are treated medically and their condition may represent end-stage illness. Cardiac transplantation may be an option.

Medical treatment is aimed at improving myocardial function, increasing oxygen supply and reducing its demands, removing excess water and sodium, balancing electrolytes, correcting metabolic abnormalities, and promoting general health maintenance.

Home health care is primarily concerned with client assessment, identification, and resolution of potential or existing problems and caregiver instruction on medication administration, decreasing cardiac demands and maintaining optimal output, promoting nutritional intake with the least effort, prevention, recognition and management of distress or complications, and emotional and educational support.

Nursing diagnosis

Ineffective family coping: compromised
Related factors: situational, maturational crises; mourning loss of healthy child
Defining characteristics: confusion, anger, guilt, loss of control, emotional immobility, overt concerns about child's condition, nonverbal stress behaviors, somatic complaints, underlying fear of sudden death, overprotective parenting, continual focus on prognosis

OUTCOMES

Short-term
Adequate coping evidenced by verbalization of feelings, needs; decreased stress behaviors; receptivity to health care teaching (expected in 1 to 4 weeks)

Long-term
Optimal coping evidenced by adaptation, acceptance, management of child's condition; maintenance/strengthening of family unit (expected within 1 to 3 months)

NURSING INTERVENTIONS/INSTRUCTIONS

1. Ask about and actively listen to caregiver's concerns and fears. Be sensitive to cultural nuances of eye contact, space, and touch (each visit).

2. Encourage expression of feelings. Avoid blame or criticism. Be supportive, provide factual information, and repeat as needed (each visit).
3. Assess caregiver's perception of condition, its cause, treatment, and prognosis and their role in care. Clarify misinformation. Answer questions simply and honestly. Use visual aids when appropriate (each visit).
4. Explore with family meaning of illness to family and their own sources of support and assistance. Emphasize need to meet both family's and child's needs, to incorporate child into family rather than making child central to it, and to treat child as normal as possible. Avoid focusing on child to detriment of mate and siblings (each visit).
5. Query as to coping strengths and past experiences. Affirm positive coping skills. Assist with skill development and problem solving (each visit).
6. Keep caregiver informed of child's progress and strengths based on physical examination. Point out developmental milestones/traits, characteristics, and behaviors unique to child (each visit).
7. Include caregiver in treatment plan. Affirm parenting skills (each visit).
8. Instruct caregiver on recognition of child's needs and general health care concerns such as hygiene, discipline, education, and recreation (ongoing).
9. Encourage caregiver to write list of questions for practitioner visits (first visit).
10. Encourage parenting classes/counseling as appropriate (first visit, reinforce as needed).
11. Explore sources of alternate or respite care (first visit, as indicated).
12. Assist in developing list of contacts for emergency questions or services (e.g., home health nurse, pediatric cardiologist, EMS) (first visit).
13. Instruct primary caregiver and others involved in child's care to obtain training in CPR and to establish emergency protocol (first visit, reinforce as needed).
14. Inform caregiver of community support resources (e.g., American Heart Association, Program for Children with Special Health Care Needs, local support groups) (first visit).

CAREGIVER/CHILD AND FAMILY INTERVENTIONS

1. Establishes rapport with nurse.
2. Verbalizes concerns about child's condition and progress.
3. Maintains/strengthens family unit with positive interaction and communication. Participates in family activities.
4. Participates in treatment plan as well as care of child.
5. Uses home remedies and cultural health care practices with physician's approval.
6. Actively seeks assistance.
7. Takes time for and pleasure in meeting own needs.
8. Obtains CPR certification.
9. Seeks sources of support.
10. Identifies and uses respite care.
11. Attends parenting classes and sees counselor.

Nursing diagnosis

Decreased cardiac output
Related factors: structural/functional cardiac defect, decreasing effectiveness of compensatory mechanisms
Defining characteristics: fatigue, restlessness, irritability, weak cry, inappropriate diaphoresis, feeding/eating difficulties, failure to gain weight/thrive, developmental lags, exhaustion, tachycardia, tachypnea, gallop rhythm, dyspnea, pulmonary congestion, coughing, wheezing, decreased peripheral pulses, cool extremities, head bobbing, mottled or gray coloring, cyanosis

OUTCOMES

Short-term
Adequate cardiac output evidenced by stabilization, decrease in symptoms, caregiver compliance with health care regimen that facilitates cardiac function (expected within 1 to 3 weeks)

Long-term
Optimal cardiac output within limitations of condition evidenced by ability to perform age-dependent activities without further distress, complications (expected within 1 to 4 weeks)

NURSING INTERVENTIONS/INSTRUCTIONS

1. Assess caregiver perception of child's health status including general behavior, respiratory patterns, color, feeding and feeding behavior, activity tolerance, respiratory infection, and latest developmental tasks (each visit).

2. Perform complete physical assessment; assess/instruct on oxygen saturation by pulse oximetry per physician's directive and protocol.

3. Assess circulatory status including rate, rhythm, and volume of apical pulse (1 full minute) and peripheral pulses and discrepancies; location of heart sounds; gallop rhythm; blood pressure; respiratory rate and effort; evidence of pulmonary congestion; coughing; crackles; grunting; nasal flaring; use of accessory muscles; color of skin, nails, and buccal mucosa; posturing; and weight changes. Note deviations from baseline and report to physician. Give caregiver realistic appraisal of examination and affirm positive findings and appropriate behaviors (each visit).

4. Demonstrate taking apical pulse and respirations of quiet child. Have caregiver return demonstrations. Based on performance, repeat and reinforce. Include norms and when to seek assistance. Leave agency telephone number (first visit).

5. Assess accuracy of medication administration. Instruct on purpose, dosage, schedule, delivery method, side effects and their remediation, laboratory monitoring of serum levels, and barriers to compliance (ongoing).

6. Assess and query concerning client irritability, fussiness, consolability, caregiver responses, and use of sedation (each visit).

7. Assess diet for iron content, including use of unsupplemented formula, cow's milk, or iron supplementation. Instruct caregiver on dietary sources of iron and, per physician's directive, administration of iron preparations (first visit).

8. Administer/instruct on gastrostomy feedings per physician's directive (see "Alternate Feeding Management," p. 205) (first and second visits).

CAREGIVER/CHILD AND FAMILY INTERVENTIONS

1. Reports persistent increases in pulse or respiration; changes in breathing pattern or color; low or prede- termined oxygen saturation level; decreased feeding; vomiting; activity intolerance; unusual weight gain, fever, or infection; and diarrhea.
2. Correctly takes apical pulse for 1 minute before adminis- tration of digoxin. Withholds drug if pulse is less than 100 bpm in infants or 70 bpm in children per physician's directive. Pulse-taking procedure may be stopped for less family intrusion and more accurate serum digoxin levels.
3. Administers digoxin correctly.

   - Gives at same time each morning. If more than one dose is prescribed per day, gives at regular intervals.
   - Gives 1 hour before or 2 hours after feeding; does not give with bottlefeeding.
   - Gives missed dose only if less than 3 hours have elapsed.
   - Withholds second dose if child vomits; withholds drug completely and contacts physician for persistent vomit- ing, decreased appetite, or slow/irregular pulse.
   - Enforces general drug and child safety protocols.
   - Returns to laboratory for digoxin serum level tests as ordered.

4. Holds, cuddles, and comforts child; sedates, per physi- cian's directive, as necessary.
5. Uses iron-fortified formula or iron supplementation and gastrostomy feeds per physician's directive; prepares well- balanced, nutritious meals that include palatable sources of iron. Correctly administers iron preparation between meals, with a vitamin C-fortified juice. Anticipates pos- sible side effect of dark, black stools and constipation; gives prune juice in 1-oz increments for latter.

Nursing diagnosis

Ineffective breathing pattern
Related factors: pulmonary congestion

Defining characteristics: tachypnea, dyspnea, orthopnea, chronic hacking cough, hoarseness, wheezing, gasping, grunting, nasal flaring, retractions, irritability, feeding difficulties

OUTCOMES

Short-term
Adequate breathing pattern evidenced by satisfactory ease and rate of respirations; decrease in dyspneic episodes, irritability; improved feeding (expected within 1 to 2 weeks)

Long-term
Optimal breathing pattern within limitations of condition (expected within 1 month)

NURSING INTERVENTIONS/INSTRUCTIONS

1. Perform complete physical assessment. Assess pulmonary system of sleeping/resting child. Note preferred posture; note ease, rate, and depth of respirations and signs of pulmonary congestion. Include caregiver in examination by instructing on findings; report deviations from baseline to physician (each visit).
2. Query caregiver regarding client history of respiratory difficulties during feeding, adequacy, duration of feeding, sleep-wake pattern, positioning for comfort, and activity tolerance; integrate with physical findings (each visit).
3. Instruct caregiver on measures to facilitate child's breathing (each visit).
4. Instruct caregiver on use of supplemental oxygen. Include rate of flow, indications for use/increase, comfort and safety measures, and logistics of ordering (first and second visits).
5. Instruct caregiver on need and measures to prevent respiratory infections (first visit).

CAREGIVER/CHILD AND FAMILY INTERVENTIONS

1. Facilitates infant's respirations by raising mattress head 10 to 30 degrees. Provides several allergy-free pillows for older child; positions older infant in cardiac chair.
2. Stays calm. Cuddles, rocks, caresses, and consoles child; allows other family members to assist in care. Sedates

child, per physician's order, for persistent fussiness or irritability.
3. Correctly administers supplemental oxygen with humidification per physician's order; if hood, tent, or croupette is used, prevents chilling and ensures child is kept dry. Appropriately cleans and maintains equipment. Monitors respirations; increases oxygen flow per physician's directive during feedings and other high-stress activities. Notifies physician if symptoms do not resolve. Maintains oxygen safety precautions.

- Has oxygen installed in a well-ventilated area.
- Posts "oxygen in use/no smoking" signs.
- Avoids open flame, sparks, aerosols, oil, and grease.
- Keeps oxygen supplier's telephone number and emergency backup plan in prominent place.

4. Uses health measures to prevent respiratory infections.

- Provides adequate rest, nutrition, and hygiene.
- Uses good handwashing technique.
- Properly cleans oxygen delivery apparatus.
- Controls exposure to known allergens and respiratory contaminants.
- Avoids exposure to infected persons.
- Reports fever, vomiting, diarrhea, difficulty breathing, and signs of infection to physician.

Nursing diagnosis

Fluid volume excess
Related factors: decreased renal blood flow, increased sympathetic stimulation, reduced glomerular filtration rate, increased serum aldosterone
Defining characteristics: oliguria, weight gain, edema, ascites, pleural effusion, distended jugular veins, hepatomegaly

OUTCOMES
Short-term
Satisfactory fluid balance evidenced by diuresis, reduced edema (expected within 1 to 4 days)

Long-term
Optimal fluid balance within limitations of condition evidenced by stabilization of renal function, absence of edema, appropriate age-dependent weight gain (expected within 1 month)

NURSING INTERVENTIONS/INSTRUCTIONS

1. Query regarding renal function including weekly weight checks; perceived intake; proportionate output; decreases in number of diaper changes, presence of periorbital edema; dependent edema in sacrum, scrotum, legs, and feet; and deterioration of respiratory function. Report deviations to physician and instruct caregiver in same (each visit).
2. Instruct/observe caregiver on administration of diuretic. Include, as appropriate, supplemental potassium if potassium-wasting diuretics are prescribed (first and second visits).
3. Assess for diuresis, hypokalemia, and concurrent digitalis toxicity. Report alterations to physician; instruct caregiver on signs and symptoms that need to be reported (each visit).
4. Instruct caregiver on diet and, per physician's directive, on moderately sodium-restricted diet (first visit).

CAREGIVER/CHILD AND FAMILY INTERVENTIONS

1. Weighs child weekly, more often if weight gain is observable. Reports edema, inappropriate weight gain, decrease in number of diaper changes, persistent increase in dyspnea, and orthopnea to physician.
2. Administers diuretic early in day if child is toilet trained; maintains calendar or checklist if dose is given on alternating days or several times a week.
3. Provides well-balanced, high-calorie, nutritious meals, offered in small, frequent amounts. Uses low-sodium formula per physician's order. Avoids table salt and high-sodium foods such as fast foods, snack products, hot dogs, lunch meats, and convenience packs.
4. Includes rich sources of potassium in diet (e.g., bananas, other fruit juices, cereals, and legumes). Administers potassium elixir in small amount of juice.

5. Reports signs of potassium depletion (increasing irritability, fatigue, apathy, muscle weakness or cramping, and persistent change in pulse) and digitalis toxicity (bradycardia and persistent vomiting) to physician.

Nursing diagnosis

Activity intolerance
Related factors: imbalance between oxygen supply, metabolic demands
Defining characteristics: fatigue, irritability, weakness, tachycardia, exertional dyspnea, tachypnea in response to activity, falling asleep while feeding, self-imposed rest, verbal complaints

OUTCOMES

Short-term
Satisfactory activity tolerance evidenced by decreased hypoxic responses, minimal increases in baseline vital signs (expected within 1 week)

Long-term
Optimal activity tolerance evidenced by stabilized endurance within limitations of underlying condition (expected within 1 month)

NURSING INTERVENTIONS/INSTRUCTIONS

1. Assess color, respirations, and position of sleeping/resting child (each visit).
2. Identify activities that tire client (e.g., multiple visitors or trips out), self-comforting techniques of child, comfort measures used by caregiver (each visit).
3. Instruct caregiver to respond quickly to fretfulness and to avoid letting infant cry for more than 10 minutes (first visit, as needed).
4. Instruct caregiver to structure and pace activities so there are rest periods for child and caregiver (each visit).
5. Instruct caregiver on measures that decrease oxygen consumption when holding and feeding child (e.g., gavage feeds per physician's order). Concurrently instruct

another family member to prevent caregiver exhaustion (first visit).
6. Assist child and caregiver on acceptable play activities (ongoing).
7. Instruct caregiver to allow child to reasonably set own pace and to rest when child chooses (first and second visits).
8. Refer to infant stimulation and education programs (first visit).

CAREGIVER/CHILD AND FAMILY INTERVENTIONS

1. Responds quickly to child's cues of need; does not wait for child to cry before intervening.
2. Structures daily activities and provides rest periods for self and child.
3. Elevates head of bed or crib; uses cardiac chair for older infant.
4. Feeds child smaller, high-calorie amounts more frequently with times integrated into child's own sleep-wake pattern (every 2 to 3 hours during the day, every 4 hours at night). Positions child in upright position when feeding, burps infant frequently, and uses soft nipple.
5. Gavage feeds or alternates gavage feeds with bottlefeedings, per physician's directive, and gastrostomy tube-feeds whatever is left after 15 to 20 minutes of bottle-feeding (see "Alternate Feeding Management," p. 205).
6. Avoids overstimulating environments or those activities that tire child. Monitors activity and provides for quiet play; child stops and rests as needed.
7. Maintains optimal environmental temperature and avoids sudden thermal changes.
8. Consults with physician before travel or vacation.
9. Contacts developmental stimulation specialist and local schools for special education information.
10. Uses rehabilitative services (e.g., occupational therapy).

Nursing diagnosis

Altered growth and development
Related factors: effects of chronic illness; environmental,

stimulation deficiencies; inadequate parental caregiving; prescribed dependence; nutritional deficit

Defining characteristics: delay, difficulty in performing skills (motor, social) typical of age group; altered physical growth; inability of child to perform self-care activities

OUTCOMES

Short-term
Adequate growth/development behavior, activities evidenced by absence of deficits, delays, regression of functioning; performance of age-appropriate growth/development within limits imposed by illness (expected within 6 to 12 weeks)

Long-term
Progressive age-appropriate steady growth/development advances; achievement of normal physical, emotional, social parameters

NURSING INTERVENTIONS/INSTRUCTIONS

1. Assess expected growth/developmental level for age and extent of deficits. Include fine and gross motor skills, language/social development, psychosocial development, interpersonal skills, and cognitive development (see "Growth and Developmental Assessment," p. 31, for guidelines) (every visit).
2. Assess caregiver, family, and environment for stressful events and ability to provide love and caring, adequate stimulation, and appropriate play activities (each visit).
3. Assess for caregiver overprotection or negligence (each visit).
4. Instruct on normal growth/development patterns for child's age and possible lag in development caused by illness (first visit).
5. Assist caregiver and family to develop goals and to participate in care to achieve optimal development potential (ongoing).
6. Instruct caregiver to monitor child's activity tolerance. Collaborate to develop plan to provide visual, auditory, and tactile stimulation; gross motor skills for infant; time with child for talking or play activities; and self-care activities (ongoing).

7. Provide encouragement and support for efforts made by child and caregivers (each visit).
8. Provide early referral to professional resources such as special education teacher, psychosocial counselor, or social worker to assist child in specific areas of need (any visit).

CAREGIVER/CHILD AND FAMILY INTERVENTIONS

1. Complies with provision of age-related activities to enhance stimulation, independence, and developmental progression (cognitive, psychomotor, and psychosocial).
2. Sets realistic goals for growth/developmental achievement.
3. Maintains consistent caregiver and schedule of care/activities.
4. Provides an organized, consistent program of daily activities that includes mobiles, music, toys, books, other learning tools.
5. Provides time for talking and playing with other children and family members.
6. Holds, rocks, and cuddles child to provide touch and loving care.
7. Provides opportunity to participate in self-care activities including dressing, bathing, eating, and toileting with adaptations as needed.
8. Attends parenting classes for child stimulation, growth/developmental milestones, and age-related discipline and expectations.
9. Identifies and uses specialized services to assist with growth/developmental lags.

SAMPLE DOCUMENTATION INCLUSIONS

1. Specific assessment
   Assess peripheral and apical pulses (rate, volume, and rhythm); pulse deficit; location of heart sounds; murmurs; thrill; gallop; ease, rate, and depth of respirations; breath sounds; signs of respiratory distress; activity tolerance; feeding behavior; postural preference; weight; color; developmental milestones; and signs of complications (edema, increasing pulmonary congestion, hypokalemia, and digitalis toxicity).

2. Specific care/teaching
   Teach taking of pulse, respirations, and pulse oximetry; administering oxygen, digitalis, diuretic, iron preparation; feeding and holding; energy conservation techniques; diet; activity restrictions; health maintenance activities; coping strategies; recognizing and managing symptoms; referrals; and emergency protocols.
3. General
   Note responses to care, teaching, changes in plan, and progression/regression of illness status.
4. See "Documentation and Family Home Record Keeping" in Appendix for required documentation components for all home care visits.

 Surgical Repair

Surgical repair of congenital heart defects includes open-heart procedures such as shunt placement, bonding, or interventional cardiac catheterization. Generally cardiac output is improved, symptoms are resolved, and functional status is enhanced and maintained. Normal life expectancy and full cardiac function can be restored with certain congenital defects, such as patent ductus arteriosus or atrial septal defect. Surgical intervention for more complex conditions may be palliative in nature and may eventually require repeated surgery or pacemaker insertion. Outcome depends on the complexity of the underlying defect, coexisting anomalies, the client's age, cardiac reserve, and functional status. The postsurgical care of the child is the sole focus of this care plan. The reader is urged to review the nursing care plan, "Congenital Heart Defects," p. 133, for general management of the child. The special care plan, "Hospital Follow-up Home Care," p. 370, is also recommended.

Home care is primarily concerned with assessment of the postoperative course, recognition and resolution of existing or potential problems, and teaching of a health care regimen to prevent complications, enhance healing, and foster wellness.

Nursing diagnosis

Ineffective family coping: compromised

Related factors: prolonged disease, intensity of hospital experience, uncertainty of outcome, caregiver exhaustion

Defining characteristics: caregiver's expressions of inability to cope; somatic complaints; regressive behaviors; strained family relationships; feelings of inadequacy, anger, guilt, exhaustion

OUTCOMES

Short-term
Adequate coping evidenced by verbalization of feelings, decreased stress behaviors, participation in child care, receptivity to health care teaching (expected in 1 to 3 weeks)

Long-term
Optimal coping evidenced by adaptation, management of child's condition, maintenance/strengthening of family relationships (expected in 1 month)

NURSING INTERVENTIONS/INSTRUCTIONS

1. Establish/maintain rapport with family (each visit).
2. Assess living environment, family's present stressors, coping strengths, and level of adjustment. Affirm strengths and facilitate development of coping skills and problem resolution (each visit).
3. Assess caregiver's perceptions of child's condition; its cause, therapy, and prognosis; their role in care; and effect of illness on family. Clarify misinformation; reinforce information on condition and care needs (each visit).
4. Ask child to describe condition and recount hospital experience. Observe caregiver's response to child (noting acceptance, rejection, denial, and overprotection) and to each other (first visit).
5. Provide written and verbal instructions on child care including specific information on significant health behav-

iors and when to seek medical attention (first visit, repeat as needed).

6. Demonstrate procedures; have caregiver return demonstration until competency is attained (first visit, repeat as needed).
7. Inform caregiver of community support resources (e.g., local support groups, respite services, American Heart Association) (as needed).
8. Encourage parenting classes and refer to social services for counseling as appropriate (first visit).

CAREGIVER/CHILD AND FAMILY INTERVENTIONS

1. Establishes rapport with nurse.
2. Verbalizes concerns, actively participates in planning, and modifies child's care.
3. Demonstrates competence in treatments and in health care protocols.
4. Displays fewer stress behaviors and more positive family environment.
5. Identifies problem areas. Obtains community and professional assistance as needed.

Nursing diagnosis

Knowledge deficit related to postoperative care
Related factors: inadequate discharge teaching, lack of readiness to learn, situational crisis
Defining characteristics: demonstrates need for information about wound care, activity, nutrition, possible complications

OUTCOMES
Short-term
Adequate knowledge evidenced by identification of, compliance with, and understanding of health care regimen (expected within 1 to 2 weeks)

Long-term
Adequate knowledge evidenced by compliance with postoperative regimen to achieve optimal functioning (expected within 2 to 4 weeks)

NURSING INTERVENTIONS/INSTRUCTIONS

1. Review postoperative medical regimen and hospital discharge plan; note written instructions given to family. Query caregiver on understanding of condition and care to be given including use of medical equipment (e.g., oxygen, pulse oximetry, and apnea monitor) (see "Nursing Care Plan," "Apnea," p. 57) (first visit, reinforce as needed).

2. Assess caregiver's readiness to learn, learning style, coping mechanisms, cues of fatigue, and family support system. Adapt instruction per individual (each visit).

3. Perform complete physical assessment. Assess cardiovascular and respiratory status (see "Cardiovascular System Assessment," p. 11, and "Pulmonary System Assessment," p. 10). Compare vital signs to established baselines; note deviations and report to physician (each visit).

4. Instruct caregiver, as appropriate, on taking resting child's apical pulse daily for 1 full minute and to report to physician tachycardia greater than 160 bpm and persistent changes in rate or rhythm (first and second visits).

5. With pacemaker insertion, reinforce importance of pulse check. Instruct on signs and symptoms indicating malfunction or wear including significant changes in pulse rate or rhythm or evidence of decreased cardiac output. Concurrently instruct on safety protocols and need for regular medical follow-up (each visit).

6. Assess incision for redness, swelling, drainage, approximation of wound edges, and presence of sutures. Instruct caregiver to keep area clean and dry and to diaper well below incisional line. When outdoor activity is permitted, keep scar covered to avoid injury from sunburn or play (each visit).

7. Assess for incisional pain (generally minimal) and self-imposed immobilization, guarding, or decreased chest expansion. Instruct caregiver on administration of analgesics per physician's directive (first and second visits).

8. Observe/instruct caregiver on safe administration of medications. Include need for continuity, purpose, dos-

age, schedule, route, food/drug interactions, side effects and their remediation, what to report to physician, and barriers to compliance. Have caregiver give return demonstration (first visit, reinforce as needed).

9. Assess activity/exercise tolerance (child may lag in gross motor development because of underlying defect and ensuing decrease in motor activity). Instruct caregiver, per physician's directive, to restrict child to home and routine activities for approximately 1 month. Instruct to rest as needed and to avoid any activity that could injure chest wall (e.g., bicycle riding or roughhousing). Instruct to resume further activity gradually and to return to school with surgeon's approval in approximately 6 weeks. Participation in physical education may be allowed; competitive or contact sports should be avoided (second to fourth visits, reinforce as needed).

10. Instruct caregiver, per physician's directive, on high-calorie, iron-supplemented, nutritionally adequate diet high in protein and vitamin C. Feed smaller amounts frequently (each visit).

11. Instruct caregiver on infection prevention and management (each visit).

   • Use good handwashing technique.
   • Continue wound care and dressing changes.
   • Provide good oral hygiene.
   • Take child to dentist for regular checkups; inform of condition, especially before procedures, so antibiotic can be implemented.
   • Promptly report fever, vomiting, or any signs of infection.

12. Instruct caregiver to notify physician of signs and symptoms of complications: nonspecific or constitutional symptoms or chills, fever, weight loss, dyspnea, tachycardia, splenomegaly, embolic phenomena (infective endocarditis), fever, and chest pain (postcardiotomy syndrome); changes in behavior, activity tolerance, and color; increasing pulse rate; respiratory difficulties; low oxygen saturation levels; vomiting; excessive sweating; and resumption of upright posture preference (first visit).

13. Support caregiver in recognition of signs of good cardiac function (e.g., strong, regular pulses, good output, improved feeding, good skin color, warm extremities, longer sleep periods, decreased irritability, and increased activity) (each visit).
14. Instruct caregiver to give child identifying information including medical/surgical conditions, pacemaker profile, and medications being taken. Instruct on how to activate EMS (first visit, reinforce as needed).
15. Emphasize importance of physician follow-up and laboratory testing. Identify possible barriers to compliance (e.g., transportation difficulties and finances) (first visit, reinforce as needed).
16. Refer to social service agencies or community resources as required (first visit).

CAREGIVER/CHILD AND FAMILY INTERVENTIONS

1. Monitors daily apical pulse and reports aberrations to physician.
2. Weighs child weekly. Reports significant or inappropriate changes.
3. Keeps incision clean and dry. Protects it from injury or contamination.
4. Comforts child. Medicates child for operative pain.
5. Administers prescribed medications per physician's order.
6. Monitors pacemaker function by regular pulse evaluation and by telephone check, per recommended schedule.
7. Child sleeps for increasing periods and rests at will. Gradually resumes full activity, including attending school. Avoids strenuous exercise, contact or competitive sports.
8. Child consumes nutritious, high-quality foods in increasing amounts without respiratory distress or undue fatigue.
9. Evaluates good cardiac function and notifies physician of signs of decreased function or complications. Verbalizes emergency activation plan.
10. Informs other health care providers of medical/surgical background, pacemaker insertion, and medication profile.

11. Child wears identifying medical information at all times.
12. Returns for physician follow-up and laboratory testing.
13. Uses community and government resources (support groups, developmental stimulation specialists, counselors, Comprehensive Care Program, and WIC).

SAMPLE DOCUMENTATION INCLUSIONS

1. Specific assessment
   Assess vital signs, weight, condition of incision, evidence of discomfort, color, posture, activity tolerance, behavior, growth/development status, and adaptive responses of family.
2. Specific care/teaching
   Teach wound and pacemaker care, nutrition, activity, medication administration, pulse taking, symptom recognition, medical follow-up, referrals/resources, and coping strategies.
3. General
   Note responses to care, teaching, changes in plan, and progression/regression of illness status.
4. See "Documentation and Family Home Record Keeping" in Appendix for general required documentation components for all home care visits.

Neurologic system

 ## Cerebral Palsy

Cerebral palsy (CP) is a broad term used to describe a constellation of chronic, nonprogressive syndromes that are characterized by motor function deficit. Acquired and genetic factors have been implicated in its cause. Although the cause is unknown, etiology has been associated with perinatal asphyxia and ischemia. Other antecedents include low birth weight, prematurity, cerebral and noncerebral congenital malformations, congenital and perinatal infections, and metabolic disorders. Table 4 includes the classification and description of the common CP syndromes and their clinical manifestations. In addition to impaired movement and posture and resulting contractures, clinical features frequently include seizure disorders, mental retardation, visual impairment, hearing loss, speech deficits, and hyperactivity coupled with a short attention span. Outcome depends on the type and severity of the disorder, age of onset, presence of associated debilitating conditions, and cognitive and behavioral levels.

CP is the most common pediatric physical disability and the most frequent neurologic disorder encountered in pediatric home health care. Home health care is primarily concerned with offering emotional support to the family and assisting the family in developing the physical, emotional, intellectual, and psychosocial potential of the child and fostering, as much as possible, eventual independence and autonomy. These goals are accomplished through instruction to the family on establishing posture, motor control, and locomotion; preventing injury, contractures, and associated problems of immobility; establishing speech and communication; managing seizures; correcting or minimizing sensory deficits and enhancing sensorimotor experiences; facili-

Table 4 Classification of Cerebral Palsy Syndromes

Type	Occurrence	Focus	Characteristics
Spastic	Most common (approximately 70%)	Upper motor neuron involvement	Hypertonicity of involved musculature, underdevelopment of affected limb, decreased spontaneous movement on affected side, alternating muscular rigidity/relaxation, tendency to contracture, weakness, exaggerated reflexes, astereognosis May affect one side of body (hemiplegia, most common), both legs (paraplegia), all limbs (quadriplegia, tetraplegia, most severe); predominant lower limb involvement (diplegia) Toe walking, scissors gait May be mild or severe With quadriplegia: impaired swallowing, tongue protrusion, defective speech (dysarthria)
Dyskinetic (athetoid)	Relatively rare (approximately 15%-20%)	Lesions of basal ganglia	Abnormal movement that is purposeless, uncontrolled, generally symmetric Slow, writhing, generally symmetric involuntary movements (athetosis); involves all extremities, face, neck, and trunk; choreoathetosis involves abrupt, jerky, irregular, distal movement Symptoms decrease with relaxation, disappear during sleep, and are aggravated by stress Tongue thrust, head lag, drooling, dysarthria; nerve deafness and conjugate upward gaze with kernicterus-associated athetosis
Ataxic	Least common (approximately 5%-10%)	Static lesions of cerebellum or its pathways	Weakness, lack of coordination Rapid, repetitive, fine motor movements difficult Wide-based gait

tating social interaction; and referring to educational and training programs and to support groups and services. Case management is essential to coordinating a multidisciplinary health care team that may include the home health care nurse, physician, physical and occupational therapists, speech pathologist, social worker, education specialist, counselors, and psychologists.

Nursing diagnosis

Ineffective family coping: compromised
Related factors: situational/maturational crises, mourning loss of healthy child, burden of disability on family, lack of support/resources
Defining characteristics: fatigue, other somatic complaints; nonverbal stress behaviors; concern about daily care, long-term needs

OUTCOMES

Short-term
Adequate coping evidenced by verbalization of feelings, needs; decreased stress behaviors; identification of sources of support, assistance (expected in 2 to 4 weeks)

Long-term
Optimal coping evidenced by adaptation and management of child's condition, maintenance/strengthening of family unit (expected within 1 month)

NURSING INTERVENTIONS/INSTRUCTIONS

1. Ask and actively listen to caregiver's concerns and fears. Be sensitive to cultural nuances of eye contact, space, and touch (each visit).
2. Assess caregiver's perception of condition, its cause, treatment, and prognosis and their role in care. Clarify misinformation. Answer questions simply and honestly (each visit).
3. Query as to coping strengths and past experiences. Affirm positive coping skills. Assist with skill development and problem solving (each visit).

4. Instruct caregiver on recognition of child's needs and general health care concerns such as hygiene, discipline, education, and recreation (first visit, ongoing).
5. Encourage parenting classes/counseling as appropriate (first visit).
6. Explore sources of alternate or respite care; encourage use (first visit).
7. Inform caregiver of community support resources (e.g., Program for Children with Special Health Care Needs, United Cerebral Palsy Association, Special Olympics, and local support groups) (first visit, as needed).

CAREGIVER/CHILD AND FAMILY INTERVENTIONS

1. Verbalizes concerns about child's condition and progress.
2. Maintains/strengthens family unit with positive interaction and communication. Participates in family activities.
3. Actively seeks assistance.
4. Takes time for and pleasure in meeting own needs. Identifies and uses respite care.
5. Seeks sources of support.

Nursing diagnosis

Knowledge deficit related to child care
Related factors: inadequate instruction; lack of readiness to learn, help/support, experience, information on available resources
Defining characteristics: expresses concerns about daily care of child, fears of hurting child; verbalizes feelings of inadequacy, fatigue, isolation, guilt

OUTCOMES
Short-term
Adequate knowledge evidenced by caregiver's ability to describe activities that meet daily needs of child (expected within 2 to 4 weeks)

Long-term
Adequate knowledge evidenced by implementation of care plan to meet daily needs of child (expected in 1 to 3 months)

NURSING INTERVENTIONS/INSTRUCTIONS

1. Assess caregiver's readiness to learn, learning style, ethnic/cultural background, assimilation of past instruction, and family support systems (each visit).
2. Assess caregiver's knowledge of disorder and implications. Query caregiver as to what care is perceived to be needed (first visit).
3. Demonstrate all care activities, including activities of daily living (ADL). Have caregiver repeat demonstration. Reinforce positive outcomes. Repeat as necessary (each visit).
4. Instruct caregiver on general maneuvers to handle child, including use of lifts and other devices. Concurrently instruct another family member to minimize caregiver exhaustion (first and second visits).

   • When moving child, work as closely as possible, keeping caregiver's body in good alignment. Use longer, stronger muscles of arms and legs rather than back muscles.
   • Keep child in proper alignment. Avoid asymmetric positioning or abnormal posturing.
   • Perform range-of-motion (ROM) exercises at least twice daily. Support joint being handled; never forcibly manipulate.
   • Use splints and braces as necessary/ordered.
   • Work in unhurried, relaxed manner.
   • Use play to facilitate relaxation.

5. Observe child being fed. Instruct caregiver and other family members on feeding techniques (first and second visits, as needed).

   • Feed in normal feeding/eating position (i.e., semireclined for infant; head, arms, and shoulder flexed slightly forward in child; avoid hyperextension of head and neck).
   • Support cheeks and control jaw as necessary. Position formula/food in mouth so child has to actively retrieve it.
   • Make mealtime relaxed and pleasant. Use play to promote hand-eye coordination and independence.
   • Advance diet gradually.
   • Use feeding aids and appliances as appropriate.

6. If child is unable to feed orally, feed by gastrostomy tube or other method as ordered (see "Alternate Feeding Management," pp. 205-215, for guidelines).
7. Consult with physical therapist for ongoing assessment and treatment plans (ongoing).
8. Refer to support groups and agencies for assistance and information (first visit).

CAREGIVER/CHILD AND FAMILY INTERVENTIONS

1. Develops and adapts care plan in consultation with home health nurse and physical therapist.
2. Positions, handles, and transfers child using good body mechanics and sound techniques.
3. Feeds child with measures that ensure safety and facilitate mobility and independence.
4. Experiments with assorted nipple sizes and shapes. Uses appropriate appliances (e.g., coated, swivel spoons; lipped plates; suction bowls; weighted utensils).
5. Seeks assistance and information from local support groups and United Cerebral Palsy Association.

Nursing diagnosis

Impaired physical mobility
Related factors: neuromuscular impairment, perceptual/ cognitive impairment
Defining characteristics: inability to purposely move within physical environment, limited range of movement, decreased muscle strength, impaired coordination, paraplegia, quadriplegia, sensory deficits

OUTCOMES
Short-term
Adequate physical mobility evidenced by participation in activities program to preserve function, prevent complications (expected within 1 month)

Long-term
Optimal physical mobility evidenced by ability to participate in/carry out ADL (expected ongoing)

NURSING INTERVENTIONS/INSTRUCTIONS

1. Perform complete physical assessment. Assess neuromuscular status (see "Neurologic Assessment," p. 12, and "Musculoskeletal Assessment," p. 21). Include posture, coordination, mobility, gait, developmental milestones, ADL, cognitive ability, behavioral response, and ability to comply/participate in medical regimen (each visit).
2. Instruct caregiver on positioning child to prevent/control contractures (each visit).

   • General stability
   • Alignment and symmetry
   • Head control

3. Discuss with caregiver developmental milestones and measures to facilitate motor activity (e.g., crawling and walking) (ongoing).
4. Demonstrate and instruct, per consultation with physical therapist, on performance of stretching exercises and active and passive ROM exercises and use of adaptive devices (first and second visits).
5. Instruct caregiver on general care measures of hygiene, nutrition, and rest that enhance endurance and performance (first and second visits).
6. Consult with or refer child to orthopedic specialist and physical therapist for appliances (e.g., braces, crutches, motorized wheelchair, customized seats, wheeled scooter boards, and standing devices) (first visit, as needed).
7. Discuss and prepare caregiver for neurosurgical or orthopedic procedures to relieve spasms and correct contractures (as needed).
8. Instruct caregiver on administration of medications to reduce spasticity (first visit, reinforce as needed).
9. Refer to developmental/occupational specialists and educational centers (first visit).

CAREGIVER/CHILD AND FAMILY INTERVENTIONS

1. Provides nutritious, well-balanced, high-calorie diet and supplements per physician's directive.
2. Incorporates exercises into ADL (e.g., bathing, diapering, grooming, and playing).

3. Performs full ROM and stretching exercises when child is rested and as can be tolerated. Pauses when child becomes fatigued or frustrated.
4. Correctly positions child.

   - Uses cushions, pillows, rolls, bolsters, and self-adhesive straps to position and stabilize child.
   - Keeps child neutrally aligned in all positions (i.e., supine, side-lying, and seated).
   - Does not favor one side or position.
   - Supports head in midline position. Adequately supports all body parts.
   - Discourages abnormal posturing.
   - Uses chest supports and harnesses for safety and support.
   - Always uses wheelchair seat belt.
   - Avoids infant walkers, W-sitting, molded, and flexible seats.
   - Uses abductor and thigh supports to manage leg adduction and increased external rotation.
   - Applies braces and splints.

5. Encourages activity.

   - Stimulates and assists for movement and activity.
   - Uses wide variety of toys for therapeutic play.
   - Places toys out of child's reach to entice. Stimulates child to use upper extremities.
   - Provides locomotion aids.

6. Correctly administers all medications, including diazepam, dantrolene, and baclofen.
7. Consults with physical/occupational therapists. Follows their recommendations.

Nursing diagnosis

Self-care deficit: bathing/hygiene, dressing/grooming, toileting
Related factors: neuromuscular disorder
Defining characteristics: inability to carry out ADL; sensory, motor, cognitive, perceptual, behavioral impairment; inexperienced caregiver

OUTCOMES

Short-term
Adequate self-care evidenced by participation in regimen to promote independent activity (expected in 2 to 4 weeks)

Long-term
Optimal ability for self-care, within limitation of condition evidenced by ability to carry out ADL (expected in 1 to 3 months)

NURSING INTERVENTIONS/INSTRUCTIONS

1. Observe caregiver bathing and dressing child. Note ability with activity, caregiver-child interaction, measures used to promote independence, and degree of frustration exhibited by child and caregiver (first and second visits).
2. Assess child's sensory, motor and perceptual status and behavior (see "Neurologic Assessment," p. 12). Include vision, hearing, speech, and cognitive ability to follow instructions (each visit).
3. Consult with or refer child to occupational therapist to assist and adapt self-help skills (every 3 to 4 visits).
4. Instruct caregiver on measures to promote child's independence (each visit).

   - Consider age-specific developmental tasks.
   - Make activity pleasant. Incorporate toys and preferred play into activity.
   - Encourage child to participate in activity. Encourage caregiver to hold, touch, and talk to child.
   - Establish routine and allow extra time for activities.
   - Teach from simple to more complex (e.g., teach undressing before dressing; dress affected extremity, then unaffected one).
   - Use adaptive clothing when possible (e.g., larger sizes, fuller styles, elastic waistbands, self-adhering closures, or diapers, as necessary).
   - Toilet after each feeding and approximately every 3 hours during day.
   - Avoid pressuring or unduly frustrating child. Praise improvements and accomplishments.

5. Refer child to specialists for evaluation of vision, speech, and hearing (first visit).
6. Instruct caregiver on measures to facilitate sensory experiences (each visit).

   • Speak to child before touching.
   • Face child when speaking.
   • Speak slowly and distinctly; describe what you are doing.
   • Keep play area uncluttered. Position toys in child's visual field; move toys to encourage exploration.
   • Continue feeding techniques that strengthen mouth movement and facilitate speech.
   • Provide variety of sensory stimuli.

7. Instruct caregiver on modalities to further enhance communication (first visit).

   • Refer child to speech therapist.
   • Enlist child in special play groups or special education classes.
   • Acquire specialized equipment (e.g., computers and amplification devices).
   • Use nonverbal communication.

CAREGIVER/CHILD AND FAMILY INTERVENTIONS

1. Encourages self-directed activity and self-care.
2. Selects appropriate toys to stimulate motor activity and sensory awareness.
3. Includes child in family activities.
4. Promotes social interaction through special play groups and school attendance.
5. Encourages independence through continual teaching of functional skills.
6. Works to develop appropriate skills with therapists (e.g., physical, occupational, or speech therapist).

Nursing diagnosis

Risk for injury
Related factors: neuromuscular impairment, sensory deficits, perceptual/cognitive impairment

Defining characteristics: muscle weakness, instability, lack of coordination, seizure activity

OUTCOMES

Short-term
Minimal or absence of injury evidenced by safe physical environment; knowledge of, compliance with seizure protocol (expected immediately)

Long-term
Absence of injury evidenced by integrity of skin, mucous membranes, bone (expected ongoing)

NURSING INTERVENTIONS/INSTRUCTIONS

1. Assess home for safety of physical environment (see "Environmental Assessment," p. 37). Based on observations, instruct caregiver on measures to promote safety (each visit).

   - Keep play and sleep areas free of sharp, pointed objects.
   - Avoid scatter rugs and lightweight or unstable furniture.
   - Use bed side rails or crib padding.
   - Use lap belt in wheelchair and safety restraints in car.
   - Use helmet.

2. Instruct caregiver on seizure precautions (first and second visits, reinforce as needed).

   - Keep seizure record for practitioner. Include medication schedule/changes, presence of aura, time of onset, duration, description, and postictal behavior.
   - Administer prescribed anticonvulsants.
   - During seizure, keep calm and stay with child, support child to soften fall, place pad under head, do not restrain or attempt to immobilize, do not place anything in mouth, position child on side if possible, and allow to rest or sleep afterward.

CAREGIVER/CHILD AND FAMILY INTERVENTIONS

1. Maintains safe home environment.
2. Applies appropriate restraints and equipment.

3. Supports and protects child during seizure activity.
4. Correctly administers prescribed anticonvulsant.
5. Keeps log of seizure activity. Informs physician per directive.

Nursing diagnosis

Altered growth and development

Related factors: effects of chronic illness, environmental/ stimulation deficiencies, nutrtional deficit

Defining characteristics: delay, difficulty in performing skills (motor, social, expressive); altered physical growth; inability of child to perform self-care, self-control activities

OUTCOMES

Short-term

Growth/development of behavior, activities evidenced by absence of deficits, delays, regression of functioning; exhibition of adequate growth/development within limits imposed by illness (expected within 6 to 12 weeks)

Long-term

Progressive, steady, growth/development advances; achievement of normal physical, emotional, social parameters (expected ongoing)

NURSING INTERVENTIONS/INSTRUCTIONS

1. Assess expected growth/developmental level for age and extent of deficits. Include fine and gross motor skills, language/social development, psychosocial and interpersonal skills, and cognitive development (see "Growth and Developmental Assessment," p. 31, for guidelines) (every visit).
2. Assess caregiver, family, and environment for stressful events and ability to provide love and caring, adequate stimulation, and play activities (each visit).
3. Assess for caregiver overprotection or negligence (each visit).

4. Instruct on normal growth/development patterns for child's age and possible lag in development caused by illness (first visit).

5. Assist caregiver and family to develop goals, to participate in care to achieve optimal development (ongoing).

6. Instruct caregiver to monitor child's activity tolerance. Collaborate with caregiver to develop plan based on this information to provide visual, auditory, and tactile stimulation; gross motor skills for infant; time with child for talking or play activities; and self-care activities (ongoing).

7. Provide encouragement and support for efforts made by child and caregivers (each visit).

8. Provide early referral to professional resources such as speech/physical therapist, special education teacher, psychosocial counselor, or social worker to assist child in specific areas of need (any visit).

CAREGIVER/CHILD AND FAMILY INTERVENTIONS

1. Complies with activities to enhance stimulation, independence, and developmental (cognitive, psychomotor, and psychosocial) progression.

2. Sets realistic goals for growth/developmental achievement.

3. Maintains consistent caregiver and schedule of activities.

4. Provides organized and consistent program of daily activities that include mobiles, music, toys, books, and other learning tools.

5. Provides time for talking and playing with other children and family members.

6. Holds, rocks, and cuddles child to provide touch and loving care.

7. Provides opportunity to participate in self-care activities, including dressing, bathing, eating, and toileting with adaptations as needed.

8. Attends parenting classes for child stimulation, growth/developmental milestones, discipline, and expectations.

9. Identifies and uses specialized services to assist with growth/developmental lags.

Nursing diagnosis

Social isolation
Related factors: alterations in physical appearance (hyperto-
nicity, contractures, drooling), mental status; altered
communication; unacceptable social behavior
Defining characteristics: evidence of physical, mental
handicap; inappropriate activities for developmental age/
stage; repetitive, meaningless actions; exists in subculture;
overprotectiveness of caregiver

OUTCOMES

Short-term
Decreased social isolation evidenced by participation in
activity outside immediate care unit (expected in 1
month)

Long-term
Minimal isolation evidenced by optimal functioning;
participation in social, recreational, educational
groups within limits of condition (expected in 1 to 3
months)

NURSING INTERVENTIONS/INSTRUCTIONS

1. Discuss with caregiver amount of social interaction occurring, expected, and projected (first visit).
2. Encourage caregiver to include child in all family activities (e.g., eating, playing, shopping, and attending
   church). Discuss perceived barriers and their remediation (ongoing).
3. Reinforce exercises/activities that promote child's self-
   sufficiency, confidence, and pleasure (each visit).
4. Refer family to agencies, organizations, and institutions
   that offer social outlets, information, and assistance (first
   visit).

CAREGIVER/CHILD AND FAMILY INTERVENTIONS

1. Child participates in self-care activities, becoming as self-
   reliant as possible.
2. Child functions as integral part of family.

3. Caregiver contacts special support groups. Child participates in play groups, educational activities, and school.

SAMPLE DOCUMENTATION INCLUSIONS

1. Specific assessment
   Assess posture; alignment; coordination; mobility; gait;
   areas of spastic flexion/extension; range-of-motion of
   muscle groups; use of adaptive appliances/devices; presence of contractures; speech, hearing, vision deficits;
   history of seizures (seizure diary); developmental
   milestones; mentation; and ability to eat, groom, toilet,
   ambulate, and socialize.
2. Specific care/teaching
   Teach ROM exercises; how to safely handle, move, position, and feed child; sensory enrichment; seizure
   protocol; referral to physical, occupational, and speech
   therapists; and procurement and use of adaptive appliances and equipment.
3. General
   Note responses to care, teaching, changes in plan, and
   progression/regression of illness.
4. See "Nurse Documentation and Family Home Record
   Keeping" in Appendix for required documentation components for all home care visits.

 Neurologic Defects

Neural tube defects (dysraphia), resulting from failed closure of the neural plate in utero, represent the most
common and serious congenital anomalies of the central
nervous system (CNS). Major defects include spina bifida,
myelocele, meningocele, myelomeningocele, encephalo-
cele, and anencephaly. Causes are unknown, although many
factors have been associated with their etiology (e.g., genetic predisposition; exposure to toxins, drugs, chemicals,
and radiation; and malnutrition involving folic acid deficiency). Symptoms, course, and prognosis depend on the

type and size of defect and the extent of neurologic involvement. (Table 5 gives definitions and descriptions of types of dysraphia.) In the absence of other serious coexisting defects or infection, surgical repair is the treatment of choice. It may be performed immediately after birth or in early infancy. Even after repair of the defect, a multidisciplinary team approach is necessary to manage long-term neurologic, urologic, and orthopedic problems.

Home health care is primarily concerned with recognizing and resolving associated conditions (increased intracranial pressure [ICP] and hydrocephalus); preventing complications (infection and shunt blockage); managing problems associated with lower limb paralysis, saddle anesthesia, and sensory/tactile defects; promoting growth and development; and instructing, supporting, and counseling the client and the caregivers.

Nursing diagnosis

Risk for infection
Related factors: dysraphic portal of entry, bowel/bladder incontinence
Defining characteristics: cerebrospinal fluid (CSF) leaks, defect, abrasion/irritation, denuded skin, infectious organisms, continuous dribbling of urine, fecal incontinence, postoperative surgical incision with continuing paralysis, saddle anesthesia

OUTCOMES
Short-term
Prevention of infection evidenced by normal temperature, undisturbed defect/operative site, caregiver compliance with prophylactic regimen (expected immediately)

Long-term
Absence of infection; early intervention and treatment of infection evidenced by clean, undisturbed operative site; postoperatively complete wound healing (expected within 2 to 4 weeks)

Table 5   Neurologic Defects: Definitions and Descriptions

Defect	Definition/Description
Spina bifida occulta	Defective closure of vertebral laminae, generally at levels L5, S1
	No overt clinical manifestation
	No neurologic involvement; no abnormalities of spinal cord, nerve roots or meninges
	May present midline dorsal skin discoloration, patch of hair, dermal sinus or lipoma
	Infrequently associated with other developmental anomalies
Spina bifida cystica	Defective closure of vertebral laminae from which protrudes the meninges (meningocele), spinal cord (myelocele), or both (myelomeningocele)
	Most common site is lumbar-sacral region
	Frequently associated with hydrocephalus; as general rule, the lower the vertebral defect, the lower the risk of hydrocephalus
	Characterized by marked neurologic involvement
	Cord or nerve protrusion causes paralysis below the innervated area; sensory, tactile deficits; impaired bowel, bladder function
	Frequently associated with orthopedic abnormalities, other congenital defects
Hydrocephalus	Accumulation of CSF in cerebral ventricular system resulting from imbalance between production or, more commonly, absorption of CSF caused by ventricular blockage
	Onset may be insidious, gradual, abrupt; progression may stop spontaneously
	Signs, symptoms reflective of increased intracranial pressure; generally requires shunting to relieve pressure
Encephalocele	Defective skull closure from which brain tissue, meninges protrude
	Occiput is most common site; anterior involvement may include frontal, nasofrontal, nasopharyngeal, parietal region
	Frequently associated with other congenital defects, hydrocephalus
Anencephaly	Absence of major portions of CNS
	Incompatible with survival

CSF, Cerebrospinal fluid; *CNS,* central nervous system.

NURSING INTERVENTIONS/INSTRUCTIONS

1. Perform complete physical assessment. Instruct caregiver to assess defect site for clear to pale yellow or purulent drainage; fever; and changes in defect integrity, size, color, and temperature. Note infant position, presence of urine or stool on or near defect, condition of dressing, changes in feeding or level of alertness, irritability, and lethargy. Notify physician of significant findings (each visit).

2. Instruct caregiver on need for meticulous infection control. Demonstrate handwashing technique and have caregiver repeat demonstration (first and second visits).

3. Instruct/monitor caregiver on positioning techniques and methods to minimize contamination from urine, stool, or other fomites (each visit).

4. Provide wound care. Per physician's directive, apply sterile, nonadhesive dressing moistened with sterile saline or antibiotic solution; cover with larger, dry sterile dressing (each visit).

5. Provide perineal care. Do not diaper over affected area. Shield site with foam donut cutout; use plastic barrier between anus and affected site (each visit).

6. Instruct/monitor caregiver, per physician's directive, on wound care (each visit).

7. Postoperatively assess and teach caregiver to assess wound healing. Note redness, changes in color or temperature, approximation of edges, swelling, drainage, and fever. Notify physician of significant findings or aberrations (each visit).

CAREGIVER/CHILD AND FAMILY INTERVENTIONS

1. Uses good handwashing techniques before tending infant or providing prescribed wound care.

2. Handles infant gently and carefully. Positions infant on side or in prone position with hips elevated and slightly flexed and leg abducted. Uses pillows, sandbags, rolled towels for support, and anchor.

3. Does not cover affected site with clothing or diapers. Cushions area around site. Tents bed linens.

4. Provides frequent perineal care. Uses plastic shield to protect sac from fecal contaminants.

5. Changes dressing when it is soiled. Uses sterile technique to gently clean and moisten affected area per physician's directive. Applies and secures dry outer dressing.
6. Reports to physician any redness, swelling, or drainage from site; fever; and change in appetite or level of alertness.

Nursing diagnosis

Risk for injury
Related factors: neurologic defect, trauma; coexisting anomalies
Defining characteristics: heat loss from defect site, poor feeding, increased ICP, seizure activity

OUTCOMES
Short-term
Absence of injury evidenced by adequate intake, maintenance of optimal temperature, control/management of deteriorating condition/complication (expected in 1 to 4 weeks, ongoing)

Long-term
Absence of injury evidenced by optimal growth, development, and functioning within limitations of condition (expected ongoing)

NURSING INTERVENTIONS/INSTRUCTIONS
1. Assess wound site; motor, sensory responses; head circumference; status of fontanels; and level of alertness (each visit).
2. Assess, observe if possible, caregiver's knowledge of feeding technique and instruct based on observed need (each visit).

- Maintain alignment in prone or side-lying position. Do not put pressure on wound site.
- Feed child in crib or on lap with head turned and head, neck, and shoulders slightly elevated.
- To avoid distracting child, touch, caress, and talk to infant before feeding. Feed slowly.

- Provide adequate fluids.
- Let child sleep afterward.

3. Assess and instruct caregiver to assess infant temperature, ambient temperature, amount of clothing, and warming methods. Instruct caregiver on techniques to maintain optimal thermal environment (first visit, as needed).
4. Instruct caregivers to regularly check soft and flat fontanels of seated, quiet infant: see and touch anterior fontanel; describe tenseness and bulging. Notify physician of latter (first and second visits).
5. Assess for signs of increasing ICP: increased head circumference; tense, bulging fontanels; widening of cranial suture lines; irritability; decreased level of alertness; change in appetite; vomiting; and downward deviation of pupils ("sunset" eyes). Report aberrations to physician (each visit).
6. Query caregiver regarding seizure activity. Instruct on management of seizures (first visit, as needed).

   - Provide crib rail padding.
   - Clear away toys and any harmful, interfering objects.
   - Maintain side-lying or prone position.
   - Do not restrain. Do not place anything in mouth.
   - Loosen clothing.
   - Allow time postictally for reorientation, rest, or sleep.
   - Notify practitioner if activity is new or changes significantly in frequency or duration.
   - Maintain seizure diary.

7. Refer to local support groups and national organizations (e.g., Spina Bifida Association of America) for information, assistance, and support (first visit).

CAREGIVER/CHILD AND FAMILY INTERVENTIONS

1. Nurtures infant and provides and maintains adequate nutrition.
2. Provides optimal temperature. Appropriately, lines crib with fleece, keeps body appropriately covered, tents blankets over affected site, and adapts for weather change.
3. Monitors for increased ICP (incipient hydrocephalus or postoperative shunt function). Notifies physician.

4. Provides for safe environment during seizure activity, monitors for changes, and contacts physician as directed.
5. Participates in support groups to learn about condition and its management and in coping.

Nursing diagnosis

Altered urinary elimination
Related factors: neuromuscular impairment
Defining characteristics: saddle anesthesia, neurogenic bladder, constant dribbling of urine, incomplete bladder emptying, lack of voluntary bladder control despite physical maturation

OUTCOMES

Short-term
Urinary elimination managed evidenced by regular mechanical emptying of bladder, absence of infection (expected in 2 to 4 weeks)

Long-term
Urinary elimination managed evidenced by ongoing urologic regimen; absence of infection, renal complication; intact kidney function (expected in 4 weeks)

NURSING INTERVENTIONS/INSTRUCTIONS

1. Assess renal status (see "Renal and Urinary Systems Assessment," p. 22). Note age, ability to voluntarily control bladder, color and odor of urine, and fever (each visit).
2. Instruct caregiver on prescribed bladder control program and clean intermittent catheterization approximately every 3 to 4 hours (age-dependent). Demonstrate procedure. Provide opportunity for caregiver to return demonstration and perform procedure during subsequent visits. Teach child as soon as old enough and willing to participate (first visit, reinforce as needed).
3. Instruct caregiver on measures to minimize urinary tract infection (UTI) (first and second visits).

   - Encourage adequate fluid intake; include acid-ash producing foods (e.g., cranberries, plums, prunes, corn, breads, cereals, and meat).

- Change diapers as soon as they become soiled. Keep perineal area clean.
- If child has some sensation, toilet (age-appropriate) every 2 hours during day.
- Notify physician of fever or foul-smelling urine.
- Take child for periodic assessment of renal function, as prescribed.

4. Instruct caregiver on administration of prescribed antispasmodics, smooth muscle relaxants, urinary antiseptics, alpha adrenergics, and antibiotics (first visit).
5. After consultation with physician, discuss and explain surgical intervention (individual).

CAREGIVER/CHILD AND FAMILY INTERVENTIONS

1. Keeps genital area clean from stool.
2. Empties bladder regularly with frequent toileting, catheterization post voiding or clean intermittent catheterization (CIC).
3. Maintains infection control protocol, including fluids, appropriate diet, meticulous perineal care.
4. Monitors and reports signs of UTI to physician.
5. Takes child for prescribed testing (e.g., urine culture and analysis, serum electrolytes and creatinine, creatinine clearance, blood urea nitrogen [BUN], intravenous pyelograms, and renal ultrasound).
6. Demonstrates knowledge of surgical options to control incontinence.

Nursing diagnosis

Bowel incontinence
Related factors: neuromuscular deficit, saddle anesthesia
Defining characteristics: relaxed anal sphincter, limited anal reflex, bowel incontinence, constipation, impaction

OUTCOMES
Short-term
Beginning bowel control evidenced by regular elimination program in developmentally ready child (expected in 3 months)

Long-term
Bowel continence within limitations of condition (6 to 12 months)

NURSING INTERVENTIONS/INSTRUCTIONS

1. Assess developmental age, motor, sensory deficits, bowel function, and candidacy for bowel management program (first visit).
2. Instruct caregiver to toilet child after each meal or at given time daily (beginning when child is about 2 years of age). Use fingertip rectal stimulation as necessary (first visit, reinforce as needed).
3. Demonstrate digital evacuation of impacted bowel. Instruct caregiver on indications and technique. Have caregiver repeat demonstration (as needed).
4. Instruct caregiver on dietary measures to promote elimination (first visit).
5. Instruct caregiver on administration of prescribed bulk formers, stool softeners, laxatives, and suppositories (first visit).

CAREGIVER/CHILD AND FAMILY INTERVENTIONS

1. Has diet with adequate fluids, roughage, and fiber.
2. Uses potty/toilet at same time every day.
3. Caregiver monitors evacuations and modifies diet accordingly; tests for impaction when there has been no evacuation, deviation from established schedule, fecal incontinence around hardened retained stool; and removes impaction manually.

Nursing diagnosis

Impaired physical mobility
Related factors: neuromuscular deficit, musculoskeletal defects
Defining characteristics: varying degrees of paralysis; sensory, motor deficits; skeletal anomalies (kyphosis, scoliosis, subluxation of hips, or club foot), contractures

OUTCOMES

Short-term
Adequate mobility evidenced by preservation of current function and participation in orthopedic/occupational health regimen (expected in 2 to 4 weeks)

Long-term
Optimal mobility to perform motor activities within limitations of condition (expected within 4 to 6 weeks)

NURSING INTERVENTIONS/INSTRUCTIONS

1. Assess musculoskeletal/neurologic status, including areas innervated for sensation and motion and presence of anomalies, defects, and contractures (each visit).
2. Confer with primary care physician and health care team (including physical/occupational therapists) to develop program of exercises and activities (first visit).
3. Observe and instruct caregiver on measures to preserve and improve muscular function (first visit, reinforce as needed).

   - Perform passive ROM exercises with affected extremities.
   - Assist child in active ROM exercises with unaffected extremities; progress through resistance exercises per team conference.
   - Incorporate all exercises into ADL (e.g., bathing and changing). Use play as enticement for motion and stimulation.
   - Maintain good body alignment.
   - Adapt positioning based on defect, time since repair, and presence of coexisting defects.
   - Encourage and reward progressive activity such as weight bearing and continued use of adaptive devices (e.g., scooter boards, walkers, and motorized or manual wheelchairs).

4. Assist with physical therapy program. Observe and instruct caregiver and older child on safe and proper use of splints, braces, crutches, and wheelchairs and care of cast as applicable (each visit).

5. Observe and instruct caregiver on measures to preserve skin integrity (each visit).

   - Inspect pressure areas for redness, blanching, excoriation, and change in temperature or sensation.
   - Keep bed linens smooth and dry. Use sheepskin or eggcrate mattresses, as indicated.
   - Provide good skin care and massage.
   - Pad/cushion areas under/around cast, braces, and traction.
   - Provide sturdy shoes with good support.

CAREGIVER/CHILD AND FAMILY INTERVENTIONS

1. Works with health team to develop, implement, and adapt physical therapy program.
2. Maintains skin integrity, motor function through integrated plan of play, hygiene, and exercise.
3. Correctly uses adaptive devices to facilitate child's activity and bolster self-confidence.
4. Uses educational/recreational outlets outside home to enhance learning and mobility.

Nursing diagnosis

Altered growth and development
Related factors: effects of chronic condition, environmental/stimulation deficiencies, inadequate parental caregiving, prescribed dependence, nutritional deficit
Defining characteristics: delay/difficulty in performing skills (motor, social, expressive); altered physical growth; inability of child to perform self-care, self-control activities

OUTCOMES

Short-term
Adequate growth/development of behavior, activities evidenced by absence of deficits, delays, regression of functioning; performance of age-appropriate growth/development within limits imposed by condition (expected within 6 to 12 weeks)

Long-term
Progressive growth/development advances; achievement of normal physical, emotional, social parameters within limitations imposed by condition (expected ongoing)

NURSING INTERVENTIONS/INSTRUCTIONS

1. Assess expected growth/developmental level for age and extent of deficits. Include fine and gross motor skills, language/social development, psychosocial and interpersonal skills, and cognitive development (see "Growth and Developmental Assessment," p. 31, for guidelines) (each visit).
2. Assess caregiver, family, and environment for stressful events and for ability to provide love, caring, adequate stimulation, and play activities (each visit).
3. Assess for caregiver overprotection or negligence (each visit).
4. Instruct caregiver on normal growth/development patterns for child's age and possible lag in development caused by condition (first visit).
5. Assist caregiver and family to develop goals and to participate in care to achieve optimal development potential (ongoing).
6. Instruct caregiver to monitor child's activity tolerance. Collaborate to develop plan to provide visual, auditory, and tactile stimulation; gross motor skills for infant; and time with child for talking, play, and self-care activities (ongoing).
7. Provide encouragement and support for efforts made by child and caregivers (each visit).
8. Provide early referral to professional resources such as physical therapist, special education teacher, psychosocial counselor, or social worker to assist child in specific areas of need (any visit).

CAREGIVER/CHILD AND FAMILY INTERVENTIONS

1. Complies with provision of activities to enhance stimulation, independence, and developmental (cognitive, psychomotor, and psychosocial) progression.
2. Sets realistic goals for growth/developmental achievement.

3. Maintains consistent caregiver and schedule of activities.
4. Provides organized and consistent program of daily activities that include mobiles, music, toys, books, and other learning tools.
5. Provides time for talking and playing with other children and family members.
6. Holds, rocks, and cuddles child to provide touch and loving care.
7. Provides opportunity to participate in self-care activities, including dressing, bathing, eating, and toileting with adaptations as needed.
8. Attends parenting classes for child stimulation, growth/developmental milestones, discipline, and expectations.
9. Identifies and uses specialized services to assist with growth/developmental lags.

Nursing diagnosis

Altered family processes
Related factors: situational crisis, altered family dynamics, ineffective problem solving
Defining characteristics: family feelings of anxiety, tension, distress, powerlessness, vulnerability; child's feelings of being different; inadequate understanding, knowledge of disorder, how to manage it

OUTCOMES
Short-term
Enhanced family processes evidenced by stabilization, reduction of negative feelings, behaviors (expected in 1 month)

Long-term
Optimal family processes evidenced by verbalization, demonstration that all basic individual and family needs are being met (expected in 1 to 3 months)

NURSING INTERVENTIONS/INSTRUCTIONS
1. Assess family dynamics (see "Family Assessment," p. 41), roles, responsibilities, expectations, adaptive capacity, and emotional/economic resources (each visit).

2. Assess family's perception of disability; its cause, prognosis, and treatment; role of health care practitioners; and ethnic/cultural beliefs and practices (first visit, as needed).
3. Encourage expression of feelings. Facilitate dialogue about condition and its impact on family members (each visit).
4. Explain condition to caregiver using visual aids or other appropriate learning modalities. Use models to demonstrate treatment (first visit).
5. Instruct family to incorporate child into family unit and to treat as normally as possible. Reinforce that child's self-esteem and self-perception are directly related to caregivers' attitudes and behaviors. Act as positive role model (each visit).
6. Allow each family member time to express and progress through phases of shock, denial, confusion, anxiety, guilt, and depression, to ultimate acceptance and adaptation (each visit).
7. Assist family in identifying strengths, positive coping strategies, and problem resolution. Direct family to services that offer information, assistance, support, and respite care (ongoing).
8. Explain need to maintain/enhance individual and family health (e.g., wellness strategies and social/recreational outlets) (each visit).

CAREGIVER/CHILD AND FAMILY INTERVENTIONS

1. Family members establish rapport with nurse and openly share their feelings, concerns, hopes, and misgivings.
2. Treat child not as center of, but rather part of family.
3. Individual and family progress through stages of adjustment and ultimately achieve realistic view of disabled child.
4. Family demonstrates positive, cohesive family relationships.
5. Family participates in variety of growth-promoting activities and contacts religious and community agencies, governmental organizations, physical therapist, occupational therapist, health care services, and educational institutions for information, support, and assistance.

SAMPLE DOCUMENTATION INCLUSIONS

1. Specific assessment
   Assess vital signs; status of fontanels and scalp veins; head circumference; location, extent, and characteristics of CNS defect; signs of leakage, infection, breaks in integrity; coexisting anomalies; sensory/motor deficits; degree of disability; use of assistive aids and appliances; developmental age; bowel/bladder control; and history/signs of increased ICP, seizures, irritability, lethargy, and poor feeding.
2. Specific care/teaching
   Teach wound care; infection control; handling and positioning infant; ROM exercises; use of assistive aids and appliances; bladder/bowel control programs; management/resolution of complications (early hydrocephalus, shunt obstruction, and seizure activity); and compliance with regimens to promote locomotion, growth, development, and stimulation.
3. General
   Note responses to care and teaching.
4. See "Nurse Documentation and Family Home Record Keeping" in Appendix for required documentation components for all home care visits.

 Seizure Disorders

Seizure disorders are a symptom complex of CNS dysfunction. The involuntary, paroxysmal, convulsive disorder may be characterized by abnormal motor activity, altered consciousness, and sensory or behavioral disturbances. Although the cause is frequently unknown, the abnormal firing patterns of cerebral neurons may be associated with a variety of conditions. These include perinatal hypoxia, genetic defects and developmental anomalies, metabolic disorders, intracranial neoplasms, hemorrhage or infection, cerebral trauma, edema, hypoxia, degenerative CNS disease or infection, febrile illness, toxic agents, anaphylaxis, or drug withdrawal.

Seizures are classified according to their clinical manifestations and electroencephalographic features. Proper classification is essential in determining cause and ascribing treatment. Broad classifications include partial, generalized, and unclassified seizures. Simple, partial seizures are focal or localized in origin, and consciousness is maintained; in complex partial seizures, consciousness is altered. Generalized seizures are classified as absence, general tonic-clonic, tonic, clonic, myotonic, atonic, and infantile spasms. Motor activity and consciousness are affected. Seizures may be acute and nonrecurrent or chronically recurrent. Clinical manifestations vary widely and reflect the size and extent of the cerebral insult. Prognosis depends on the classification of the seizure, its cause and accompanying neurologic disease or damage, the age of onset, the family history, and the client's responsiveness to drug therapy. Outcome is frequently good (i.e., seizures are controlled by medication or are self-limiting by virtue of their association with a treatable medical or neurologic condition). Outcome is less optimistic for recurrent seizures resistant to pharmacotherapy or for sequelae associated with anoxia or degenerative processes. Treatment is directed at determining and correcting the underlying condition and at controlling seizures through medication or surgical intervention.

Home health care is primarily concerned with instruction on seizure management, injury prevention, maintenance of a safe environment, administration of anticonvulsant medication, and family support.

Nursing diagnosis

Risk for injury

Related factors: CNS dysfunction, loss of consciousness

Defining characteristics: ill-defined preseizure aura, loss of motor control, convulsive activity, altered consciousness, cyanosis, sensorimotor alteration, trauma from falls, asphyxia

OUTCOMES

Short-term
Minimal or no injury evidenced by integrity of bone and soft tissue and intact motor, respiratory, cognitive functions (expected immediately, maintained throughout seizure)

Long-term
Absence of injury evidenced by seizure prophylaxis and control (expected ongoing)

NURSING INTERVENTIONS/INSTRUCTIONS

1. Perform complete physical examination, including neurologic, renal, and hepatic systems (see "Physical Assessment Guide," pp. 12, 22, and 26). Note vital signs, growth and development, developmental milestones, congenital anomalies, motor skills and responses, ocular response, and level of alertness (first visit).
2. Assess/query caregiver about child's seizure activity. If caregiver is more comfortable, instruct to act out impression of seizure (each visit).
3. Instruct caregiver to keep log of all seizure activity (each visit). Record the following information:

   • Date and time of seizure. Length of time since last seizure.
   • Perceived precipitating factors (sleep deprivation, sensory stimuli, and stress) and concurrent fatigue, fever, infection, stress, and sensory stimulants.
   • Presence of aura, using child's verbal description if possible.
   • Description of seizure (type of movement, duration, state of consciousness, presence of automatism, muscle tone, color, respirations, and loss of urinary or bowel function).
   • Postictal behavior (confused, sleepy, difficult to rouse or normal/preictal).

4. Instruct caregiver on care during seizure activity (first visit, repeat as needed).

   • Stay calm. Remain with child.
   • Clear harmful objects from immediate environment.

- If child is not in bed, gently slide to floor, position on side, and gently hyperextend neck and jaw if possible.
- Place padding under child's head.
- Loosen constrictive clothing.
- Do not restrain child.
- Do not pry open child's mouth or place anything in it.
- Allow seizure to run its course.
- Comfort child after seizure. Allow time to sleep if difficult to rouse or sleepy. Check approximately every ½ to 1 hour until awake.

5. Instruct caregiver to immediately notify physician if following conditions exist (first visit, reinforce as needed):

- Continuous seizures that last longer than 30 minutes (or predetermined, established time) and recurrent seizures from which child does not regain consciousness or return to preictal state (status epilepticus or medical emergency)
- Significant change in type, frequency, or duration of seizure
- Vomiting and inability to retain anticonvulsant medications

6. Instruct caregiver on the following measures to promote child safety (first and second visits).

- Promote safe, age-dependent activity.
- Avoid dangerous play (e.g., tree climbing and bike riding without helmet).
- Supervise bathing, swimming, and water sports.
- Apply lap belt when in infant seat, high chair, or wheelchair.
- Enforce use of helmet (activity-dependent and condition-dependent).
- Enforce continual wear of identifying medical information.
- Inform those who need to know about condition and seizure protocol.

CAREGIVER/CHILD AND FAMILY INTERVENTIONS

1. Provides safe home environment.
2. Observes safety protocols during seizure activity.

3. Maintains accurate record of seizure activity.
4. Notifies physician of significant changes.
5. Educates teachers, day-care workers, and babysitters about condition and its management.
6. Child wears identifying medical tags.

Nursing diagnosis

Knowledge deficit
Related factors: lack of information about disorder, lack of readiness to learn
Defining characteristics: verbalize need for information about disorder, its control with medication, cannot answer questions, express self regarding child care

OUTCOMES
Short-term
Adequate knowledge evidenced by caregiver's ability to verbalize cause, course, prognosis of disorder, medication, health regimen (expected within 1 to 2 weeks)

Long-term
Adequate knowledge evidenced by compliance with medication, medical regimens to achieve optimal growth, development, health (expected within 1 month)

NURSING INTERVENTIONS/INSTRUCTIONS
1. Assess caregiver's readiness to learn, learning style, ethnic/cultural background, coping mechanisms, and family support systems (each visit).
2. Inform caregiver of course of seizure activity, if known, and implication for regular follow-up care (i.e., laboratory testing, neurologic examination, and regular physical examinations) (first visit).
3. Instruct caregiver on allowable home and school activities (each visit).
4. Direct caregiver in identification of factors that precipitate seizures and their management (each visit).
5. Instruct caregiver on correct administration of anticonvulsant medication, including time, dosage, route, food/drug interactions, safety precautions, side effects, and ne-

cessity of laboratory testing (first visit, reinforce each visit).

6. Instruct caregiver on prescribed ketogenic diet, as applicable, in vitamin and mineral supplementation (first visit).

7. Instruct caregiver on need for scrupulous dental hygiene, especially if child is taking phenytoin. Include instructions for care and need for regular dental checkups (first visit).

8. Refer to organizations for information and support (first visit).

CAREGIVER/CHILD AND FAMILY INTERVENTIONS

1. Child engages in appropriate activities, gets adequate rest, and exercises in moderation.

2. Takes child for regularly scheduled visits to pediatrician, neurologist, and dentist. Reminds practitioner of seizure disorder before administration of pertussis immunization.

3. Minimizes conditions that may precede/precipitate child's seizures.

   • Provides for adequate sleep and rest.
   • Immediately treats fevers.
   • Sees physician for infections.
   • Appropriately manages stressors.
   • Avoids known sensory stimulants (e.g., flashing lights).

4. Correctly administers anticonvulsant medications.

   • Thoroughly mixes suspension and advances to tablets per physician directive.
   • Adjusts time to fit child's and family's schedule.
   • Does not skip doses.
   • Does not abruptly stop/discontinue drug, even in absence of seizures.
   • Has child tested, per physician's directive, for serum levels and metabolic influences of medication.
   • Takes vitamin D supplements, per physician's directive, with phenytoin or phenobarbital drug regimen.
   • Refers sexually active females taking teratogenic anticonvulsants to family planning services.

5. Reports unusual side effects of medications, including rash; fever; sore throat; easy bruising/bleeding; visual disturbances; headache; dizziness; changes in alertness, motor activity, cognition, or behavior; and gastrointestinal disturbances to physician.
6. Performs/supervises tooth brushing, flossing, and gum massage.
7. Consumes carbohydrate-restricted and protein-restricted, high-fat diet, per physician directive, to increase seizure threshold and reduce medication toxicity. Takes vitamin-mineral supplements containing calcium, iron, and vitamins B, C, and D.
8. Has ordered serum drug levels, complete blood count (CBC), prothrombin time, BUN, urinalysis, and liver function studies performed on a regular, continuing basis.
9. Contacts Epilepsy Foundation of America or National Epilepsy League for information and assistance.

Nursing diagnosis

Anxiety
Related factors: situational crisis; apprehension about disorder, its implications; altered health concept
Defining characteristics: display of generalized uneasiness; uncertainty concerning perceived intermittent, unpredictable course of disorder; social isolation; helplessness during seizure activity; social stigma

OUTCOMES
Short-term
Decreased anxiety evidenced by more relaxed posture, statements that feelings of anxiety and helplessness are reduced and that caregiver has more control over management of disorder (expected within 2 to 4 weeks)

Long-term
Anxiety at optimal level to manage stress and facilitate learning and growth (expected within 1 to 3 months)

NURSING INTERVENTIONS/INSTRUCTIONS

1. Assess anxiety level, perceptions, and implications of disorder; coping strengths; impact of condition on family, social relationships, school, work, and finances; and level of support and assistance (each visit).
2. Discern perception of disorder and its cause, control, course, and outcome. Provide pertinent, factual information (each visit).
3. Allow expression and acceptance of feelings (each visit).
4. Ask family what will most help them cope. Assist in resolving their self-identified needs (each visit).
5. Assist family in measures to reduce anxiety and facilitate coping (each visit).
6. Refer to family counseling as indicated (any visit).

CAREGIVER/CHILD AND FAMILY INTERVENTIONS

1. Openly shares knowledge of/feelings about disorder.
2. Uses variety of activities and techniques to promote wellness and control anxiety.
3. Maintains social/work relationships. Child has positive self-image.
4. Seeks counseling as needed.

SAMPLE DOCUMENTATION INCLUSIONS

1. Specific assessment
   Assess neurologic, renal, and hepatic systems; vital signs; motor and ocular responses; weight; growth; development; developmental milestones; congenital anomalies; level of alertness; resumption of ADL; play and school activities; seizure activity; evidence of injury; seizure log; demonstration of medication administration and seizure protocol; home safety; side effects of medications; and adaptive family response.
2. Specific care/teaching
   Teach information and administration of medications, home safety, management of seizures, seizure log, diet, physician and laboratory follow-up, and referrals to social services.

3. General
   Note responses to care, teaching, changes in plan, and progression/regression of illness status.
4. See "Nurse Documentation and Family Home Record Keeping" in Appendix for general required documentation components for all home care visits.

Gastrointestinal system

 ## Alternate Feeding Management

Alternate feeding methods are used to provide optimal nutrition, to correct altered metabolic function, or to treat congenital, chronic, or debilitating diseases that affect gastrointestinal (GI) function. These methods result in imposed restriction of or inability to maintain oral nutritional intake and growth and developmental needs.

Enteral nutrition is used if the GI tract is able to absorb nutrients to maintain status. Specially prepared liquid formula enters the GI tract through a small-bore gastric tube inserted through the nose or mouth into the stomach (nasogastric or orogastric) or into the duodenum or jejunum (enteral gavage). For long-term enteral nutrition, a surgically placed retention-type catheter is inserted in the stomach through an abdominal incision (gastrostomy). Sometimes a gastrostomy button containing an antireflux valve may be used to administer the formula. Feedings are usually delivered intermittently but continuously and slowly if the formula is administered into the small intestine to prevent the dumping syndrome. Conditions that may warrant home enteral nutrition include cystic fibrosis, congenital anomalies (cleft palate, or esophageal or tracheoesophageal atresia, fistula, or stricture), prematurity, failure to thrive, and neurologic conditions that cause difficulty in swallowing or sucking. Children with severe gastroesophageal reflux may receive a fundoplication procedure to prevent reflux and aspiration.

Home total parenteral nutrition (HTPN) provides long-term or life-time nutritional support via a central venous line (Broviac/Hickman) inserted into the jugular or subclavian vein to the superior vena cava. It can also be administered via a right atrial catheter at the chest site. The nutritional composition of the formula is developed to meet the individual child's needs. It is usually provided in a cyclic manner when administered at home. Conditions that may warrant HTPN include short bowel syndrome, inflammatory bowel disease, congenital bowel defects, pancreatitis, malignancy, and refractory diarrhea or opportunistic candida infections of human immunodeficiency virus.

Home care is primarily concerned with posthospitalization nutritional maintenance, including environmental, nutritional, clinical disorder status assessments, and teaching of central line and nasogastric or gastrostomy care, administration of enteral (nasogastric, orogastric, or gastrostomy tube) and parenteral (total parenteral nutrition [TPN]) nutrition, as well as monitoring metabolic (fluid volume and electrolyte and glucose imbalances), GI (diarrhea, nausea, vomiting, cramping, and distention), infection (catheter or formula), and mechanical (infusion pump) complications associated with these therapies. As with any technology-dependent situation in child care, psychosocial issues should be addressed in the specific care plan that may be cross-referenced with these procedures.

Nursing diagnosis

Altered nutrition: less than body requirements/ineffective infant feeding pattern

Related factors: inability to ingest/absorb nutrients because of biologic factor of illness, feeding aversion

Defining characteristics: inadequate oral intake (prematurity, inability to suck/swallow); low–birth-weight status; congenital, acquired physical pathologic condition; protein, vitamin, mineral deficits; muscle wasting; edema; weakness; irritability; dullness; lethargy; dermatitis; hair loss

OUTCOMES

Short-term
Adequate daily nutritional intake by nasogastric, orogastric, gastrostomy, HTPN feedings evidenced by weight gain, improved clinical profile, thriving child (expected within 1 week)

Long-term
Nutritional status for optimal growth/development demonstrated by adequate feedings; appropriate weight maintenance/gains at recommended level for age, sex; safe administration of alternate feeding method; absence of signs, symptoms of nutritional deficits, complications associated with feeding method; progression to oral feeding if possible, as applicable (expected within 1 to 3 months)

NURSING INTERVENTIONS/INSTRUCTIONS

1. Review discharge plans and teaching before first visit.
2. Assess ability of caregiver to perform procedures and to adapt to changes in lifestyle, family relationships, and home modifications. Assess availability of resources needed to provide TPN solution, supplies, and equipment for alternate feeding methods (before or during first visit).
3. Collaborate with caregiver in reviewing discharge teaching performed and demonstration of proficiency in enteral or HTPN therapy. Have caregiver repeat demonstration (first visit).
4. Perform complete physical assessment. Assess nutritional requirement for age and weight, needed caloric intake, and weight deviation from standard for age; consult with nutritionist as needed (see "Gastrointestinal Assessment," p. 16, for guidelines) (first visit).
5. Assess and inform of rationale for therapy; type/route of alternate feeding to be administered; estimated length of time of feedings; and presence of gastrostomy button/tube, nasogastric tube, and neck or chest venous catheter site (first visit, reinforce as needed).
6. Support participation of caregiver and family in alternate feeding procedures, provide written instructions for all teaching components, and assist in developing teaching sheet to guide all aspects of care related to type of alternate feeding prescribed. Provide agency telephone number and assure of 24-hour availability (each visit).
7. Instruct to weigh child daily or every 3 to 7 days to assess for change, and note intake and output (I&O) ratio for fluid volume balance (first visit).

8. Collaborate with caregiver to plan, prepare, and administer tube feeding to child at as normal mealtime as possible (first visit).

9. Instruct on formula preparation and storage. Provide written instructions to follow or obtain home referral of nutritionist for instructions (first visit, reinstruct as needed).

10. Demonstrate and instruct on delivery of commercially prepared or home blenderized formula feedings (rate, frequency, amount, and dilution ordered) to child, how to increase/decrease rate, and dilution as tolerated via gastrostomy or nasogastric tube (first and second visits).

11. Instruct to check gastrostomy or nasogastric tube patency and placement; to vent gastrostomy tube or button; to check residual volume as applicable before feeding (flushing and closing tubing after feeding); to elevate head of bed before and after tube feedings; to change tube according to protocol; and to perform daily gastrostomy or nasogastric site and tube, mouth, and oral care for cleanliness and lubrication (first visit, as needed).

12. Instruct to observe for complications associated with tube feedings, including nausea, vomiting, diarrhea, abdominal cramping, constipation, and actions to prevent/treat these conditions (change of formula, change in rate, and administration of medications) (first visit, as needed).

13. Collaborate with family to plan, prepare, and administer HTPN (amount, rate, frequency, and specifically prepared solutions) that includes the type/site of central venous catheter or implanted port, scheduling, use of tubing, filters, and infusion pump (standard or ambulatory) (see "Medication Administration and Teaching Guidelines," pp. 450-463), procurement and handling of supplies/equipment, and disposal of used supplies (first visit, continue as needed).

14. Instruct on and demonstrate preparation, set-up, and delivery of ordered formula and lipid solutions by cyclic, continuous, and piggyback infusions. Instruct on and demonstrate protocols for changing intravenous (IV) tubing, filters, and extension sets (first visit, as needed).

15. Instruct to assess and note implications of HTPN daily, including I&O balance (fluid volume), electrolyte balance (hyponatremia, hyperkalemia, hypokalemia, and hyperphosphatemia), and glucose changes (hyperglycemia and hypoglycemia); laboratory testing weekly or monthly (blood urea nitrogen, electrolytes, creatinine, glucose, proteins, and complete blood count [CBC]); glucose testing every 8 to 12 hours; and daily assessment of signs and symptoms related to any alteration. Instruct on actions to take to prevent/treat these conditions as ordered by physician (change in solution constituents or concentrations) (each visit).

16. Instruct on abdominal tube site or button and central venous insertion site wound care, including cleansing around tube area, applying dressings, and securing dressings in place with nonirritating tape (button does not need dressing) (first and second visits, as needed).

17. Instruct to observe for discomfort caused by tubing or leaking around tubing or catheter; loss of patency of tube, button, or catheter; and procedure to irrigate or heparinize. Report to physician for dislodgement or repair if appropriate (each visit).

18. Initiate social services referral for assistance in obtaining supplies and equipment for tube feedings or HTPN procedures (appropriate visit).

CAREGIVER/CHILD AND FAMILY INTERVENTIONS

1. Adjusts lifestyle to include activities related to need for enteral/parenteral nutritional procedures.

2. Safely prepares, administers, and provides total care in all procedures necessary to meet caloric and nutritional requirements via gastrostomy or nasogastric tube or HTPN methods.

3. Provides pacifier to infant for nonnutritive sucking if fed via gastrostomy or nasogastric tube.

4. Holds and cuddles infant or small child during or after tube feedings.

5. Maintains patency of gastric tube by instillation of 10 to 30 ml of water after feeding or medication administration; changes tube (orogastric/nasogastric) every 4 to 8 weeks according to established protocol; irrigates or heparinizes depending on catheter; and makes changes

in set-up, tubing, and bags of solution according to protocol.

6. Obtains weight using same scale, with child wearing same clothing, at same time on specified days and measures daily I&O.

7. Uses infusion pump with rate or volume changes/ corrections, programs small portable infusion pump, and checks alarm systems on pump.

8. Maintains flow sheet to document important aspects and untoward effects of alternate feeding method.

9. Reports glucose abnormalities, signs and symptoms of fluid or electrolyte imbalance, and other complications to physician.

10. Complies with laboratory testing and physician appointments for monitoring and follow-up examinations.

11. Obtains financial, informational, and support resources if needed.

Nursing diagnosis

Risk for infection

Related factors: inadequate primary defenses (broken skin), invasive procedures (gastrostomy, central venous line insertion), aspiration of enteral formula, insufficient knowledge of caregiver to avoid exposure of child to pathogens

Defining characteristics: contaminated/unrefrigerated formula causing diarrhea, vomiting, cramping; contamination during procedures at venous, gastrostomy insertion site, redness with edema, pain, tenderness, drainage; change in color of sputum (aspiration pneumonia); temperature instability; chills; headache; lethargy; hyperirritability with sepsis

OUTCOMES

Short-term

Minimal risk for signs, symptoms of local/systemic infection, respiratory infection, GI tract complications evidenced by optimal respiratory parameters; airway patency maintained; afebrile status; absence of abdominal discomfort, changes in appearance at catheter insertion site; or absence of headache, fever, chills, malaise indicating septicemia (expected at initiation of therapy, with daily assessment)

Long-term
Adaptation to lifestyle that promotes clean, safe environment; performs measures to minimize risk for infection evidenced by optimal nutritional status via alternate feeding method without complication; early detection, reporting, treatment of infectious process (expected ongoing)

NURSING INTERVENTIONS/INSTRUCTIONS

1. Assess home and living conditions for safety and long-term therapy (see "Environmental Assessment," p. 37, for guidelines) (first visit, follow-up for additional modifications on second visit).
2. Maintain universal precautions (each visit).
3. Assess for and instruct to assess for changes in respiratory rate, depth, and ease and change in color/odor of pulmonary secretions (each visit).
4. Assess temperature for increase and instruct on taking axillary (oral for child) temperature (first visit, reinforce as needed).
5. Assess and instruct to assess catheter insertion site for redness, edema, tenderness, or drainage. Assess for fever, headache, weight loss, and malaise and report these to health care provider or physician immediately (each visit).
6. Instruct on administration of prescribed oral liquid antibiotic and antipyretic in proper form or adding IV medication to IV system (see "Medication Administration and Teaching Guidelines," pp. 450-463) (first visit, reinforce as needed).
7. Instruct on sterile or clean technique as appropriate for care procedures at skin site, handling catheter tips, catheter manipulation, and all components of IV system (containers, tubing, connections) (each visit until proficient).
8. Instruct on proper handling/storage of formula or infusion solution and cleansing of supplies/equipment used for procedures (first and second visits).

9. Instruct on precautions to prevent infection such as washing hands and avoiding contact with those with infections and on importance of rest (ongoing).
10. Obtain sputum, if possible, insertion site drainage specimens for culture, blood specimens for CBC and glucose level if ordered (any visit).

CAREGIVER/CHILD AND FAMILY INTERVENTIONS

1. States and performs measures to reduce possibility of infection (sterile or clean technique, handwashing, and avoidance of contact with infections in others).
2. Assesses catheter insertion site daily for signs of infection or leakage. Notifies physician of complications.
3. Assesses GI system for signs and symptoms of infection.
4. Changes tubing, filter (usually every 24 hours), and feeding containers according to protocol.
5. Covers and secures catheter. Minimizes young child's access to catheter.
6. Stores properly labeled enteral feedings in refrigerator. Administers feedings and solutions at room temperature.
7. Takes oral or axillary temperature if sputum changes color, respirations change, or signs and symptoms of local/systemic infection appear. Reports changes to physician.
8. Administers antibiotic therapy correctly until all medication is taken or infused.
9. Properly disposes of or cleanses all articles/supplies used in performing procedures according to universal precautions.
10. Complies with laboratory testing for glucose, CBC, and other ordered tests.

Nursing diagnosis

Risk for impaired skin integrity
Related factors: external factors of pressure, irritation at tube (gastrostomy, nares), IV sites; contamination of feedings, solutions, insertion sites
Defining characteristics: tissue damage, disruption of skin at insertion sites, redness, irritation of nasal mucous membranes

OUTCOMES

Short-term
Skin, mucous membranes protected from irritation, minimal tube movement or pressure to susceptible tissue sites evidenced by clean, dry, intact areas free of redness or other color changes, predisposition to breakdown (expected within 1 to 2 days)

Long-term
Intact skin; mucous membranes free from infection, discomfort, breakdown at gastrostomy, nasal site, catheter site; perianal site maintained (expected within 1 week)

NURSING INTERVENTIONS/INSTRUCTIONS

1. Assess and instruct to assess gastrostomy tube site for redness, drainage, edema, rash, irritation, tension/ movement of tube, use of tape/dressing to ensure secure placement of tube; nares mucosa for dryness, cleanliness, redness, crusting, lesions, breaks, or tension/friction caused by nasogastric tube (each visit).
2. Assess and instruct to assess catheter insertion site for redness, irritation from manipulation, or pressure of catheter (each visit).
3. Instruct to apply petrolatum around gastrostomy tube site, use diaper to cover site, apply bandage to prevent tube manipulation, use water-soluble lubricant to nares, and correct taping to secure tube without placing pressure on nares or skin (first and second visits).
4. Suggest using only small amount of tape to secure tube, place tape on gauze square, and then tape to skin (first visit, as needed).
5. Apply and instruct on ointment or cream (antimicrobial or corticosteroid) to tube site if ordered for rashes or breaks in skin at gastrostomy site or venous catheter insertion site (first and second visits).
6. Instruct caregiver to report any irritation or soreness at tube/catheter areas to physician immediately (first visit).

CAREGIVER/CHILD AND FAMILY INTERVENTIONS

1. Assesses perigastrostomy skin site and nares mucosa daily. Gently washes and pats dry, avoiding excess

movement/tension of tubes on tissues. Lubricates sites with appropriate preparations.

2. Assesses venous catheter site for tension, irritation, and breakdown. Avoids manipulation of catheter when changing dressing.

3. Assesses perianal site if diarrhea is present for skin irritation. Gently cleanses and dries following each elimination. Applies protective ointment.

4. Prevents pulling on tube or catheter by child and tangling with movement or activity of child.

5. Applies ointments at gastrostomy/nares site, and gauze, dressing around tube if needed. Tapes sparingly or secures in place with diaper, as appropriate.

6. Exposes irritated sites to air during day if possible.

7. Reports any reddened areas, drainage, swelling, or breaks in skin at tube or venous catheter sites to physician.

SAMPLE DOCUMENTATION INCLUSIONS

1. Specific assessment
   Assess caregiver's and family's ability to perform therapy, teaching; discharge plan; nutritional status; short-term or long-term administration and care; complexity of regimen; ability for independence in care; insertion site status; skin; infection; metabolic, mechanical, and GI complications; need for home modifications; child and family coping skills; anxiety level related to home management; and need for assistance.

2. Specific care/teaching
   Teach delivery method and administration of feeding regimen to include type, route, amount, frequency, times of day, and composition of nutritional formula/solutions; addition of medications; use of infusion pump; special considerations of basic needs and comfort measures; imposed restrictions; procedures to be performed; monitoring of essential components of care; use and care of supplies, equipment used for therapy/care procedures; and recognition of signs and symptoms of complications that necessitate additional visits or reporting to physician.

3. General
   Note responses to feeding and teaching; goal achievement; changes/modifications of plan, supplies, or procedures; abilities of caregiver and family to manage child's complete care; resources for acquiring medication; and all supplies/equipment needed for therapy.
4. See "Nurse Documentation and Family Home Record Keeping" in Appendix for general required documentation components for all home care visits.

 Bowel Diversion

Bowel diversion refers to surgical procedures (colostomy or ileostomy) that bypass the diseased gut and correct or alleviate disorders or defects of the lower GI tract. The resulting abdominal stoma, the outlet for bowel evacuations, is formed from intact intestine brought to and sutured to the skin's surface. An intraabdominal reservoir pouch, a continent ileostomy, is a surgical option for selected candidates. Bowel diversion may be permanent or temporary. Permanent ostomies are frequently associated with inflammatory bowel disease in the older child who no longer responds to medical treatment. Temporary, palliative ostomies, seen more frequently in children, may be performed before more definitive corrective surgery to allow the gut to rest. Some authorities believe corrective surgery should be postponed until optimal nutritional status has been established or a predetermined weight and age have been reached. Conditions that may require bowel diversion include necrotizing enterocolitis, imperforate anus, congenital aganglionic megacolon (Hirschsprung's disease), inflammatory bowel disease, and multiple trauma.

Home health care is primarily concerned with instruction on ostomy care; recognition and resolution of complications; and promotion of the child's growth, development, and self-image.

Nursing diagnosis

Risk for impaired skin integrity
Related factors: artificial anus on abdominal skin surface, poor nutritional state
Defining characteristics: stoma on delicate skin, frequent fecal skin contamination, irritating nature of fecal excreta, inexperienced caregiver

OUTCOMES
Short-term
Decreased/absent risk of skin disruption evidenced by caregiver/client demonstration of ostomy care; intact, supple skin around stoma (expected within 1 week)

Long-term
Optimal skin integrity evidenced by fully functioning ostomy with healthy stoma; intact, supple surrounding tissue; no signs of impaired skin integrity (expected within 1 month)

NURSING INTERVENTIONS/INSTRUCTIONS

1. Review postoperative discharge instructions with caregiver. Have caregiver demonstrate ostomy care. Note ability, reaction to procedure, and parent-child interaction. Based on observed need, instruct caregiver on ostomy care. Enlist child's assistance (age-dependent) and progress to self-care as appropriate (each visit).
2. Confer with enterostomal therapist to devise and adapt treatment plan; include caregiver (first visit, follow up as needed).
3. Maintain universal precautions (each visit).
4. Perform complete physical assessment, including GI and integumentary assessments (see "Assessments," pp. 16 and 22). Note placement and condition of dressings; characteristics of stool; condition of stoma; skin integrity surrounding site; and evidence of redness, skin breaks, rashes, excoriation, irritation, bleeding, and purulent discharge. Report significant findings to physician. Concurrently instruct caregiver on how to assess same and what to report to physician (each visit).

5. Instruct caregiver on measurements of 24-hour stool and to report diarrhea, unrelieved constipation, or any change in established stooling pattern to physician (first and second visits).

6. Instruct caregiver on infant ostomy care (not using appliance) as appropriate (first visit, reinforce as needed).

   • Wash hands before and after changing dressing. Use nonsterile gloves per recommendation.
   • Change dressing after each stooling.
   • Remove soiled dressing. If dressing adheres to stoma, moisten before attempting further removal.
   • Remove stool and wash area thoroughly with mild soap and soft washcloth. Rinse and dry completely.
   • Apply prescribed nonporous skin protection.
   • Cover with recommended dressing. Secure with stretchable wrap, Montgomery straps, or diaper.

7. Instruct caregiver and child on ostomy care with appliance as appropriate (first visit, reinforce as needed).

   • Wash hands before and after changing appliance. Use nonsterile gloves per recommendation.
   • Change appliance on regular schedule or if torn, leaking, or nonadhering.
   • Gently remove appliance. Empty, if necessary, and discard.
   • Remove stool and remaining skin protection from skin.
   • Cleanse skin with mild soap and water.
   • Thoroughly dry; hair dryer on cool/low setting may be used.
   • Paint skin around stoma with recommended skin sealant. Let dry completely.
   • Apply karaya powder, stoma adhesive, or approved product to further protect skin and facilitate appliance adherence.
   • Apply correctly sized appliance. Clamp distal portion.
   • Between changes, empty pouch/appliance by unclamping distal portion and letting stool drain into toilet. Rinse, dry, and reclamp.

8. If child has central venous access line or gastrostomy, instruct or demonstrate to caregiver to prevent cross con-

tamination by following aseptic techniques, sequencing dressing changes appropriately, and meticulously performing ostomy care to keep stool away from central line and gastrostomy incision site. Have caregiver repeat demonstration (each visit until proficient).
9. Instruct caregiver on dietary measures that relieve constipation and promote growth, healing, and function (first visit, as needed).

CAREGIVER/CHILD AND FAMILY INTERVENTIONS

1. Assists health care team in developing treatment plan.
2. Provides aseptic wound care to central line or gastrostomy site before starting ostomy care.
3. Changes dressing after each infant stooling, maintains clean technique, and preserves skin integrity.
4. Child assists in ostomy care, working at own level. Assists with supplies, paints skin, and progresses to full self-care.
5. Notifies enterostomal specialist of skin breakdown or other related problems. Notifies physician of alterations in established bowel pattern.
6. Provides age-appropriate well-balanced, frequent, high-calorie, high-protein, nourishing meals. Uses recommended vitamin and mineral supplements.
7. Promotes intake by offering preferred foods, feeding smaller amounts more frequently, and making eating experiences pleasant.
8. Feeds via gastrostomy or administers TPN as prescribed to chronically debilitated child who fails to thrive (see "Alternate Feeding Management," pp. 205-215, for guidelines).

Nursing diagnosis

Self-esteem disturbance
Related factors: negative feelings about physical/psychosocial capabilities
Defining characteristics: embarrassment; verbalized shame, guilt, negative feelings about self; differences in lifestyle from that of peers; hesitant to try anything new, deal with events; difficulty making decisions; denial; projection, rationalization of problems/failures

OUTCOMES

Short-term
Begins to develop positive feelings/perceptions of differences in lifestyle caused by chronic illness evidenced by reduction in self-negating statements, identification of problems that decrease feelings of self-worth, verbalization of need for treatments that differentiate them from others (expected within 4 to 6 weeks)

Long-term
Maintains positive self-esteem; accepts awareness of limitations imposed by condition evidenced by adjustment to condition, its associated risks; engages in peer group activities that increase feeling of belonging, acceptance, development of positive relationships with family/friends; participates in plans; achieves goals that enhance physical health, lifestyle changes (expected within 3 months)

NURSING INTERVENTIONS/INSTRUCTIONS

1. Assess child's age, cognitive status, other developmental parameters, understanding of condition, situational factors, extent of disturbance, negative or other feelings of perceived differences caused by condition, influences of family on child's perceptions, ability to become involved in and take control of own daily care, and specific social activities (first visit, as needed).
2. Display positive attitude of acceptance and communication with child; avoid judgmental, intrusive attitude (each visit).
3. Encourage and listen to verbalizations of feelings about condition, other therapies, and limitations in activities (each visit).
4. Encourage and listen to verbalizations of feeling different, how peers perceive differences and feel about the condition, and experiences that encourage feelings of well-being and success with peers and family (each visit).
5. Acknowledge expressed feelings. Facilitate sharing of feelings by child with family and health team (any visit).
6. Assist and allow child to identify positive feelings, strengths noted in dealing with experiences, and coping

behaviors learned that decrease negative feelings (each visit).

7. Encourage independent, constructive thinking and activities allowed by condition. Allow child to make choices and participate in care when desirable (each visit).

8. Promote praise for any goal achievement and interest and participation in care plan (any visit).

9. Incorporate play into building confidence, reinforcing positive behaviors, and improving self-esteem (each visit).

10. Suggest community resources for support and introduction to peers with same disorder.

CAREGIVER/CHILD AND FAMILY INTERVENTIONS

1. Expresses feelings about therapy, being different, and difficulties/limitations imposed by condition.

2. Displays positive behaviors. Facilitates improved self-esteem.

3. Develops coping skills to adjust to home and school routines and satisfactory family and peer relationships.

4. Allows time for necessary changes in lifestyle with promotion of flexibility and insight by family. Avoids negative remarks or behaviors.

5. Verbalizes feelings of independence and control. Becomes involved in self-care when appropriate.

6. Uses opportunities for contact with peers who have adjusted to similar problems.

7. Family investigates community resources for information, support, acceptance, guidance, and supervised activities (camps, schools, and playgrounds).

Nursing diagnosis

Altered family processes
Related factors: resistance to treatment/procedure, inadequate coping skills, situational crisis
Defining characteristics: family system unable to meet physical needs of members; verbalization of distaste, reluctance to perform physical care; inability to adapt to

change, deal with trauma effectively; perceived offensive-
ness of condition

OUTCOMES

Short-term
Progressive adaptation, acceptance of child evidenced by
verbalization, overt signs of positive coping, family interactions (expected within 2 to 4 weeks)

Long-term
Optimal adaptation, acceptance evidenced by family health
(expected within 4 to 6 weeks)

NURSING INTERVENTIONS/INSTRUCTIONS

1. Assess family dynamics, roles, and responsibilities; adaptive and coping behaviors; limitations; knowledge deficit;
   internal strengths; and external resources (first visit).
2. Serve as positive role model in dealing with and caring
   for ill child (each visit).
3. Instruct family on underlying disorder and its expected
   progression and prognosis. If ostomy is temporary, focus
   on its healing role and limited nature (first visit, as
   needed).
4. Instruct and reinforce that parental reactions and behaviors directly affect child's perception of self and condition (each visit).
5. Inform and encourage activities that promote family
   health (e.g., wellness modalities and recreational/social
   outlets) (first visit).
6. Instruct family on need to treat child normally, to make
   child integral part of, not exclusive focus of, family activity (first visit).
7. Include child in treatment plan. Assist with skill development and self-care activities (each visit).
8. Instruct caregiver to inform school nurse, teacher, day-
   care workers, or those with need to know about child's
   condition. Provide extra ostomy supplies and change
   of clothing (first visit).
9. Refer to organizations for information and assistance
   (e.g., United Ostomy Association). Confer with enterostomal therapist and provide opportunities to meet

children of similar age and condition (first visit, as needed).

CAREGIVER/CHILD AND FAMILY INTERVENTIONS

1. Verbalizes misgivings, questions, and concerns.
2. Initiates/maintains activities in which whole family can participate.
3. Adapts to and accepts child's condition and family's evolving roles.
4. Provides effective care.
5. Participates in support group activities.

SAMPLE DOCUMENTATION INCLUSIONS

1. Specific assessment
   Assess chronologic age; weight; temperature; developmental milestones; location and condition of stoma; evidence of stricture, prolapse, bleeding, retraction, or infection; intake and retention; characteristics of stool; stooling pattern; and ability and compliance with ostomy care.
2. Specific care/teaching
   Teach ostomy care, diet, nutrition, intake, output, and referrals.
3. General
   Note responses to care and teaching.
4. See "Nurse Documentation and Family Home Record Keeping" in Appendix for required documentation components for all home care visits.

 Cleft Lip and Palate Repair

Cleft lip and palate are the most common facial malformations caused by defective development of the oral cavity in utero. They may occur singularly or in combination. Cleft lip, the most cosmetically distressing, results from an incomplete fusion of the medial nasal and maxillary processes. It is evident at birth and may vary in presentation from a small unilateral or bilateral notch at the lip's upper border to a wide fissure extending to the nostril. Cleft palate results from incomplete fusion of the palatine plates. It may involve the uvula and the soft and hard palates. Both defects may be associated with other malformations and syndromes. Problems include feeding difficulties, impaired speech acquisition, dental anomalies, recurrent infection, otitis media, and hearing loss. Surgical correction of the cleft lip is generally performed at 2 months of age with possible revisions performed later. Cleft palates are frequently repaired by 2 years of age, although the size and extent of the deformity may require a more individualized surgical response. Residual speech, hearing, dental, and cosmetic impairments may persist postoperatively and require long-term rehabilitation with a multidisciplinary health care team.

Home health care is primarily concerned with instruction on feeding; wound care; prevention of injury and infection; and management of psychologic, speech, hearing, and dental problems through instruction and referrals.

Nursing diagnosis

Risk for injury
Related factors: surgical repair, spontaneous movement
Defining characteristics: incisional site on lip or oral cavity; drainage, formula/food remnants at surgical site; wound pressure from crying; trauma from hands, toys, feeding utensils; inexperienced caregiver

OUTCOMES

Short-term
Minimal/absent injury evidenced by caregiver compliance with postoperative regimen; intact, healing surgical site (expected in 1 week)

Long-term
Absence of injury evidenced by intact, healed surgical site; optimal growth, development, function (expected in 6 to 8 weeks)

NURSING INTERVENTIONS/INSTRUCTIONS

1. Review discharge plan, caregiver's knowledge, facility with feeding, and positioning techniques (first visit).

2. Perform complete physical assessment. Assess operative site for integrity, redness, swelling, presence of drainage, formula/food, and presence and condition of lip protective device (each visit).

3. Assess child's level of alertness, fussiness, irritability, responsiveness, and distractibility. Note caregiver-child interaction (each visit).

4. Demonstrate and have caregiver repeat demonstration of wound care. Gently clean lip repair with gauze or cotton swab moistened with normal saline or as recommended. Apply lubricant, antibiotic, or steroid cream as prescribed (first visit, repeat as needed).

5. Instruct/reinforce instruction to caregiver on measures to promote healing and prevent injury (first visit, follow up as needed).

   - Monitor integrity of lip protection device (Logan's bow).
   - Anticipate needs to minimize crying. Do not let child cry vigorously or for protracted periods. Provide comfort, consolation, and distraction.
   - Restrain infant with elbow cuffs and older child with cuffs and jacket restraint. Alternate releasing restrained arms. Stay with child while arms are unrestrained. Note color and condition of skin, joints, and prominences. Perform range-of-motion (ROM) exercises, massage, and caress.
   - Remove hard, angular, or pointed toys. Avoid toys that require sucking or blowing.

6. Weigh child weekly. Compare with standardized measures and preoperative weight. Observe caregiver feeding child; based on observed need, instruct on feeding techniques (each visit).

   - Provide quiet, comfortable environment with no distractions.
   - Feed slowly. Allow extra time for feedings.

- Provide water before and after feedings.
- Feed infant with lip repair with medicine dropper or plastic-coated spoon. Burp after every ½ to 1 oz.
- Feed older child with wide, coated spoon (do not insert into mouth) or cup. Do not use fork or straws.
- Advance diet as directed. Give formula (infant) and semisoft food (older child) as tolerated by 3 weeks after the procedure.
- Avoid hard foods (e.g., toast, tostadas, and cookies).
- After feeding, position infant with lip repair on side, preferably right. Position child with palate repair on abdomen.

7. Inform caregiver that feeding and activity restrictions described in #6 are relaxed based on status of wound healing (generally 4 to 6 weeks for palate repair, less for lip repair) (each visit).

CAREGIVER/CHILD AND FAMILY INTERVENTIONS

1. Maintains injury-free incisional site.
2. Uses appropriate restraining devices properly to prevent injury.
3. Provides physical contact. Holds, caresses, rocks, and talks to child.
4. Administers age-appropriate diet in safe manner.
5. Provides wound care to lip repair. Rinses mouth with water before and after feedings.

Nursing diagnosis

Knowledge deficit
Related factors: lack of information about postoperative course, readiness to learn; fatigue of preoperative wait and child care; lack of support, assistance
Defining characteristics: requests for information about/inability to answer questions concerning general care, implications, complications of long-term care; inability to recognize, accept need for information; lack of respite care/support

OUTCOMES

Short-term
Adequate information evidenced by verbalization of long-term problems of speech, hearing, infection, sources of assistance, therapy (expected in 1 week)

Long-term
Adequate information evidenced by compliance with health care regimen, participation in needed therapies (expected in 4 to 6 weeks)

NURSING INTERVENTIONS/INSTRUCTIONS

1. Confer with multidisciplinary health care team to establish long-term treatment plan (before first visit). Make appropriate referrals during course of treatment.
2. Assess caregiver's readiness to learn, emotional climate of home, family relationships, levels of adjustment, coping strengths, and sources of support/assistance. Pace teaching on caregiver's receptivity and need to know (first visit).
3. Instruct caregiver on child's susceptibility to middle ear and sinus infections and to report fever, unexplained irritability, tugging at ears, upper respiratory infections, and green or yellow sputum to physician (first visit).
4. Assess hearing. Instruct caregiver to monitor for deficits (lack of response to auditory stimuli [startle reflex], indifference to sound, preference for gesturing requests rather than verbalization, and impaired speech). Refer for hearing evaluations as needed (each visit).
5. Assess child's age-appropriate speech acquisition. Note hypernasality and difficulty with explosive sounds (e.g., *P, B, D, T, H, Y*) or sibilants (e.g., *S, SH, CH*). Refer to speech therapist as needed (each visit).
6. In keeping with physician's and speech therapist's treatment plan, encourage caregiver to promote child's speech development (each visit).

   - Encourage face-to-face position and age-appropriate verbal interaction.
   - Use word play (e.g., repetitive rhymes and sing-alongs).
   - Incorporate chewing, swallowing, and blowing exercises into games (e.g., Simon says).

- Praise accomplishments. Do not nag, ridicule, belittle, or ignore.

7. Instruct caregiver on child's increased susceptibility to dental caries and need for meticulous mouth care. Instruct on care of speech appliances and dental prostheses and need for regular dental and orthodontic care (second and third visits, ongoing).
8. Refer to agency providing respite care (as needed).

CAREGIVER/CHILD AND FAMILY INTERVENTIONS

1. Verbalizes potential problems and sources of assistance.
2. Focuses on child's abilities and interests.
3. Uses games to encourage speech development.
4. Monitors for infection and deficits. Reports to physician.
5. Provides and teaches care of mouth and teeth.
6. Consults with hearing and speech therapists, primary care physician, pediatric dentist, orthodontist, prosthodontist, otolaryngologist, and plastic surgeon as needed.
7. Uses respite care.

Nursing diagnosis

Altered family processes
Related factors: situational crisis, immaturity, inadequate coping skills
Defining characteristics: verbalization of reluctance to feed child, provide wound care; rigidity in function, roles; family system unable to meet emotional needs of members

OUTCOMES

Short-term
Progressive adaptation to/acceptance of child evidenced by overt signs of positive coping, family interactions (expected in 1 to 2 weeks)

Long-term
Optimal adaptation/acceptance evidenced by family health (expected in 2 to 4 weeks)

NURSING INTERVENTIONS/INSTRUCTIONS

1. Assess family dynamics, roles, and responsibilities; adaptive and coping behaviors; internal strengths; and external resources (first visit).
2. Be positive role model in dealing with and caring for child (each visit).
3. Instruct and reinforce that parental reactions and behaviors directly affect child's perception of self (each visit).
4. Inform and encourage activities that promote family health (e.g., wellness modalities and recreational/social outlets) (first visit).
5. Instruct family on need to treat child normally, to make child an integral part of, not exclusive focus of, family activity (first visit).
6. Refer to specialty organizations for information and assistance (e.g., American Cleft Palate Association, Cleft Palate Foundation, March of Dimes). Provide opportunities to meet children of similar age and condition (first visit, as appropriate).

CAREGIVER/CHILD AND FAMILY INTERVENTIONS

1. Verbalizes misgivings, questions, and concerns.
2. Initiates or maintains activities in which whole family can participate.
3. Adapts to and accepts child's condition and family's evolving roles. Child's positive self-esteem evolves.
4. Provides effective care.
5. Participates in support group activities.

SAMPLE DOCUMENTATION INCLUSIONS

1. Specific assessment
   Assess chronologic age, weight, developmental milestones, condition of lip repair and protective dressing, use of restraining devices, feeding and positioning techniques, level of alertness, degree of fretfulness, hearing, and speech development.
2. Specific care/teaching
   Teach wound care, feeding and positioning techniques, injury protection, speech exercises, hearing assessment, and referrals.

3. General
   Note responses to care and teaching.
4. See "Nurse Documentation and Family Home Record Keeping" in Appendix for required documentation components for all home care visits.

 ## *Inflammatory Bowel Disease*

Inflammatory bowel disease (IBD) includes the clinical entities ulcerative colitis (UC) and Crohn's disease (regional enteritis and granulomatous enterocolitis). UC primarily affects the rectum and the colon although the entire colon may be affected. It is characterized by diffuse and extensive inflammatory lesions of the intestinal mucosa. Severe, recurrent bloody diarrhea results. Crohn's disease primarily affects the distal ileum and the colon although the transmural, segmented, asymmetric lesions may involve any area from the mouth to the anus. Diarrhea and, frequently, abdominal pain result. Enteric fistulas and perianal disease are common.

UC and Crohn's disease are marked by periods of unpredictable exacerbations and remissions. Onset generally occurs in late childhood or early adolescence. Systemic, nonintestinal problems are common to both. These may include fever, general malaise and fatigue, weight loss, persistent growth problems, or failure to thrive; arthritis of the larger joints, skin lesions, and eye irritation may also occur. Prognosis depends on age and rapidity of onset, extent and severity of lesions, and response to therapy.

Home health care is primarily concerned with instruction in control and management of distressing GI symptoms; recognition and resolution of complications; maintenance of optimal fluid, electrolyte, and nutritional status to support growth and development; and counseling and support to assist in coping and self-concept development.

Nursing diagnosis

Diarrhea
Related factors: GI inflammation, irritation, genetically determined immune response
Defining characteristics: multiple loose/liquid stools, bloody or mucoid stools, fecal urgency, abdominal cramping, explosive stools, tenesmus

OUTCOMES
Short-term
Maintenance of baseline bowel remission pattern evidenced by decrease in frequent, unformed stool (expected in 1 to 2 weeks)

Long-term
Decrease/absence of diarrhea evidenced by soft, formed stools eliminated in individual, baseline remission pattern (expected in 2 to 4 weeks)

NURSING INTERVENTIONS/INSTRUCTIONS
1. Perform complete physical assessment (first visit, as needed).
2. Assess bowel activity and elimination (see "Gastrointestinal System Assessment," p. 16, for guidelines). If possible, note stool characteristics (each visit).
3. Instruct client or caregiver to maintain log of bowel elimination including color, consistency, frequency, odor, amount, presence of mucus or blood, and aggravating factors. Review. Report significant changes to physician (each visit).
4. Instruct to notify physician of following (first visit):

   - Increase in frequency/severity of stooling
   - Increase of or beginning of blood in stools or rectal bleeding
   - Marked changes in consistency of stools or constipation
   - Anorexia or vomiting
   - Tense, hard, swollen abdomen; tenderness, pain
   - Fever

5. Instruct on and monitor compliance with administration of prescribed antidiarrheals antispasmodics, antiinflammatory and antisecretory agents, bulk formers, and antibiotics. Demonstrate instillation of corticosteroid retention enemas (first visit, as needed).

CAREGIVER/CHILD AND FAMILY INTERVENTIONS

1. Maintains log of bowel elimination.
2. Administers medications as prescribed.
3. Notifies physician of significant changes.

Nursing diagnosis

Altered nutrition: less than body requirements
Related factors: malabsorption, increased caloric needs, decreased intake
Defining characteristics: anorexia; malaise; abdominal pain exacerbated by eating, poor dietary intake, weight loss, failure to thrive or failure to mature

OUTCOMES

Short-term
Adequate nutrition, evidenced by compliance with dietary management, increased intake, weight maintenance (expected in 1 week)

Long-term
Optimal nutrition evidenced by adequacy of food intake, weight gains to support growth/development (expected in 1 month)

NURSING INTERVENTIONS/INSTRUCTIONS

1. Assess nutritional status (see "Nutritional Assessment," p. 17, for guidelines). Include serial weights, compare with standardized growth/development charts; and vital signs; explore food preferences, cultural, religious prescriptions/restrictions, and alleviating/aggravating foods (each visit).
2. Assess hydration status, including approximate intake, output, skin turgor, and condition of mucous mem-

branes. Instruct on need to maintain adequate fluid intake (each visit).

3. Instruct on/reinforce need for prescribed diet (high-calorie, high-protein, low-fat, low-residue, and occasionally lactose-restricted for milk intolerance) (first visit, reinforce as needed).

4. Instruct on administration of recommended vitamin/mineral supplements, especially iron for anemia and folic acid for deficiency associated with sulfasalazine therapy (first visit).

5. Instruct on measures to facilitate eating (first visit, reinforce as needed).

    *   Eliminate noxious odors.
    *   Provide relaxed atmosphere; do not emphasize or force food issues.
    *   Administer antispasmodic and analgesic drugs ½ to 1 hour before meals as prescribed and sulfasalazine after meals to decrease GI upset.
    *   Provide/assist with mouth care before meals.
    *   Include client in meal planning.
    *   Provide smaller, more frequent meals. Include preferred foods and beverages.
    *   Encourage nutritious snacks.
    *   Do not punish child for not eating.

6. Demonstrate and instruct on administration of prescribed gastrostomy or TPN feedings (see "Alternate Feeding Management," pp. 205-215, for guidelines) (each visit).

7. Instruct on need for regular laboratory follow up to monitor electrolytes, glucose, CBC, and other prescribed tests (first visit, as needed).

8. Refer to nutritionist as indicated.

CAREGIVER/CHILD AND FAMILY INTERVENTIONS

1. Assists in menu selection and meal preparation. Seeks assistance of nutritionist as needed.

2. Eats variety of nutritious foods and snacks. Avoids known irritants; highly seasoned, fatty, or fried foods; raw fruits and vegetables; and milk and milk products as indicated.

3. Supplements diet with vitamins, minerals, and high-protein and high-calorie snacks.
4. Gains weight. Maintains ideal weight according to standardized measures.
5. Maintains hydrated state.
6. Assists with/administers prescribed gastrostomy feedings or nocturnal TPN.
7. Keeps scheduled laboratory visits.

Nursing diagnosis

Knowledge deficit
Related factors: lack of information, inadequate teaching, lack of readiness to learn
Defining characteristics: verbalization of need for information about condition and its cause, care, implications

OUTCOMES
Short-term
Adequate knowledge evidenced by verbalization of condition's long-term course, management of symptoms, daily care (expected in 1 to 3 weeks)

Long-term
Adequate knowledge evidenced by compliance with health care regimen, optimal GI functioning (expected in 1 month)

NURSING INTERVENTIONS/INSTRUCTIONS
1. Assess client's and family's knowledge of condition, levels of adjustment, readiness to learn, and support systems. Base instruction accordingly and repeat as needed (each visit).
2. Instruct family on basic knowledge of disease, anatomy, physiology; need for ongoing care; unpredictability of exacerbations; and strategies to minimize/prevent episodes and complications (first visit).
3. Instruct family on general health care management, including getting adequate sleep and exercise; nutritious, well-balanced diet; and adequate hydration and participating in educational/social activities (first visit).

4. Instruct on management of abdominal pain and cramping as indicated (first and second visits).

   - Provide periods of uninterrupted rest, especially during exacerbation. Assume position of comfort.
   - Judiciously use heating pad on low setting.
   - Administer analgesic and antiinflammatory medications as prescribed.
   - Provide lighter meals. Scrupulously avoid known irritants. Maintain hydration.
   - Promote quiet activity.
   - Inform physician of pain pattern, increasing severe pain, distention, and fever.

5. Instruct on skin care as indicated (first and second visits).

   - For perianal lesions, provide sitz baths twice daily, after each elimination, and as desired.
   - Keep perineal and rectal areas clean and dry. Apply skin protectant or topical anesthetic to perianal area.

6. Instruct on surgical interventions, if imminent. Use visual aids (e.g., dolls to explain ostomy procedure, its implications, and care) (as needed).

7. Instruct on need for continuing regular medical checkups to monitor growth/development, for laboratory testing (CBC with differential, sedimentation rate, electrolyte panel, and serum protein), and for diagnostic screenings (stool hematest, culture, scopic examinations, and biopsies) to evaluate status (first visit).

CAREGIVER/CHILD AND FAMILY INTERVENTIONS

1. Maintains full, satisfying lifestyle.
2. Incorporates health measures for rest, exercise, diet, and stress control into lifestyle.
3. Manages symptoms.
4. Reports significant changes to physician.

Nursing diagnosis

Ineffective individual coping
Related factors: situational crisis, maturational crisis, vulnerability

Defining characteristics: verbalization of inability to cope, inability to ask for help, alteration in societal participation, change in usual communication pattern

OUTCOMES

Short-term
Adequate coping, evidenced by verbalization or demonstration of need for assistance in adapting to chronic condition (expected in 2 to 4 weeks)

Long-term
Effective coping evidenced by compliance with health care regimen, acceptance, adaptation to condition (expected in 1 to 3 months)

NURSING INTERVENTIONS/INSTRUCTIONS

1. Establish rapport and create ambience that facilitates trust and dialogue (each visit).
2. Compare chronologic age with developmental level. Note coping behaviors and readiness/willingness to participate in health care (each visit).
3. Be role model. Include child and family in treatment plan. Elicit and incorporate suggestions. Provide positive feedback (each visit).
4. Discuss developmental/educational issues and possible resolutions (each visit, as indicated).

   • Delayed growth/development — most readily corrected by diet. Discuss importance of rest, adequate exercise, and medication regimen.
   • Frequent school absences — consult with faculty and school nurse. Explain alternate educational plans.
   • Peer support — encourage school/recreational outlets. Refer to local support groups.
   • Possible surgery (colostomy) — encourage expression of fears.
   • Provide information and expand support group.

CAREGIVER/CHILD AND FAMILY INTERVENTIONS

1. Asks questions. Openly discusses feelings and fears.
2. Participates in self-care planning and treatment.

3. Identifies lifestyle issues. Explores options for resolution or remediation.
4. Develops positive self-concept and self-esteem.
5. Participates in support groups with others of comparable age and condition.

SAMPLE DOCUMENTATION INCLUSIONS

1. Specific assessment
   Assess vital signs; age; weight; developmental level and changes; frequency and pattern of bowel elimination; amount, color, odor, and consistency of stools; accompanying related GI symptoms; presence of blood or mucus in stools; presence of perirectal fistulas; factors that alleviate or aggravate condition; presence of complications (e.g., infection, obstruction, or hemorrhage) or extraintestinal manifestations (e.g., renal calculi, arthritis, and skin lesions); nutritional and hydration status; and compliance, facility with medication administration, and alternate feeding methods.
2. Specific care/teaching
   Teach information about and administration of medications and feeding modalities; management of diet and activity; skin care; need for regular follow-up visits, testing, and cancer screening; referrals to support groups; educational options; and preoperative care.
3. General
   Note responses to care and teaching.
4. See "Nurse Documentation and Family Home Record Keeping" in Appendix for required documentation components for all home care visits.

 Liver Transplant

Orthotopic (placed in normal anatomic position) liver transplantation is a surgical option for end-stage liver disease. Conditions for which it is indicated include extrahepatic biliary atresia, metabolic disorders (e.g., alpha$_1$ antitrypsin deficiency, Wilson's disease, and tyrosinemia), bile duct hypoplasia, familial cholestasis, and hepatitis. Surgical candidates must meet defined criteria. Full-sized, matched-donor organs or reduced-size adult livers may be used. Although there have been dramatic increases in survival rates, long-term (>5 years) prognosis has yet to be established. Retransplantation is sometimes required. There is the potential for alteration in oxygenation and cardiovascular, renal, or neurologic status in the immediate postoperative period. Graft rejection and infection are the predominant postoperative complications. Postoperative course is influenced by the underlying, premorbid condition and its clinical profile, extent of surgical manipulation, and immunosuppressive drug response.

Home health care is primarily concerned with instruction on administration of medications; monitoring for signs and symptoms of organ rejection; the prevention, recognition, and management of complications; and counseling for emotional support, information, and financial assistance.

Nursing diagnosis

Anxiety
Related factors: situational crisis, chronic illness, rejection, role transitions, financial strain
Defining characteristics: verbalization of feelings, fears, concerns, misgivings; somatic complaints; behavioral changes; regressive behaviors

OUTCOMES

Short-term
Decreased anxiety evidenced by more relaxed attitude, behavior, conversation (expected in 1 to 4 weeks)

Long-term
Minimal level of anxiety evidenced by compliance with health care regimen, sense of control, acceptance of/adaptation to condition (expected in 1 to 3 months, highly variable)

NURSING INTERVENTION/INSTRUCTIONS

1. Develop trusting relationship. Establish and maintain therapeutic relationship (each visit).
2. Assess family's and child's anxiety levels, current stressors, coping abilities, internal strengths, and external resources. Do not be reactive, but provide feedback (each visit).
3. Facilitate communication. Actively listen to concerns about illness, possible organ rejection, complications, disruption of/stress on family life, financial burden of traveling to transplant center, accommodations, and frequent hospital visits (each visit).
4. Provide clear, accurate, current information about treatments and progress. Repeat as needed (a handbook, *Resuming Life after Transplantation: A Handbook for Liver Transplant Recipients,* may be used to complement other teaching materials per transplant team/physician recommendation; free to transplant recipients; telephone 800-725-6818) (each visit).
5. Assure family of support. Provide agency telephone number (any visit).
6. Refer to social services for sources of financial assistance (each visit).
7. Refer for support and information to American Liver Foundation and Transplant Recipients International Association (any visit).

CAREGIVER/CHILD AND FAMILY INTERVENTIONS

1. Openly and honestly discusses fears, concerns, and misgivings.
2. Seeks assistance from health care providers.
3. Develops sense of control. Manages anxiety.
4. Participates in support groups. Sees counselor, if needed.
5. Explores services of government agencies, social services, foundations, and specialty groups, especially peer groups of those with transplants.

Nursing diagnosis

Knowledge deficit
Related factors: lack of information about health care regimen, lack of readiness to learn

Defining characteristics: requests for information about general care, medication regimen, signs of complications; inability to answer questions, recognize/accept need for information; lack of support/finances

OUTCOMES

Short-term
Adequate information evidenced by caregiver's verbalization of health care regimen, demonstration of medication protocol (expected in 1 to 3 weeks)

Long-term
Adequate information evidenced by caregiver's compliance with entire prescribed health care protocol and client's optimal levels of healing, growth, development (expected in 1 to 3 months)

NURSING INTERVENTIONS/INSTRUCTIONS

1. Assess caregiver's readiness to learn, emotional climate of home, family relationships, levels of adjustment, coping strengths, and sources of support and assistance (each visit).
2. Review transplant team's discharge plan. Identify name and telephone number of transplant coordinator; confer as needed (first visit).
3. Perform complete physical assessment of client. Inform client and caregiver of focus, results of examination, and significant findings (each visit).
4. Use assessment data as basis for teaching. Introduce basic information first; reinforce and supplement at later visits (each visit).
5. Assess operative site and degree of wound healing (may be weeks before client is discharged from transplant/rehabilitative centers). Note wound color, size, temperature, approximation of edges, presence of bleeding, and infection (each visit).
6. If T tube is present, concurrently assess type and amount of drainage (should be minimal to absent), condition of surrounding skin, presence of leakage, redness, swelling, warmth, purulent discharge, and change in tube length. Instruct caregiver on normal findings and care of operative and drain sites. Report significant

findings to physician. Inform caregiver of aberrations to report (each visit).

7. Assess for clinical signs and symptoms of graft rejection (fever, fatigue, decreased alertness, hepatic tenderness, jaundice, light or clay-colored stools, and dark-colored [yellow or orange] urine) (each visit).

8. Demonstrate temperature-taking and abdominal girth measurement. Have caregiver repeat demonstration (report and instruct caregiver to report significant findings) (first visit, reinforce as needed).

9. Stress to caregiver that signs of rejection do not necessarily mean that transplant will be lost; change in anti-rejection medication may be effective. Reinforce need for prompt attention to adverse clinical manifestations (each visit).

10. Demonstrate/instruct caregiver on medication administration of immunosuppressive agents, generally, cyclosporin, methylprednisolone, and azathioprine; include name, purpose, dose, frequency, routes, and side effects of drugs. Instruct not to skip doses or discontinue drugs (each visit).

11. Instruct on need for prescribed laboratory testing of drug serum levels and screens for graft function (especially direct bilirubin, alkaline phosphase, AST, ALT, GGTP, and coagulation times) (each visit).

12. Assess client for adverse effects of medications, including increased susceptibility to infection, delayed growth/development, weight gain, cushingoid appearance, marked GI irritation, hyperglycemia, hypertension, tremors, sensitivity to ultraviolet light, decreased visual acuity, acne, altered hair growth, hepatotoxicity, nephrotoxicity, bone marrow suppression, increased risk of malignancy, and personality changes. Report significant findings to physician (each visit).

13. Assess and instruct caregiver to monitor for early signs of infection and susceptibility from immunosuppressive drugs, including fever (persistent low-grade, episodic spiking fevers), tachycardia, and tachypnea (each visit, as needed).

14. Assess sources of opportunistic infection (e.g., wound sites, lungs, kidney, mouth, and skin). Report significant findings to physician (each visit).

15. Instruct client and caregiver on measures to avoid infection (first visit, follow up as needed).

- Maintain nutritious diet with vitamin and mineral supplementation.
- Use good hygienic practices (frequent bathing and handwashing after toileting and before wound care).
- Clean T tube site daily with prescribed antimicrobial.
- Perform meticulous oral hygiene and use oral antifungal medications as instructed. Obtain regular dental care (antibiotic should be used prophylactically for dental procedures).
- Avoid infected individuals, especially those with upper respiratory infections and those with children who are infected with childhood diseases.
- Avoid animal excreta.
- Eat only thoroughly cooked meats.
- Receive influenza and pneumococcal vaccines or immune globulins as needed. Avoid active live virus immunizations.
- Use safer sex practices (older, sexually active client).

16. Instruct client and caregiver on health promotion activities (second visit, as needed).

- Get adequate rest. Progress to full activity. Exercise in moderation. Attend school; avoid competitive or contact sports.
- Maintain a well-balanced, nutritious diet modified to correct premorbid nutritional deficits.
- Get regularly scheduled cataract and glaucoma screening examinations.
- Regularly examine entire body, including mouth and lips for skin lesions. Report new or ulcerated lesions, sores that do not heal, and moles that increase in size to physician. Limit exposure to sun; use sunscreen.

17. Instruct client to wear identifying medical information at all times (first visit, reinforce as needed).
18. Initiate referrals to social services and service organizations as needed (first visit).
19. Instruct caregiver to inform health care professionals of transplant profile (e.g., local physician, dentist, pharmacist, and immunization nurse) (first visit, as needed).

CAREGIVER/CHILD AND FAMILY INTERVENTIONS

1. Correctly administers prescribed medications. Monitors for and reports adverse effects.
2. Performs aseptic care to biliary drain.
3. Monitors wound healing. Reports signs of infection.
4. Maintains list or verbalizes signs and symptoms of graft rejection. Reports promptly to physician.
5. Engages in variety of health promoting activities to enhance healing and growth and to decrease possibility of infection, rejection, and malignancies.
6. Keeps regularly scheduled appointments with laboratory, physician, dentist, and transplant team.
7. Informs all health care providers of condition, date of surgery, and medications being taken.
8. Wears identifying medical information.
9. Participates in support group. Enlists aid of health care team for information, support, and assistance.

Nursing diagnosis

Altered growth and development
Related factors: effects of condition; environmental, stimulation deficiencies; inadequate parental caregiving; prescribed dependence; nutritional deficit
Defining characteristics: delay/difficulty in performing skills (motor, social, expressive) typical of age group; altered physical growth; inability of child to perform self-care, self-control activities

OUTCOMES

Short-term
Adequate growth/development of behavior, activities evidenced by absence of deficits, delays, regression of functioning; exhibition of age-appropriate growth/development within limits imposed by illness (expected within 6 to 12 weeks)

Long-term
Progressive growth/development advances; achievement of normal physical, emotional, social parameters (expected ongoing)

NURSING INTERVENTIONS/INSTRUCTIONS

1. Assess expected growth/developmental level for age and extent of deficits. Include fine and gross motor skills; language/social development; psychosocial and interpersonal skills; and cognitive development (see "Growth and Developmental Assessment," p. 31, for guidelines) (every visit).
2. Assess caregiver, family, and environment for stressful events and ability to provide love, caring, adequate stimulation, and appropriate play activities (each visit).
3. Assess for caregiver overprotection or negligence (each visit).
4. Instruct on normal growth/development patterns for child's age and possible lag in development caused by illness (first visit).
5. Assist caregiver and family to develop goals and to participate in care to achieve optimal development potential (ongoing).
6. Instruct caregiver to monitor child's activity tolerance. Collaborate to develop plan to provide visual, auditory, and tactile stimulation; gross motor skills for infant; and time with child for talking, playing, and self-care activities (ongoing).
7. Provide encouragement and support for child's and caregivers' efforts (each visit).
8. Provide early referral to professional resources such as special education teacher, psychosocial counselor, or social worker to assist child in specific areas of need (any visit).

CAREGIVER/CHILD AND FAMILY INTERVENTIONS

1. Complies with provision of activities to enhance stimulation, independence, and developmental progression (cognitive, psychomotor, and psychosocial).
2. Sets realistic goals for growth/developmental achievement.
3. Maintains consistent caregiver and schedule of activities.
4. Provides organized, consistent program of daily activities that include mobiles, music, toys, books, and other learning tools.
5. Provides time for talking and playing with other children and family members.

6. Holds, rocks, and cuddles child to provide touch and loving care.
7. Provides opportunity to participate in self-care activities, including dressing, bathing, eating, and toileting with adaptations as needed.
8. Attends parenting classes for child stimulation, growth/developmental milestones, discipline, and expectations.
9. Identifies and uses specialized services to assist with growth/developmental lags.

SAMPLE DOCUMENTATION INCLUSIONS

1. Specific assessment
   Assess vital signs, including temperature; weight; head circumference; abdominal girth; condition and characteristics of operative and drain sites; color of skin, urine, and stools; diet; activity; growth/developmental status; compliance with medical regimen; and laboratory findings.
2. Specific care/teaching
   Teach medication administration; wound care; signs of rejection, infection, and complications; measures to minimize and what to report to physician; and referrals to medical social worker/services.
3. General
   Note responses to care and teaching.
4. See "Nurse Documentation and Family Home Record Keeping" in Appendix for required documentation components for all home care visits.

Endocrine system

 ## Diabetes Mellitus

Diabetes mellitus is a metabolic dysfunction involving a deficit of insulin secretion by the pancreas. Associated etiologic factors include a genetic predisposition, autoimmune defect, and infectious and environmental factors. Insulin normally affects the metabolism of carbohydrates, fats, and proteins by promoting glucose entry into the muscle and fat cells and storage of glucose as glycogen in the liver and muscle cells. The loss of these physiologic functions when insulin is lacking or inefficient results in a concentration of glucose in the blood. The onset of the disorder in childhood is known as insulin-dependent diabetes mellitus (IDDM) and manifests the most common symptoms of polydipsia, polyphagia, and polyuria with nocturia and bedwetting. Although people of all ages can be affected, the peak incidence in children is 5 to 7 years of age. Care of the child with IDDM requires insulin replacement, planning, and management for instructions, interventions, and monitoring of dietary intake, exercise and daily activities, personal hygiene, effects of illnesses, stressors and emotional events, and growth and developmental changes. The prevention of long-term complications is a primary goal of a complete diabetes mellitus therapeutic regimen.

Home care is concerned with the multiple assessments, concerns, and teaching needs (diet, exercise, and insulin administration) of the child and family. The long-term nature of the disease requires ongoing, in-depth home teaching and assistance in the adjustments and interventions needed to achieve self-care and compliance to control the disease and prevent complications (blindness, renal disease, and peripheral vascular disease).

Nursing diagnosis

Knowledge deficit (complete management/care of child with newly diagnosed diabetes mellitus)

Related factors: lack of exposure to/misinterpretation of specific information regarding disease, cognitive limitations, lack of request for information

Defining characteristics: request for information; misconceptions about disease; denial; lack of readiness for learning; fear/anxiety about health status, performing therapeutic regimen

OUTCOMES

Short-term
Development of attitude that is conducive to learning; adequate basic knowledge, understanding of diabetes and treatment regimen evidenced by verbalization of definition of diabetes; components of care plan; interrelationship among insulin, food, exercise; demonstration of administration/monitoring of insulin; dietary, exercise requirements; blood, urine testing; personal hygiene needs; recognition of acute complications (expected within 2 weeks)

Long-term
Adequate, continuing in-depth knowledge, counseling, performance of complete therapeutic regimen evidenced by progressive self-care; adaptation to lifestyle changes; modification of plan as needed to achieve/maintain normoglycemia, prevent long-term complications associated with diabetes; participation in continuing education; routine monitoring by health care provider (expected within 2 months)

NURSING INTERVENTIONS/INSTRUCTIONS

1. Assess caregiver, family, and child for health beliefs; learning readiness; educational and developmental levels; competency; understanding for implementing therapeutic plan; best methods and approach for teaching and learning; and techniques required (ongoing).

2. Assess home environment for learning; space for storage of supplies/medications; area to practice procedures; facilities for handwashing, cleansing, and disinfecting supplies; area for food preparation and personal hygiene needs; and need for financial assistance (see "Environmental and Financial Assessments," pp. 37 and 41, for guidelines) (first visit).

3. Start care plan and perform procedures to allow family and child time to observe and adjust to new diagnosis. Collaborate with caregiver and family to develop teaching plan (initial visits until teaching can begin).

4. Plan for and allow sufficient time during each visit (15 minutes for child, 30 minutes for caregiver and family) for instruction, demonstration, return demonstration, and discussion of information, assessment, and procedures of care management program (each visit).

5. Use varied teaching strategies (play therapy with kit containing articles to be used in care) and educational materials (visual aids, pamphlets, pencil, and paper) (each visit teaching/evaluation is performed).

6. Use language that is content appropriate for the level of the learners. Allow time for learners to respond and ask questions for clarification (each visit).

7. Include child and encourage all family members to attend instruction sessions. First, define type of diabetes, source of insulin and how it affects health status, importance and benefits of controlling disease, and how to achieve good control (first visit, when teaching takes place).

8. Explain initial treatment regimen that includes insulin administration, meal planning, and exercises and how these influence diabetes control (first visit).

9. Instruct on dietary planning; importance of proper nutrition; maintaining consistency in calories; and percentages of carbohydrate, fat, and protein. Include types and amounts of foods, how to modify meals during illness, increased exercise, use of sugar substitutes, and eating at social activities and school. Assist to plan written menus that contain amounts and exchanges of food groups and calories, considering family cultural preferences, and conform to child's needs (each visit).

10. Explain benefits of exercise, its influence on glucose levels, types of exercise to include in plan, timing of exercises, need for regulation of insulin, and food intake before and after exercises (ongoing).

11. Instruct on action of insulin in body; administration; type (onset, peak, and duration); action and effect on glucose level; times and rotated sites of injections; prevention of lipoatrophy/hypertrophy; and possible adjustment in insulin dosage based on written guidelines. Demonstrate and allow for repeat demonstration of correct preparation of insulin (single or mixed) in syringe; technique for subcutaneous injection in thigh or arm using doll for young children for practice until confidence is achieved; use of portable insulin pump for continuous administration (see "Medication Administration and Teaching Guidelines," pp. 450-463); and care of supplies (ongoing).

12. Instruct on testing blood glucose by finger puncture; using commercial glucometer to determine acceptable range of 80 to 120 mg/dl; scheduling to perform tests; how to interpret results; adjusting insulin, meal, and exercise plan based on results; urine ketone testing and, if blood glucose is >240 mg/dl or if child is ill, using teststrips; how to interpret results; caring for supplies/ equipment used to perform monitoring procedures; and contacting health provider when abnormal levels persist. Allow for return demonstrations until confidence is established (ongoing).

13. Instruct on importance of daily bathing; foot care; care of cuts, scratches, or other skin breaks because child is more susceptible to infection; and periodic dental and eye examinations (second or third visit, reinforce).

14. Instruct on recommendations to follow for sick days, including insulin adjustments to compensate for decreased appetite; blood and urine testing every 2 or more hours; continuing with meals unless vomiting or anorexic; adding carbohydrate in liquid form; and notification of health care provider if vomiting persists (second or third visit).

15. Instruct on acceptable record keeping procedure to document insulin; diet intake; exercise level; blood

and urine test results; and illness, stressors, or significant signs and symptoms of hyperglycemia or hypoglycemia (any visit after initial instructions).

16. Direct child to wear identification that notes condition and telephone numbers of caregivers and health providers (first visit).

17. Provide follow-up plan for laboratory testing; visits to health provider; and referral to nutritionist, counselor, and community resources to provide continuing education (any visit).

CAREGIVER/CHILD AND FAMILY INTERVENTIONS

1. Participates in all teaching sessions on diabetes management.

2. Defines diabetes and cause. Explains insulin and dietary and exercise components of treatment protocol.

3. Plans, prepares, modifies, and provides meals of measured volumes of food for age, growth, and development needs that maintain control of disease and energy requirements (carbohydrate 55% to 60%, protein 0.08 g/kg, fat 30% with <300 mg/day cholesterol). Refers to food groups and exchange lists recommended by the American Diabetes Association. Obtains evaluation of dietary plan by nutritionist every 6 months.

4. Ingests food according to planned menus at consistent times and includes snacks. Increases or decreases food intake depending on physical activity or illness.

5. Tests blood and urine at appropriate times. Analyzes results for adjustments in insulin, food intake, and exercise.

6. Exercises daily. Maintains constant day-to-day program.

7. Administers insulin correctly and in timely manner. Uses insulin pump correctly if appropriate. Adjusts dosage based on glucose monitoring as prescribed by physician if sliding scale is used, food intake, and level of exercises. Properly disposes of supplies.

8. Maintains rotation injection site record, allowing for 4 to 6 injections in one area about 1 inch apart. Uses paper doll for child to mark sites.

9. Performs consistent, meticulous foot care with daily bathing; wearing clean cotton socks and good-fitting

shoes; trimming nails straight across; avoiding wearing sandals, wearing shoes without socks, and walking barefoot; performing personal hygiene measures, including daily bathing and dental brushing.

10. Allows child to progress to self-care as appropriate for age, motivation, and dexterity; ability to adjust insulin, diet, and activities to blood testing results.

11. Maintains record of dietary intake; need for changes, weight changes, insulin dosage, exercises, blood and urine monitoring results, and adjustments made to achieve control of disease.

12. Investigates for resources available and uses best value in purchasing supplies for care procedures.

13. Consults podiatrist, ophthalmologist, and dentist for specific monitoring of long-term disease process.

14. Informs all health care providers and prescribers of diagnosis and care regimen (dentist and surgeon).

15. Wears or carries identification information.

16. Returns to school with schedule that includes glucose testing, insulin administration, meals and snacks plan, and allowances in physical education class and other activities.

Nursing diagnosis

Risk for injury

Related factors: internal biochemical regulatory dysfunction (insulin deficit, excess)

Defining characteristics: hypoglycemia (irritability, shaky, hungry feeling, mood swings, dizziness, pallor, sweating, tachycardia, shallow respirations, tremor), hyperglycemia (lethargy, confusion, nausea, vomiting, thirst, weakness, flushed, weak pulse, fruity breath, Kussmaul's respirations, abdominal pain)

OUTCOMES

Short-term

Risk for insulin deficit/excess minimized evidenced by replacement of insulin as prescribed, appropriate ingestion of carbohydrate based on blood glucose level, testing of blood glucose for deviations from normal levels (expected within 1 week)

Long-term
Remains free of complications of hypoglycemia or hyperglycemia; maintains optimal health by compliance with therapeutic regimen evidenced by normal blood/urine test results, mood, mental status, respirations, pulse, neurologic/gastrointestinal status, stable growth pattern, weight gain (expected within 2 weeks)

NURSING INTERVENTIONS/INSTRUCTIONS

1. Perform complete physical assessment. Assess for signs and symptoms of hypoglycemia and possible causes (excess insulin administration, excessive exercise, or inadequate/inappropriate dietary intake) and hyperglycemia and possible causes (inadequate insulin production/administration, excessive carbohydrate dietary intake, or sedentary lifestyle) (first visit, as needed).

2. Instruct caregiver and child on early signs and symptoms of impending hypoglycemia or hyperglycemia; how to monitor for these complications; and effect illness has on maintaining control of disease with modification of regimen as needed (first visit, reinstruct on second visit).

3. Assess for caregiver and child understanding of therapeutic regimen, type of measures to take, and when to implement them to prevent complications (first and second visits).

4. Explain and instruct on treatment of hyperglycemia by checking blood glucose levels before breakfast and dinner or 2 hours after last meal; administering insulin as prescribed before breakfast and during day based on blood glucose levels, and adhering to exercise program (first and second visits, as needed).

5. Instruct on treatment of hypoglycemia by checking blood glucose levels; severity of signs and symptoms with ingestion of rapidly absorbed sugar (orange juice, milk, sugar cube, candy, or honey, if mild; Instaglucose, if moderate) that can be repeated every 10 to 15 minutes as necessary followed by longer lasting carbohydrates (crackers or bread) or protein (cheese); and administration of

prescribed recommended dosage of glucagon if severe (first and second visits, as needed).

6. Encourage exercise that is important for growth/development and reduction in need for insulin. Instruct to eat snack before exercise to prevent sudden drop in blood glucose (first visit).

7. Stress importance of compliance with treatment regimen, not to stop when feeling better, and need for ongoing monitoring and supervision (first visit).

8. Explain how and when to notify health care provider during acute episode of hyperglycemia or hypoglycemia (first visit).

CAREGIVER/CHILD AND FAMILY INTERVENTIONS

1. Verbalizes understanding of causes of complications, signs, and symptoms.

2. Assesses and performs monitoring procedures to identify signs and symptoms of hyperglycemia or hypoglycemia. Checks blood levels 3 to 4 times/day as ordered by physician.

3. Intervenes early to prevent/correct episode of hyperglycemia or hypoglycemia by adjusting insulin, food, and activity.

4. Complies with therapeutic regimen. Maintains monitoring by health prescriber.

5. Communicates with school nurse and teacher regarding child's special needs (limit setting, time to test blood, and ingestion of carbohydrate snack).

Nursing diagnosis

Altered family processes

Related factors: situational crisis of child with newly diagnosed diabetes mellitus

Defining characteristics: fear/anxiety about chronic illness, providing long-term care; family unable to meet physical/emotional needs of members; denial; lack of information, knowledge about disease; inability to express/accept feelings of child and family members, adapt to child's needs; inability to investigate sources for and to accept assistance/support

OUTCOMES

Short-term
Progression toward family acceptance of/adaptation to child with chronic disease evidenced by open communication among family members regarding understanding of disorder, discussion of fears/concerns about child's long-term special needs, ability to provide care, effect on family (expected within 2 to 3 weeks)

Long-term
Development of positive behaviors, attitudes, interactions that support child and family members; lifestyle changes evidenced by demonstration of effective coping skills, confidence in child's and family's abilities; ability to set goals, plan care, seek information/understanding/support (expected within 1 to 2 months)

NURSING INTERVENTIONS/INSTRUCTIONS

1. Assess level of development as family and of caregiver and family members; ethnic/cultural beliefs; stressors on family and extended family; impact of child's chronic illness on behaviors of parents and siblings (protective, nurturing, supportive, disruptive, neglectful, use of coping mechanisms); and ability to adjust to diagnosis and participate in care planning (see "Family Assessment," p. 41, for guidelines) (first and second visits).

2. Assess feelings of all family members, including siblings, and allow them to express their concerns (fears, anxiety, guilt, grief, threatened, complex therapeutic regimen) about responsibilities involved in providing care/support to one another (each visit).

3. Encourage open communications among family members. Inform them of importance of maintaining own health and social activities (first visit).

4. Discuss family's reaction to child and disease. Emphasize positive family relationships and coping mechanisms. Discuss child's positive abilities, potential, and limitations (each visit).

5. Inform family that disease is ongoing and requires lifetime care and monitoring (first visit).

6. Suggest referral of family to family counselor, local agencies, support group, and financial resources (any visit).

CAREGIVER/CHILD AND FAMILY INTERVENTIONS

1. Verbalizes feelings and concerns. Resolves reactions and negative behaviors toward child and among family members.
2. Identifies problems within family, role changes, and types of assistance needed and works together (immediate, long-term).
3. Promotes and demonstrates adjustment and adaptation to diagnosis and its implications for family.
4. Reduces own anxiety about chronic illness, therapies, fear of future complications, and possible death of child.
5. Gains confidence in ability to set goals and cope with child's needs and effect on family.
6. Demonstrates positive growth-promoting behaviors in family members and child by interacting with other families and seeking support from community resources.

Nursing diagnosis

Self-esteem disturbance
Related factors: negative feelings about physical/psychosocial capabilities
Defining characteristics: verbalizes shame, guilt, negative feelings about self; differences in lifestyle from that of peers; hesitant to try new things, deal with events; difficulty making decisions; denial; projection; rationalization of problems/failures

OUTCOMES

Short-term
Begins to develop positive feelings, perceptions of differences in lifestyle caused by chronic illness evidenced by reduction in self-negating statements; identifies problems that decrease feelings of self-worth; verbalizes need for treatments (expected within 1 to 2 weeks)

Long-term
Maintains positive self-esteem; accepts awareness of limitations imposed by disease evidenced by adjustment to disease, its associated risks; engages in peer group activities

that increase feelings of belonging, acceptance; develops positive relationships with family and friends; participates in plans, achieves goals that enhance physical health/lifestyle changes (expected within 1 month)

NURSING INTERVENTIONS/INSTRUCTIONS

1. Assess child's age, cognitive status, development, understanding of disease, situational factors, extent of disturbance, feelings of perceived differences caused by illness, influences of family on child's perceptions, and ability to become involved in and take control of own daily care and specific social activities (each visit, as needed).

2. Display positive attitude of acceptance and communication with child. Avoid judgmental, intrusive attitude (each visit).

3. Encourage and listen to feelings about disease, pain (injections), and other therapies (interruptions for blood tests, meals, and snacks and limitations in activities) (each visit).

4. Encourage and listen to feelings of being different, how peers perceive differences, and experiences that encourage feelings of well-being and success with peers and family (each visit).

5. Acknowledge expressed feelings. Facilitate sharing of feelings by child with family and health team (any visit).

6. Assist and allow child to identify positive feelings and strengths noted in dealing with experiences and coping behaviors learned that decrease negative feelings (each visit).

7. Encourage independent, constructive thinking and activities allowed by condition. Allow child to make choices and participate in care when desirable (each visit).

8. Praise all goal achievement, interest, and participation in care plan (any visit).

9. Incorporate play into building confidence, reinforcing positive behaviors, and improving self-esteem (each visit).

10. Suggest community resources for support and introduction to peers with same disorder (American Diabetes Association).

CAREGIVER/CHILD AND FAMILY INTERVENTIONS

1. Expresses feelings about therapy, being different, and difficulties/limitations imposed by disease.
2. Displays positive behaviors that facilitate improved self-esteem.
3. Develops coping skills to adjust to home/school routines and satisfactory family and peer relationships.
4. Allows time for necessary changes in lifestyle with promotion of flexibility and insight by family. Avoids negative remarks or behaviors.
5. Verbalizes feelings of independence and control. Becomes involved in self-care.
6. Uses opportunities for contact with peers who have adjusted to similar problems.
7. Family investigates community resources for information, support, acceptance, guidance, and supervised activities (camps, schools, and playgrounds).

Nursing diagnosis

Ineffective management of therapeutic regimen: family and individual

Related factors: complexity of therapeutic regimen; excessive demands made on individual or family; family decisional conflicts; social/economic support deficits; knowledge deficits; age, developmental level of child

Defining characteristics: choices of daily living, inappropriate family activities for effective meeting of goals of treatment/prevention program, verbalizes difficulty with regulation/integration of prescribed regimens, prevention of complications, acceleration of illness with exacerbation of symptoms

OUTCOMES

Short-term
Daily compliance with therapeutic regimen by caregiver, family, child evidenced by ability to interpret/follow instructions; adherence to specifics of treatment plan with absence of complications (expected within 2 to 3 weeks)

Long-term
Effective adherence to long-term health regimens evidenced
by regulated lifestyle with progressive performance of self-
care techniques, restrictions of behaviors that adversely
affect health status, absence of consequences of noncompliance to treatment plan, growth/development within expected ranges for child, resumption of normal activities
(school, play, social activities), acceptance of support/
assistance from community resources (expected within 1 to 2
months)

NURSING INTERVENTIONS/INSTRUCTIONS

1. Assess and review caregiver's and child's understanding
   of treatment plan, ability to adhere to requirements by
   interviewing and observing behaviors and techniques,
   documentations in log, and checking blood and urine for
   normoglycemic status (each visit).
2. Be nonjudgmental and accepting. Encourage expression
   of perceptions of disease and responsibilities (each visit).
3. Evaluate knowledge and understanding of role, adherence to therapeutic plan, and modifications (any visit,
   depending on problems).
4. Include caregiver and child in planning and adjustments,
   if needed, to comply with personal characteristics and
   needs (each visit).
5. Assist to develop program with goals that are easily
   achieved, including foods and activities that child prefers.
   Reward each positive behavior change or improvement
   (any visit).
6. Offer written agreement with expected change and specific reward (toy, money, or special event) (first visit, revise on second visit if needed).
7. Instruct caregiver to perform all therapeutic activities for
   1 day to give child relief from multiple responsibilities.
8. Consider referral to counselor for those with more complex behavioral or medical problems to promote adherence (any visit).

CAREGIVER/CHILD AND FAMILY INTERVENTIONS

1. Participates in all planning and implementation of health
   care.

2. Adjusts lifestyle to comply with daily specific requirements of therapeutic regimen.
3. Demonstrates facility in performance of self-care as appropriate.
4. Records observations and care in diary to evaluate compliance.
5. Maintains normoglycemic state.
6. Obtains routine follow-up health care. Continues with education of diabetes.
7. Attends school. Participates in family routines within identified limitations.

SAMPLE DOCUMENTATION INCLUSIONS

1. Specific assessment
   Assess general health status, stressors of caregiver and child, effect on treatment regimen, family's and child's coping ability to comply with long-term management, possibility of self-monitoring, signs and symptoms of complications, need for reinstruction of aspects of care, and need for referrals (counselor or nutritionist).
2. Specific care/teaching
   Teach disease, signs and symptoms, insulin dosage, preparation and administration; injection site rotation; dietary inclusions and exclusions; blood glucose testing; urine testing for ketones; exercise regimen; personal hygiene; foot care; dental care; signs and symptoms of complications; and interventions.
3. General
   Note responses to care and teaching; goal achievement; changes in plan; progression/regression of health status; adaptation of caregiver, family, and child to long-term care; change in lifestyle; self-care abilities; resources for acquiring medication, supplies, equipment for care; maintenance of log to record test results and treatments; and need for monitoring by health care provider.
4. See "Documentation and Family Home Record Keeping" in Appendix for general required documentation components for all home care visits.

Hematologic system

 Acquired Immunodeficiency Syndrome/Pediatric Acquired Immunodeficiency Syndrome

Acquired immunodeficiency syndrome (AIDS)/pediatric acquired immunodeficiency syndrome (PAIDS) is a fatal viral disorders characterized by marked cellular and humoral mediated immune dysfunction that is unexplained by congenital defect or drug suppression. AIDS is the seventh leading cause of death in children 1 to 4 years of age. The cause is the human immunodeficiency virus, HIV-1, a retrovirus. It is present in blood, semen, vaginal fluids, amniotic fluid, and other body fluids and, in lower concentrations, breast milk, tears, and saliva. AIDS is the final phase of a biologic process that includes inoculation, seroconversion, variable latency, and progressive symptoms. Profound immunosuppression results in recurrent and/or severe opportunistic and, frequently, treatment-resistant infections from bacteria, viruses, fungi, or protozoa and in malignancies and autoimmune disorders. Overwhelming infection, commonly from *Pneumocystis carinii* pneumonia (PCP), is the major cause of death. Almost all current pediatric HIV infection is the result of vertical transmission from an HIV-infected mother. Clinically asymptomatic and undiagnosed HIV-infected women are a major source of infection, and the infant may be the first in the family unit to present clinical manifestations. Other high-risk maternal groups include women who are intravenous drug users, who have had multiple sex partners, who have been recipients of blood products (before 1985 AIDS blood screening programs), or whose sexual partners are at high risk. These populations are frequently poor, undereducated, unemployed, and from unstable families, which make health care and child care problematic. AIDS occurs disproportionately in the African-American and Hispanic populations. Heterosexual transmission has increased significantly. Older children and adolescents are at risk when they become sexually active and engage in high-risk behaviors or if they received blood transfusions before 1985 or have had blood sharing activities since. No population is exempt. A universal approach to disease prevention and control is appropriate.

The HIV transmission rate from mother to infant is about 30%. Azidothymidine (AZT, ZDV) administration to select, diagnosed HIV-infected women has resulted in a two-thirds reduction in transmission rate, and its use may be recommended. Optimally, all women would be voluntarily and routinely tested before or during early pregnancy and then counseled, treated, and followed. Mild self-resolving infant anemia is the only known short-term adverse effect of AZT therapy. Long-term effects have yet to be established.

Three mutually exclusive, prognostically significant categories have been established in the classification of pediatric HIV infection: infection status (Table 6), immunologic status (Table 7), and clinical status (Table 8).

Medical management is directed at disease prevention and at early recognition and aggressive treatment of life-threatening opportunistic infections, encephalopathies, wasting, and malignancies.

Home health care is primarily concerned with client advocacy and identification and protection of the high-risk infant; instruction in the prevention of infection and disease transmission and health maintenance activities, in treatment of infection; and in the support of the family. A multidisciplinary team is necessary to support and assist the family to meet its health, psychosocial, and financial needs.

Nursing diagnosis

Risk for injury
Related factors: caregiver negligence, abuse; lack of health
care, basic services; drug use of mother, her partner;

(*Text continued on p. 265.*)

Table 6   *Diagnosis of HIV Infection in Children*

Diagnosis	Criteria
HIV infected	a) Child < 18 months of age who is known to be HIV seropositive or born to HIV-infected mother *and* has positive test results on two separate determinations (excluding cord blood) from one or more HIV detection tests (HIV culture, HIV polymerase chain reaction, HIV antigen [p 24]); or meets criteria for AIDS diagnosis based on the 1987 AIDS surveillance case definition b) Child ≥ 18 months of age who is born to HIV-infected mother or any child infected by blood, blood products, or other known modes of transmission (e.g., sexual contact) who is HIV-antibody positive by repeatedly reactive EIA and confirmatory test (Western blot, IFA) *Or* meets any of the criteria above in a
Perinatally exposed	Child who does not meet previously mentioned criteria, is HIV seropositive by EIA and confirmatory test (Western blot, IFA), is < 18 months of age at time of test or has unknown antibody status, but was born to mother infected with HIV
Seroreverter	Child who is born to HIV-infected mother, has been documented as HIV-antibody negative (i.e., two or more negative EIA tests performed at 6-18 months of age or one negative EIA test after 18 months of age), *and* has had no other laboratory evidence of infection (has not had two positive viral detection tests if performed) has not had an AIDS-defining condition

From Centers for Disease Control and Prevention: *Morbid Mortal Wkly Rep* 43/RR-12:1-10, 1994.
HIV, Human immunodeficiency virus; *AIDS,* acquired immunodeficiency syndrome; *EIA,* enzyme immunoassay; *IFA,* immunofluorescence assay.

Table 7   Immunologic Categories Based on Age-Specific CD4+ T-lymphocyte Counts and Percent of Total Lymphocytes

	Age of child					
	<12 months		1-5 yr		6-12 yr	
Immunologic category	µl	%	µl	%	µl	%
No evidence of suppression	≥1500	(≥25)	≥1000	(≥25)	≥500	(≥25)
Evidence of moderate suppression	750-1499	(15-24)	500-999	(15-24)	200-499	(15-24)
Severe suppression	<750	(<15)	<500	(<15)	<200	(<15)

From Centers for Disease Control and Prevention: *Morbid Mortal Wkly Rep* 43/RR-12:1-10, 1994.

Table 8   Clinical Categories for Children with HIV Infection

Category N: Not symptomatic

Children who have no signs or symptoms considered to be the result of HIV infection or who have only one of conditions listed in Category A.

Category A: Mildly symptomatic

Children with two or more conditions listed below but no conditions listed in Categories B and C.

- Lymphadenopathy (≥ 0.5 cm at more than two sites; bilateral = one site)
- Hepatomegaly
- Splenomegaly
- Dermatitis
- Parotitis
- Recurrent or persistent upper respiratory infection, sinusitis, or otitis media

Category B: Moderately symptomatic

Children who have conditions other than those listed for Category A or C that are attributed to HIV infection. Examples of conditions include, but are not limited to the following:

- Anemia (< 8 g/dl), neutropenia ($< 1000/mm^3$), or thrombocytopenia ($< 100,000/mm^3$) persisting for ≥ 30 days
- Bacterial meningitis, pneumonia, or sepsis (single episode)
- Candidiasis, oropharyngeal (thrush), persisting > 2 months in children > 6 months of age
- Cardiomyopathy
- Cytomegalovirus infection, onset before 1 month of age
- Diarrhea, recurrent or chronic
- Hepatitis
- Recurrent HSV stomatitis (more than two episodes within 1 year)
- HSV bronchitis, pneumonitis, or esophagitis, onset before 1 month of age
- Herpes zoster (shingles) involving at least two distinct episodes or more than one dermatome
- Leiomyosarcoma
- LIP or pulmonary lymphoid hyperplasia complex
- Nephropathy
- Nocardiosis

Centers for Disease Control and Prevention: *Morbid Mortal Wkly Rep* 36(15): 1987.

HIV, Human immunodeficiency virus; *HSV,* herpes simplex virus; *LIP,* lymphoid interstitial pneumonia.   *Continued.*

Table 8   Clinical Categories for Children with HIV Infection — cont'd

- Persistent fever lasting >1 month
- Toxoplasmosis, onset before 1 month of age
- Varicella, disseminated (complicated chickenpox)

Category C: Severely symptomatic

Children with any condition listed in the 1987 surveillance case definition for AIDS with the exception of LIP

- Serious bacterial infections, multiple or recurrent (i.e., any combination of at least two culture-confirmed infections within 2-year period), of septicemia, pneumonia, meningitis, bone or joint infection, or abscess of internal organ or body cavity (excluding otitis media, superficial skin or mucosal abscesses, and indwelling catheter-related infections)
- Candidiasis, esophageal or pulmonary (bronchi, trachea, or lungs)
- Coccidioidomycosis, disseminated (at site other than, or in addition to lungs or cervical or hilar lymph nodes)
- Cryptococcosis, extrapulmonary
- Cryptosporidiosis or isosporiasis with diarrhea persisting >1 month
- Cytomegalovirus disease with onset of symptoms at age >1 month (at site other than liver, spleen, or lymph nodes)
- Encephalopathy (at least one of following progressive findings present for at least 2 months in absence of concurrent illness other than HIV infection that could explain) (a) failure to attain or loss of developmental milestones, loss of intellectual ability, verified by standard developmental scale, or neuropsychologic tests; (b) impaired brain growth, acquired microcephaly demonstrated by head circumference measurements, brain atrophy demonstrated by computed tomography or magnetic resonance imaging (serial imaging is required for children <2 years of age); (c) acquired symmetric motor deficit manifested by two or more: paresis, pathologic reflexes, ataxia, or gait disturbance
- HSV infection causing mucocutaneous ulcer that persists for >1 month; or bronchitis, pneumonitis, or esophagitis for any duration affecting child >1 month of age
- Histoplasmosis, disseminated (at site other than, or in addition to, lungs or cervical or hilar lymph nodes)
- Kaposi's sarcoma
- Lymphoma, primary, in brain
- Lymphoma, small, noncleaved cell (Burkitt's), or immunoblastic, or large cell lymphoma of B-cell or unknown immunologic phenotype

Table 8   Clinical Categories for Children with HIV Infection — cont'd

- *Mycobacterium tuberculosis,* disseminated, extrapulmonary
- *Mycobacterium,* other species or unidentified species, disseminated (at site other than or in addition to lungs, skin, or cervical or hilar lymph nodes)
- *Mycobacterium avium* complex or *Mycobacterium kansasii,* disseminated (at site other than, or in addition to, lungs, skin, or cervical or hilar lymph nodes)
- *Pneumocystis carinii* pneumonia
- Progressive multifocal leukoencephalopathy
- *Salmonella* (nontyphoid) septicemia, recurrent
- Toxoplasmosis of brain, onset at >1 month of age
- Wasting syndrome in absence of concurrent illness other than HIV infection that could explain (a) persistent weight loss $>10\%$ of baseline or (b) downward crossing of at least two of following percentile lines on weight-for-age chart (e.g., 95th, 75th, 50th, 25th, 5th) in child ≥ 1 year of age or (c) <5th percentile on weight-for-height chart on two consecutive measurements, ≥ 30 days apart, plus chronic diarrhea (i.e., at least two loose stools per day for ≥ 30 days), or documented fever, intermittent or constant, for ≥ 30 days

caregiver distrust of health care system; family distancing from government/social services because of fear of incarceration, family separation

Defining characteristics: caregiver refusal/reluctance to answer personal questions, participate in health care; denial of problem; altered sensorium; cognitive dissonance; discrepancy between accounts of child's care, actual condition (hungry, listless, soiled, bruised, missed school, unkept medical appointments); tacit acceptance of drugs, crime cultures; reports that children are frequently left unattended; documented health care, police history of substance abuse; child neglect, abuse; domestic violence

OUTCOMES

Short-term
Absence of injury evidenced by caretaker distancing from high-risk behaviors, entry into health care system, observed child well-being (expected in 1 month)

Long-term
Absence of injury evidenced by physically/emotionally
healthy child housed in safe, nurturing environment (expected ongoing)

NURSING INTERVENTIONS/INSTRUCTIONS

1. Maintain personal safety (e.g., schedule visits during day-
   light hours and when others will be in household or
   nearby, know route to home, inform agency of visit times,
   and use agency-provided escorts as available) (each
   visit).
2. Establish and maintain rapport. Be honest and direct in
   services provided, responsibilities, and obligations (each
   visit).
3. Assess caregiver's health, social, and behavioral histories;
   lifestyle; perceived responsibilities; limitations; capabilities; decision making and coping abilities; and desire
   to change. Note congruence of attitude, behavior, and
   conversation and any discrepancies between what is being communicated by family and what is objectively
   observed (each visit).
4. Assess emotional milieu; include bonding behaviors,
   stressors, and sources of support (each visit).
5. Inform caregiver of benefits of having child and others in
   household HIV tested (first visit, reinforce as needed).
6. Assess child's overall health and general well-being. Note
   developmental level, general cleanliness, nutritional status, unusual clinging to nurse, impropriety of responses,
   history and evidence of injury, characteristics, and degree
   of healing (each visit).
7. Encourage positive parenting and lifestyle changes, reduction of high-risk behaviors, and rehabilitation efforts
   (each visit).
8. Inform caregivers of resources for respite care, family
   counseling, self-esteem workshops, vocational training,
   and substance abuse control (each visit).
9. Immediately report suspicion or evidence of abuse to
   child protective services (any visit).

CAREGIVER/CHILD AND FAMILY INTERVENTIONS

1. Interacts with health care system.
2. Recognizes personal strengths and limitations.

3. Seeks appropriate assistance for self-defined limitations.
4. Works with health care worker to define and remediate areas that need further strengthening.
5. Participates in rehabilitative/educational programs.
6. Provides safe, nurturing home for child.

Nursing diagnosis

Risk for infection
Related factors: compromised immune system
Defining characteristics: presence of endogenous flora or opportunistic pathogens (e.g., *Pneumocystis carinii, Streptococcus pneumoniae, Haemophilus influenzae, Staphylococcus aureus, Mycobacterium tuberculosis, avium* complex, *Salmonella* sp, *Escherichia coli, Camphylobacter, Candida,* cytomegalovirus [CMV], Epstein-Barr virus, *Aspergillus fumigatus*) (signs, symptoms depend on target site, offending pathogen, and immunologic status)

OUTCOMES

Short-term
Absent or minimal infection evidenced by intact baseline health parameters; absence of signs, symptoms of specific infection (depends on immune status)

Long-term
Absent or minimal infection, early intervention/treatment of infection evidenced by compliance with long-term infection prophylaxis, optimal function within limitations of condition (expected ongoing)

NURSING INTERVENTIONS/INSTRUCTIONS

1. Before visit, review referral, hospital record, and discharge plan as applicable; HIV status of client and family; immunologic profile; age; weight; and general health.
2. If child is in foster or preadoptive home, determine status of parental rights. Identify adults legally responsible for care, including health care (first visit).
3. Query caregiver about child's medical history, including episodes of unexplained fever, poor growth, weight loss,

recurrent pneumonia, otitis media, candidiasis, eczema, diarrhea, and exposure to tuberculosis or other infectious diseases (first visit).

4. Perform complete physical assessment to establish database. Include vital signs, weight, head circumference, and developmental milestones. Note especially early, nonspecific indicators of disease (i.e., weight loss >10% of baseline and not necessarily related to intake), failure to thrive, unexplained fever, diarrhea, parotitis, lymphadenopathy, and hepatosplenomegaly (each visit).

5. Assess pulmonary status. Note cough, fever, decreased/adventitious breath sounds, tachypnea, retractions, wheezing, rhonchi, and digital clubbing. Report adverse findings to physician (each visit).

6. Perform complete home assessment. Note general cleanliness, toilet and laundry facilities, and utilities (first visit). Observe universal precautions (each visit).

7. Instruct caregiver on age-appropriate child activity. Encourage normal, self-paced activity and provide rest periods and adequate sleep (first visit).

8. Instruct caregiver on need for child's personal hygiene; supervised handwashing after play and contact with soil, pets, and toileting; scrupulous oral care; and diaper/perineal care (first visit, reinforce as needed).

9. Instruct caregiver on need for high-calorie, high-protein diet as recommended. Supplement feedings with nutrient dense foods. Concurrently investigate need for possible enteral/parenteral feedings (each visit).

10. Instruct caregiver on proper food handling and preparation, including washing hands before handling food and different food items; cleaning utensils; avoiding use of unpasteurized milk, raw or undercooked eggs, fish, shellfish, and undercooked meat and poultry; washing fruits and vegetables thoroughly; and properly storing food and thoroughly heating leftovers (each visit).

11. Instruct caregiver to avoid exposing child to infectious disease and crowds. If caregiver is ill and respite care is unavailable, instruct caregiver to use surgical mask for airborne infection prevention, maximum skin cover, and gloves for dermatologic infections. Contact physician

if child is exposed to measles, chickenpox, tuberculosis, or other infectious diseases (first visit, reinforce as needed).

12. Encourage caregiver to have all family members immunized per recommended schedule and physician's directive. Include booster shots (ongoing). Immunization schedule for a seropositive child generally includes the following:

   - Diphtheria, pertussis, tetanus (DPT) and *Haemophilus influenzae* type B conjugated (HbCV, Hvb)
   - Measles, mumps, rubella (MMR)
   - Enhanced inactivated poliovirus for child and all others in household
   - Influenza vaccine after 6 months of age; annually thereafter for client and family before start of flu season
   - Pneumococcal vaccine after 2 years of age; revaccination after 3 or more years
   - Hepatitis B
   - Past exposure prophylaxis: immune globulin after measles exposure; varicella-zoster immune globulin after exposure to chickenpox
   - Tuberculin skin test (5 TU PPD by Mantoux) at 9 to 12 months of age

13. Instruct caregiver on prevention of animal-borne disease, including having pets immunized; avoiding young, sick, or stray animals and reptiles; properly handling litter boxes and pet excreta; and flea control (first visit, as needed).

14. Instruct caregiver on administration of first line chemoprophylaxis for PCP. Table 9 lists medications for treatment of opportunistic disease in HIV-infected children (see "Guidelines for Medication Administration and Teaching," pp. 450-463). Teach and reinforce recognition and management of adverse effects and systemic toxicities, aseptic technique, enforcement of universal precautions with indwelling central lines, need for regular medical follow-up, and monitoring. Instruct on administration of other medications, including immunomodulators, antiinfectives, anticonvulsants, and bronchodilators as ordered (each visit).

(Text continued on p. 275.)

Table 9 Medications for Prophylaxis for First Episode of Opportunistic Disease in HIV-Infected Infants and Children

Pathogen	Indication	Preventive regimens	
		First choice	Alternatives
Strongly recommended as standard of care			
Pneumocystis carinii*	All infants 1-4 months old born to HIV-infected women; HIV-infected or HIV-indeterminate infants <12 months old; HIV-infected children 1-5 yr old with CD4+ count of <500/μl or CD4+ of <15%; HIV-infected children 6-12 yr old with CD4+ count of <200/μl or CD4+ of <15%	TMP-SMZ, 150/750 mg/m^2/day in 2 divided doses PO tiw on consecutive days (AII); acceptable alternative schedules for same dosage (AII); single dose PO tiw on consecutive days, 2 divided doses PO qd, or 2 divided doses PO tiw on alternate days	Aerosolized pentamidine (children ≥5 yr old), 300 mg qm via Respirgard II nebulizer (CIII); dapsone (children ≥1 month old), 2 mg/kg (not to exceed 100 mg) PO qd (CIII); IV pentamidine, 4 mg/kg q2-4wk (CIII)
Mycobacterium tuberculosis Isoniazid-sensitive	TST reaction of ≥5 mm or prior positive TSTs	Isoniazid, 10-15 mg/kg (maximum, 300 mg) PO	Rifampin, 10-20 mg/kg (maximum, 600 mg) PO or IV qd × 12 months (BI)

	result without treatment or contact with case of active tuberculosis	or IM qd × 12 months or 20-30 mg/kg (maximum, 900 mg) PO biw × 12 month (BIII)	Uncertain
Isoniazid-resistant	Same as above; high probability of exposure to isoniazid-resistant tuberculosis	Rifampin, 10-20 mg/kg (maximum, 600 mg) PO or IV qd × 12 months (BII)	
Multidrug-resistant (isoniazid, rifampin)	Same as above; high probability of exposure to multidrug-resistant tuberculosis	Choice of drugs requires consultation with public health authorities	None

From Centers for Disease Control and Prevention: *Morbid Mortal Wkly Rep* 44/RR8:27-28, 1995.

HIV, Human immunodeficiency virus; *TMP-SMZ,* trimethoprim-sulfamethoxazole; *tiw,* three times weekly; *PO,* orally; *qd,* daily; *qm,* monthly; *IV,* intravenously; *TST,* tuberculin skin test; *IM,* intramuscularly; *biw,* twice weekly.

Note: Not all of recommended regimens reflect current Food and Drug Administration-approved labeling.

The Respirgard II nebulizer is manufactured by Marquest, Englewood, CO. Letters and Roman numerals in parentheses after regimens indicate strength of recommendation and quality of evidence supporting it.

*The efficacy of parenteral pentamidine (e.g., 4 mg/kg qm) is controversial. TMP-SMZ and dapsone/pryimethamine (and possibly dapsone alone) appear to be protective against toxoplasmosis, although relevant data have not been prospectively collected. Daily treatment with TMP-SMZ reduces frequency of some bacterial infections. Patients receiving sulfadiazine/pyrimethamine for toxoplasmosis are protected against *Pneumocystis carinii* pneumonia and do not need TMP-SMZ. *Continued.*

Table 9   *Medications for Prophylaxis for First Episode of Opportunistic Disease in HIV-Infected Infants and Children — cont'd*

Pathogen	Indication	Preventive regimens	
		First choice	Alternatives
Varicella-zoster virus	Significant exposure to varicella with no history of varicella	VZIG, 1 vial (1.25 ml)/10 kg (maximum, 5 vials) IM, given ≤96 hr after exposure, ideally within 48 hr (AI) (children routinely receiving IVIG should receive VZIG if the last dose of IVIG was given >14 days before exposure)	None
Various pathogens	HIV exposure/infection	Immunizations	
Recommended for consideration in all patients			
Toxoplasma gondii†	IgG antibody to *Toxoplasma* with severe immunosuppression (CD4+ count of <100/μl) (prophylaxis may be considered at higher CD4+ counts in	TMP-SMZ, 150/750 mg/m²/day in 2 divided doses PO tiw on consecutive days (CIII); acceptable alternative schedules for same dosage (CIII);	None Dapsone (children ≥1 month old), 2 mg/kg or 15 mg/m² (maximum, 25 mg) PO qd, plus pyrimethamine, 1 mg/kg PO qd, plus leucovorin,

	relevant data are available)	vided doses PO qd, or 2 divided doses PO tiw on alternate days	
Mycobacterium avium complex	CD4+ count of <75/μl	Children 6-12 yr old: rifabutin, 300 mg PO qd (BI); children <6 yr old: 5 mg/kg PO qd when suspension is available (BI)	All ages: azithromycin, 7.5 mg/kg in 2 divided doses PO qd (CIII); clarithromycin, 5-12 mg/kg PO qd (CIII)
Not recommended for most patients; indicated for consideration only in selected patients			
Invasive bacterial infections	Hypogammaglobulinemia	IVIG, 400 mg/kg qm (AI)	None
Candida species‡	Severe immunosuppression	Nystatin (100,000 U/ml), 4-6 ml PO q6h or topical clotrimazole, 10 mg PO 5×/day (CII)	Ketoconazole, 5-10 mg/kg PO q12-24h (CL); fluconazole, 2-8 mg/kg PO qd (CI)
Cryptococcus neoformans	Severe immunosuppression	Fluconazole, 2-8 mg/kg PO qd (BI)	Itraconazole, 2-5 mg/kg PO q12-24h (CIII)
Histoplasma capsulatum	Severe immunosuppression, endemic geographic area	Itraconazole, 2-5 mg/kg PO q12-24h (CIII)	Fluconazole, 2-8 mg/kg PO qd (III)

VZIG, Varicella-zoster immunoglobulin; *IVIG*, intravenous immune globulin; *IgG*, Immunoglobulin G.
†Protection against *Toxoplasma gondii* is provided by the preferred antipneumocystitis regimens. Dapsone alone cannot be recommended on basis of currently available data. Pyrimethamine alone probably provides little, if any, protection.
‡Ketoconazole and fluconazole are preferred for prophylaxis of esophagitis and severe mucocutaneous infection.   *Continued.*

Table 9 Medications for Prophylaxis for First Episode of Opportunistic Disease in HIV-Infected Infants and Children — cont'd

Pathogen	Indication	Preventive regimens	
		First choice	Alternatives
Coccidioides immitis	Severe immunosuppression, endemic geographic area	Fluconazole, 2-8 mg/kg PO qd (CIII)	Itraconazole, 2-5 mg/kg PO q12-24h (CIII)
Cytomegalovirus (CMV)§	CD4+ count of <50/µl, CMV antibody positivity	Children 6-12 yr old: oral ganciclovir under investigation	None
Influenza A virus	High risk of exposure (e.g., institutional outbreak)	Rimantadine or amantadine, 5 mg/kg qd (maximum, 150 mg) in 2 divided doses PO for children <10 yr old; for children ≥10 yr old, 5 mg/kg up to 40 kg, then 200 mg in 2 divided doses PO qd	None

§Data on oral ganciclovir are still being evaluated; durability of its effect is unclear. Acyclovir is not protective against CMV.

15. Instruct caregiver to immediately notify physician of fever, cough, tachypnea, dyspnea, mucocutaneous lesions (white, patchy or oral sores and diaper rash), failure to eat, vomiting, diarrhea, bloody bowel movements, and neurologic manifestations (first visit, reinforce as needed).

16. Instruct caregiver on need to keep appointments for medical visits, laboratory testing (blood panels; immune profiles; x-ray films; pulmonary, neurologic, and development tests), and retinal evaluations (each visit).

17. Refer to local organizations for assistance with food, finances, and respite care (first visit, as needed).

18. Inform client, as appropriate, on availability of experimental and approved treatments for HIV/AIDS (AIDS Clinical Trials Information Service, telephone 800-874-2572; HIV/AIDS Treatment Information Service, telephone 800-448-0440).

CAREGIVER/CHILD AND FAMILY INTERVENTIONS

1. Engages in full health promotion activities, including rest, diet, and diversion.
2. Keeps client and family fully immunized per physician's directive.
3. Maintains infection control protocols.
4. Recognizes and reports signs and symptoms of infection, drug reactions, and deteriorating status.
5. Administers medications as prescribed.
6. Keeps medical and laboratory appointments.
7. Uses local and national services as needed.

Nursing diagnosis

Knowledge deficit
Related factors: lack of information, lack of readiness to learn
Defining characteristics: verbalization of need for information about methods of preventing disease transmission to others, of available resources

OUTCOMES

Short-term
Adequate information evidenced by caregiver and client statements of disease transmission, prevention (expected in 1 to 4 weeks)

Long-term
Adequate information evidenced by compliance with health care regimen, lifestyle changes, viral containment, optimal family health (expected in 1 to 2 months)

NURSING INTERVENTIONS/INSTRUCTIONS

1. Assess learning needs, styles, and receptivity. Provide information in manner appropriate for culture, language, education, and age. Provide written directions. Provide adolescent clients opportunity for private instruction and demonstration. Note special needs of extended and foster families (each visit).

2. Provide agency telephone number and list of community resources (first visit).

3. Use universal precautions in delivery of nursing care (each visit).

4. Instruct on transmission modes, including sexual contact and exposure to blood, blood products, and other body fluids. Emphasize that disease cannot be spread by casual or close, nonintimate contact. Note nonverbal cues of interest. Allow time for questions (each visit).

5. Instruct clients on need to inform all health care workers (e.g., nurses, physicians, clinic personnel, and laboratory workers) of serostatus and of confidentiality requirements (first visit, as needed).

6. Explore willingness to inform sexual contacts of diagnosis and for follow up; encourage same (as needed).

7. Discourage seropositive mothers from breastfeeding and all high-risk and HIV-positive clients from blood and organ donations (first visit, reinforce as needed).

8. Instruct family members on methods to control blood-borne transmission (first visit, reinforce as needed).

    • Do not share razors, toothbrushes, or any item that may have blood on it.
    • Wear gloves when providing care; all blood and body fluids are potential sources of infection.

- Cover open cuts/sores with bandages.
- Wash hands after contact with blood, even if gloves were used.
- Handle medication needles carefully. Do not recap needles and dispose of needles in puncture-proof container.
- Store away from children and pets. Dispose of full container at local health agency per protocol. For accidental needle sticks, wash area thoroughly and immediately notify physician.
- Flush liquids or tissues containing blood, seminal fluids, or vaginal fluids down toilet; avoid splashing and lower toilet lid. Nonflushable, used dressings, latex gloves, sanitary napkins, and condoms should be securely bagged in plastic before discarding. Follow trash disposal regulations.

9. Instruct on safer sex options including abstinence and consistent/correct use of latex condoms. Explore family planning options and refer to appropriate physicians and clinics (first visit, reinforce as needed).
10. Instruct family members on housekeeping and disinfecting measures to prevent transmission (first visit).

- Wash eating utensils with hot soapy water; neither food nor utensils need to be separated from general use.
- Wear gloves to prevent contact with urine, stool, or vomit. Wash hands after removing gloves.
- Wash clothing and linens as usual (i.e., by hand, machine, or dry cleaning). Follow recommendations for cleaning agent and appliances.
- Clean blood spills with soap and water. Follow with disinfection of 1:100 solution of household bleach and water. Disinfecting solution can also be used for general cleaning and mopping. Use fresh solution every 24 hours. Use clean, intact, reusable rubber gloves.

11. Direct intravenous drug users to substance abuse programs. Instruct on bleach cleaning of needles and syringes or on needle exchange program and in not sharing drug paraphernalia (as indicated).

12. Inform clients of available resources and services (e.g., local health department or local AIDS volunteer health group). For information on local organizations, telephone 24-hour hotlines.

- English: 800-342-AIDS
- Spanish: 800-344-7432
- Deaf access: 800-AIDS-TTY

CAREGIVER/CHILD AND FAMILY INTERVENTIONS

1. Verbalizes modes of transmission and methods to prevent transmission.
2. Prevents transmission by making appropriate lifestyle changes.
3. Keeps environment noninfectious by cleaning.
4. Informs others of diagnosis on need-to-know basis.
5. Seeks rehabilitative services as needed.
6. Participates in informational, social, and support services.

Nursing diagnosis

Compromised family coping
Related factors: disability of child, caregiver; rigors of care/treatment; feelings of guilt, grief, fatigue; lack of support, interaction
Defining characteristics: emotional immobility; statements of inability to cope, distress, caregiver exhaustion, social isolation

OUTCOMES

Short-term
Adequate family coping evidenced by resolving negative feelings, statements of enhanced coping (expected in 1 month)

Long-term
Optimal coping abilities evidenced by adjustment to diagnosis, participation in educational/social activities, use of respite care (expected ongoing)

NURSING INTERVENTIONS/INSTRUCTIONS

1. Establish and maintain rapport and trusting relationship. Be nonjudgmental of family's disability, feelings, and responses (each visit).

2. Do not avoid touching. Use culturally acceptable space boundaries (each visit).

3. Encourage open expression of fears, concerns, questions, and misgivings. Assure family that they are not alone. Assign same health care worker. Leave agency telephone number (each visit).

4. Assess family interactions, roles, and responsibilities; perceived stressors; experiences with and knowledge of illness; established coping abilities; and sources of support and assistance (each visit).

5. Assess child's neurologic function, evidence of developmental delays, and participation in activities. Note trouble sleeping, regressive/alienating behaviors, reclusive/depressed behavior, and difficulty in school (each visit).

6. Assess caregiver's health; stamina; participation in health care regimen; and ability to tend to self, child, and home (each visit).

7. Encourage caregiver to discuss condition with child before child enters school. Discuss diagnosis; care implications; transmission; and possible affect on friends, family, and schoolmates. Explore past experiences, reaction of others, methods of defusing, and possible responses. Use dolls and role-playing as appropriate (each visit).

8. Encourage child's development. Treat child normally and integrate child into family. Offer emotional nurturing with embraces, holding, and kissing (do not kiss if herpes simplex is present on mouth or nose; use alternate expressions of affection) (each visit).

9. Inform caregiver of need to discipline child, limit behavior, and delay gratification. Refer to parenting classes or support groups for behavioral problems (e.g., biting) that influence transmission and social interactions (each visit).

10. Encourage entry of child into day-care or school in least restrictive environment. Stress need to inform caregiv-

ers and teachers of diagnosis and how to deal with problems such as scrapes and nosebleeds. Inform caregiver of rights of disclosure and confidentiality (each visit).

11. Include caregiver and child in planning care, setting goals, and implementing treatments. Encourage independence and adaptability (each visit).

12. Inform caregiver of resources for financial and legal assistance (first visit, as needed).

13. Assess grief and guilt reactions and facilitate resolution. Refer to counselor or spiritual adviser for psychologic support (as appropriate).

14. Explore sources of respite care. Refer to social services and to homemakers' assistance as needed.

15. Encourage support groups, AIDS information hotlines, and meeting of families with similar concerns (each visit).

CAREGIVER/CHILD AND FAMILY INTERVENTIONS

1. Establishes trusting relationship with health care worker.

2. Uses established coping mechanisms to deal with physical, psychologic, emotional, and social impact of disorder.

3. Seeks assistance in developing coping skills.

4. Plans and participates in self-care as well as child's.

5. Is expressive and open with family members.

6. Informs others who need to know of diagnosis with assurance of confidentiality.

7. Enrolls child in least restrictive learning environment after professional evaluation of developmental level and of exposure risk to self and others.

8. Participates in community activities and support groups.

9. Seeks legal, financial, or rehabilitative services as needed.

10. Uses respite care.

SAMPLE DOCUMENTATION INCLUSIONS

1. Specific assessment
   Family: Assess serostatus, symptoms, treatments, participation in health care, social and rehabilitative services, and coping ability.

Child: Assess serostatus; complete physical
assessment; infection, immunologic, and clinical profiles (per Centers for Disease Control and Prevention guidelines); safety; age; developmental level;
prophylactic regimen; health maintenance activities;
participation in activity; and medical and laboratory
follow-ups.

2. Specific care/teaching
   Teach information on infection prevention and transmission control; administration of medications; nutritional
   support; immunizations; recognition of adverse responses or progressive illness; what to report to
   physician; importance of ongoing care; and availability
   of social, rehabilitative, financial, and legal support
   and respite services.

3. General
   Note responses to care and teaching.

4. See "Documentation and Family Home Record Keeping" in Appendix for required documentation components for all home care visits.

 Anemia

Anemia, the most common hematologic condition of childhood, is not a disorder but a symptom of an underlying
pathologic process. Anemia, or subnormal numbers of red
blood cells (RBCs) or hemoglobin (Hg), may be the result of blood loss, inadequate RBC production, increased
RBC destruction, or a combination of these factors. It
should not be confused with benign, self-limiting physiologic
anemia of early infancy that results from the normal tran-
sition to extrauterine life. This nursing care plan addresses
three of the common anemias seen in home care, namely,
nutritional anemia, aplastic anemia, and sickle cell anemia.
Nutritional or iron deficiency anemia may be the result of
occult gastrointestinal (GI) losses. More commonly, the
cause is decreased stores after 4 months of age combined

with an iron-poor diet (i.e., unsupplemented breast milk, unsupplemented formula, or cows' milk with little solid food). It occurs during periods of rapid growth, generally between 9 and 24 months and in adolescence. Iron supplementation is the treatment of choice. Aplastic anemia is characterized by marked reduction of erythrocytes, platelets, and granulocytes (pancytopenia). It may be idiopathic or familial, often with other concurrent anomalies, or it may be acquired through exposure to drugs, radiation, toxins, chemicals, or infectious agents. Treatment includes immunosuppressive and antibiotic drug therapies, blood transfusions, and possible bone marrow transplantation. Sickle cell anemia, seen almost exclusively in the black population, is a chronic hemolytic condition, resulting from structurally abnormal, sickle-shaped, friable RBC. Anemia and vasoocclusive crises result. Multiple systems are involved. Treatment is symptomatic and may include rehydration, transfusions, antibiotic therapy, and analgesia.

Common to all anemias is decreased oxygen-carrying capacity of the blood. Clinical manifestations are related to the degree and duration of hypoxia. Physiologic adaptation and compensatory mechanisms may account for absent, delayed, or nonspecific early symptoms. Symptoms generally present themselves when Hg falls below 7 to 8 g/dl. Findings may include pallor of the skin and mucous membranes and increased heart rate. Progressively severe anemia may cause weakness, shortness of breath, vertigo, edema, and, if chronic, growth retardation and delayed sexual maturation. Morphologic classification (RBC number, size, and shape) is essential in determining the underlying pathophysiology and subsequent treatment.

Home health care is primarily concerned with assessment and nutrition counseling; energy conservation; prevention, recognition, and resolution of infection and complications; pain control; preparation for diagnostic tests and treatments; and referrals for financial assistance, information, support, and genetic counseling if indicated. Symptoms severe enough to warrant supplemental oxygen or transfusion require hospitalization.

Nursing diagnosis

Altered nutrition: less than body requirements

Related factors: inadequate iron intake or assimilation, growth requirements, chronic blood loss, caregiver's knowledge deficit or resistance to change, financial constraints

Defining characteristics: Pallor; listlessness; irritability; anorexia; poor feeding; poor weight gain; excessive weight gain ("milk baby"); decreased exercise tolerance, attention span; thin, brittle, concave-shaped nails; glossitis; tachycardia

OUTCOMES

Short-term

Adequate nutrition evidenced by appropriate diet alteration, iron supplementation (expected within 1 week)

Long-term

Optimal nutrition evidenced by sustained daily iron intake to promote growth/development (expected within 2 months)

NURSING INTERVENTIONS/INSTRUCTIONS

1. Review history including family history of congenital anemias and other disorders; client history of pica, blood loss, infection (especially hepatitis), and radiation; and use of drugs, chemotherapeutic agents, insecticides, and solvents (especially benzine compounds) (first visit).

2. Perform complete physical assessment (see specific system's assessment for guidelines) to determine current health status and impact of anemia (first visit).

3. Weigh unclothed child on same scale at same time of day. Plot on standardized graphs for children of equivalent ages and lengths (each visit).

4. Assess nutritional status including diet review; iron sources; cultural/religious restrictions; food preferences; and impact of caregiver's knowledge, traditions, and resources (first visit).

5. Assist caregiver in reconstructing typical 24-hour food intake recall for child. Include all foods and formula consumed, amounts, intervals, methods of preparation, and ethnic variations. Use information as basis for nutrition counseling. Retain or incorporate all safe traditional food practices (first visit).

6. After consultation with physician, instruct caregiver on well-balanced diet and iron-rich foods (first and second visits).

   - If bottlefeeding, feed infant formula instead of cow's milk for first year; whole milk may be used thereafter.
   - Begin iron-fortified formula at about 2 months in preterm infants and at 6 months in full-term infants. Supplement with iron at about 6 months for breast-fed infants.
   - Per physician's directive, slowly introduce solids to include iron-fortified cereals.
   - Advance diet to include iron, vitamin B_{12}, folic acid, and vitamin E. Add egg yolks, green leafy vegetables, meat, and liver.

7. Explore with adolescent client's typical intake, social meaning of food, and perceived importance of weight. Assist with diet planning (first visit, as needed).

8. Instruct caregiver on administration and implications of prescribed iron supplements (first visit, as needed).

   - Give single oral dose to infant 30 minutes before feeding.
   - Give in divided doses to older child between meals with vitamin-C beverage.
   - Do not give with milk, tea, or antacids.
   - Administer with straw or dropper to avoid staining teeth.
   - Advise that medication will turn stools green or tarry.
   - Administer multivitamins as recommended.

9. Verify compliance by estimating drug purchase date, amounts used, number of refills/purchases per month, and direct observation (if possible) of child's stools (as needed).

10. Instruct caregiver to keep scheduled physician and laboratory appointments for reappraisal of anemia status (first visit).
11. Refer to government and social services for milk, formula, and food provisions (e.g., women, infants, and children [WIC] and Aid to Families with Dependent Children [AFDC]) (first visit).

CAREGIVER/CHILD AND FAMILY INTERVENTIONS

1. Provides well-balanced, iron-rich diet.
2. Modifies diet only as needed to make positive changes.
3. Administers medications safely, regularly, and as instructed.
4. Keeps scheduled health care appointments and adapts dietary and medication regimens as recommended.
5. Uses community services as needed to receive food supplements.

Nursing diagnosis

Activity intolerance
Related factors: inadequate tissue oxygenation
Defining characteristics: weakness, lethargy, decreased exercise tolerance, fatigue

OUTCOMES

Short-term
Increased activity tolerance evidenced by increased appetite, decreased irritability, increased participation in activities (expected in 3 to 7 days)

Long-term
Optimal activity tolerance evidenced by full participation in social/school activities (expected in 1 to 3 months)

NURSING INTERVENTIONS/INSTRUCTIONS

1. Assess child's color, respirations, pulse, alertness, and posture at rest and during activity. Review with caregiver child's preferred activities and self-imposed changes (first visit).

2. Instruct caregiver to provide for adequate, uninterrupted sleep at night and quiet times during day (first visit).
3. Instruct caregiver to do the following (first visit):
   - Allow younger child to pace and regulate own activity.
   - Provide opportunities for quiet but challenging diversional activity.
   - Inform school officials who need to know about child's condition to exercise tolerance and limit strenuous activity.
4. Assist with referral to home infusion service for administration of prescribed blood, packed cells, and platelets (as needed).
5. After collaboration with physician and health care team, instruct caregiver and health care team on recognition of delayed transfusion reactions and to immediately report fever, toxic reactions, allergic manifestations, and symptoms of advancing anemia to physician.

CAREGIVER/CHILD AND FAMILY INTERVENTIONS

1. Devises and follows flexible plan for sleep, rest, and activity.
2. Limits activities that cause profound fatigue or exhaustion.
3. Confers with all teachers to modify school activities that cause undue stress or fatigue.
4. Receives blood products as prescribed.
5. Has written emergency protocol ready if adverse transfusion reactions occur (fever, severe headache, wheezing, noisy respirations, vomiting, diarrhea, or symptoms of progressing anemia).
6. Has anaphylaxis kit immediately available and uses it appropriately and competently.

Nursing diagnosis

Risk for infection
Related factors: leukopenia, altered splenic function; immunosuppressive therapy
Defining characteristics: fever; cough; cloudy, foul-smelling urine; purulent drainage from skin; ulcerations (sickle cell anemia)

OUTCOMES

Short-term
Minimal risk of infection evidenced by compliance
with prophylactic health care regimen (expected immediately)

Long-term
Minimal risk of infection evidenced by full immunization
status; compliance with prophylactic antibiotic regimen; recognition, resolution of incipient infection; optimal child
well-being within limits of underlying condition (expected in
1 month)

NURSING INTERVENTIONS/INSTRUCTIONS

1. Assess home environment and compliance with health
   care regimen (each visit).
2. Assess vital signs including temperature, general well-
   being of child. Assess pulmonary, GI, renal, and integumentary systems (see specific assessments for guidelines).
   Report aberrations to physician (each visit).
3. Instruct caregiver and client on measures to prevent infection (first visit, as needed).

   - Maintain good personal hygiene.
   - Receive adequate sleep/rest.
   - Maintain nutritious diet; do not eat raw/undercooked
     meats.
   - Wash hands before eating and after toileting.
   - Receive regular dental care.
   - Receive scheduled childhood immunizations and pneu-
     mococcal, *Haemophilus influenzae,* and hepatitis B vac-
     cines as prescribed.
   - Administer prescribed daily prophylactic anti-
     biotics, generally penicillin or amoxicillin (see
     "Medication Administration and Teaching Guide-
     lines," pp. 450-463).
   - Inform all health care providers of child's diag-
     nosis.

4. Instruct caregiver to notify physician of signs and symptoms of infection, especially elevated temperature. Instruct caregiver on temperature taking. Have client
   return demonstration (first visit).

CAREGIVER/CHILD AND FAMILY INTERVENTIONS

1. Maintains healthy lifestyle including proper diet, rest, and diversion.
2. Avoids infectious persons, carriers, and fomites.
3. Receives regular medical and dental care.
4. Receives scheduled and other specific immunizations.
5. Takes antibiotics as directed.
6. Immediately reports signs and symptoms of infection for early intervention to physician.

Nursing diagnosis

Knowledge deficit
Related factors: lack of information, lack of readiness to learn, denial
Defining characteristics: verbalized need for information about disorder, its cause, course, treatment, prognosis

OUTCOMES

Short-term
Adequate knowledge evidenced by caretaker's statement of prescribed health care regimen, of methods to prevent/control complications (expected in 1 to 2 weeks)

Long-term
Adequate knowledge evidenced by compliance with health care regimen to maintain optimal health, growth, function within limits of condition (expected in 1 month)

NURSING INTERVENTIONS/INSTRUCTIONS

1. Assess age, readiness to learn, perception of information already given, its source, internal coping abilities, and external resources (each visit).
2. Perform home safety assessment (see "Environmental Assessment," p. 37, for guidelines). Tactfully guide caretaker in identification and safe storage or disposal of toxins associated with anemia and child safety issues (e.g., insecticides, solvents, and medications) (first and second visits).

3. Assess knowledge of normal RBC functioning, diagnosis, its cause, course, treatment, and prognosis. Tailor teaching to specific anemia (ongoing).

4. If anemia has genetic cause (sickle cell anemia or Fanconi syndrome/congenital aplastic anemia), explore feelings of guilt and allow time for expression of feelings, concerns, and questions. Refer for genetic counseling when family seems ready (each visit).

5. If anemia is associated with poor outcome, provide time for anticipatory grieving. Instruct on measures to prevent/control complications and when to notify physician (each visit).

6. Assess for bleeding and notify physician of its presence. Instruct caregiver to notify physician of easy bruising, petechiae, epistaxis, and signs of overt bleeding (each visit).

7. Assess and instruct to assess for pain in child with sickle cell anemia. Note location, intensity, duration, and precipitating factors. Notify physician of findings of vasoocclusion (generally first seen as hand-foot syndrome); may also include fever, abdominal pain, other pain, and edema of extremities. Symptoms vary markedly in severity and frequency and may affect most systems (each visit).

8. Instruct caregiver on measures to promote oxygenation and minimize sickling (as needed).

   - Maintain adequate hydration. Encourage child to drink at least 150% of basic fluid requirements.
   - Limit strenuous exercise, extreme fatigue, and stress.
   - Avoid nicotine, alcohol, and high altitudes or low oxygen environments.
   - Prevent exposure to cold and infection.

9. Instruct caregiver on comfort measures during pain (as needed).

   - Keep child warm.
   - Apply warm packs (heating pad at low setting) to affected area as prescribed.
   - Administer acetaminophen, acetaminophen with codeine, meperidine, or morphine as prescribed. Ad-

minister around the clock rather than as needed. Do not give aspirin if thrombocytopenia is present.

- Notify physician of unrelieved severe pain (may require hospitalization for transfusions).

10. Instruct on implications of treatment modalities including antithymocyte globulin, corticosteroids, cyclosporine, and androgen (as needed).
11. Instruct caregiver to keep physician and laboratory appointments. Refer to special clinics as needed (first visit).
12. Refer to support groups and specialty organizations (e.g., National Association for Sickle Cell Disease) for information and assistance (first visit).

CAREGIVER/CHILD AND FAMILY INTERVENTIONS

1. States cause of disorder and its appropriate treatment.
2. Seeks genetic counseling as needed.
3. Maintains healthy lifestyle and complies with health care regimen to avoid hypoxia.
4. Controls pain by medicating before it becomes severe and by measures to facilitate vasodilation.
5. Keeps appointments with physician, laboratories, and clinics.
6. Seeks information, assistance, and support from self-help groups, specialty organizations, and social services.

SAMPLE DOCUMENTATION INCLUSIONS

1. Specific assessment
   Assess age, weight, total intake to include types and amounts, color, alertness, behavior, exercise tolerance, presence of bleeding, transfusion therapy, infection, hypoxic or vasoocclusive crises and measures to prevent or minimize these, growth/development status, environmental hazards, and adaptive capacity of family.
2. Specific care/teaching
   Teach nutrition counseling, energy conservation, infection prevention, pain and hypoxia control, recognition of complications, when to notify physician, and referrals to genetic counseling and specialty organizations.

3. General
   Note responses to care and teaching.
4. See "Documentation and Family Home Record Keeping" in Appendix for required documentation components for all home care visits.

 Hemophilia

Hemophilia is a generic term used to describe a group of genetically determined blood coagulation disorders resulting in deficiencies of clotting factors VIII, IX, or X. Hemophilia A (factor VIII deficiency), the classic disorder most commonly encountered, and Hemophilia B (factor IX deficiency, Christmas disease) are addressed here. Both are transmitted maternally as an X-linked recessive gene and affect males almost exclusively. Deficiency of these plasma proteins results in prolonged bleeding that may occur spontaneously or from trauma, minor or otherwise. Severity and symptoms of the disorder are determined by plasma concentration of clotting factors VIII and IX, as compared with normal plasma levels. Clinical severity includes mild (5% to 50% of normal factor VIII activity), moderate (1% to 5%), and severe (<1%). Most cases are severe and become evident by 12 to 18 months of age; less severe forms become apparent after bleeding episodes, resulting from mild injuries, minor medical procedures, or trauma. Bleeding may occur anywhere and may include skin, soft tissue, joints, muscles, abdominal organs, GI tract, peritoneal and retroperitoneal areas, and central nervous system (CNS). Sequelae of bleeding include hemarthrosis, arthropathy, musculoskeletal deformities, and degenerative changes. Mortality is associated with intracranial bleeding or with neck and mouth injuries that result in airway obstruction. Medical management is directed at swift replacement of plasma extracts with cryoprecipitate or factor VIII or IX concentrates. Problems associated with blood therapies may include transfusion reactions, factor VIII inhibition, and hepatitis. Current prognosis for the uncomplicated disorder is good. However, transfusions of pooled plasma given before 1985 have resulted in infection, and most hemophiliacs treated before 1985 are HIV positive (see "Nursing Care Plan, Acquired Immunodeficiency Syndrome," p. 259-281).

Home health care is primarily concerned with instruction on the prevention of injury, treatment and self-care during bleeding episodes, transfusion therapy and the prevention of complications and disability, promotion of physical growth and development and emotional well-being, and referrals for financial assistance for lifetime transfusion therapy and health care and for information and support. A multidisciplinary health team is often required.

Nursing diagnosis

Altered protection

Related factors: chronic blood clotting deficiency disorder, growth/development behaviors, caregiver/child reluctance to implement therapy

Defining characteristics: decreased factor VIII or IX on functional laboratory assays; prolonged partial thromboplastin time (PTT); recurrent bleeding episodes (spontaneous or after trauma); hematomas; hemarthrosis; hematuria; caregiver/child verbalization of helplessness, fear, frustration regarding management of disorder

OUTCOMES

Short-term
Adequate protection evidenced by identification of measures to prevent injury/procure medical assistance and active participation in measures to control bleeding (expected in 1 to 4 weeks)

Long-term
Adequate protection evidenced by compliance with health care practices to prevent/control bleeding episodes; statements of decreased anxiety, increased control; unhampered growth/development (expected within 1 month)

NURSING INTERVENTIONS/INSTRUCTIONS

1. Before visit, review hospital and physician records of diagnosis, bleeding or injury episode requiring treatment, and discharge teaching of injury prevention and administration of blood products.

2. Review familial history of disorder, perceptions, and experiences of protocols taught; receptivity for learning; internal coping strengths; and external resources for support and respite care (first and second visits).

3. Initiate instruction based on previously mentioned data. Progress from known data to unknown data. Include in instruction at least one other person involved in child care. Teach during remissions. Demonstrate and have caregiver repeat demonstration, and teach, in turn, alternate caregivers. Repeat information as needed. Provide written instructions of protocols and where to obtain assistance and telephone numbers of health care agency, physician, and hospital (each visit).

4. Assess home safety (see "Environmental Assessment," p. 37, for guidelines). Include layout; home contents; selection of furniture, games, and toys; play areas; suitable refrigeration for cold packs and prescribed blood products; and financial ability to make modifications (each visit).

5. Perform complete physical assessment. Assess hematologic status (see "Hematologic System Assessment," p. 20, for guidelines). Include age; vital signs; hemarthrosis; ecchymosis; areas of injury; measures taken to control bleeding; overt bleeding from skin or mucosa; history of hematuria or black, tarry stools; and pain. Report abnormal findings to physician (each visit).

6. Instruct caregiver and child on measures to promote safety (first and second visits).

   - Provide safe environment including padding of furniture, removal of scatter rugs and unstable or sharp objects, and gating of stairways.
   - Use personal safety items including protective padding, helmet, and electric shavers.
   - Supervise activity. Provide toys. Discourage roughhousing and physical contact sports.

- Have supply of prescribed blood replacement factors available for immediate use. Keep refrigerated or cooled per manufacturer's directions. Check expiration dates and replace as needed.

7. Instruct caregiver and child on measures to promote health and decrease risk of injury (first and second visits).

   - Receive regular health care supervision for preventive health care. Include recommended immunization schedule and hepatitis B vaccine per physician's order.
   - Practice good dental health including using soft toothbrush, brushing regularly, avoiding sweets, visiting dentist regularly, and factor replacement before dental procedures.
   - Maintain well-balanced, iron-rich diet with vitamin and mineral supplements as recommended. Maintain appropriate weight.
   - Avoid aspirin-containing medications.
   - Avoid taking rectal temperatures or using rectal suppositories or enemas. Maintain bowel function through diet and hydration.
   - Inform all health care providers of diagnosis. Request least invasive procedure as possible (e.g., oral medication instead of intramuscular injections and heelstick or fingerstick instead of venipuncture). Refer to primary physician as needed.
   - Wear identifying information including diagnosis and physician's name and telephone number.

8. Instruct caregiver to confer with school nurse, teachers, administrators, and those who need to know about condition, program modifications, and protocol for injuries (first visit).
9. Inform caregiver and child of measures to treat overt bleeding including sustained local pressure and application of gelfoam or fibrin. Notify physician or initiate emergency protocol as directed (each visit).
10. Inform caregiver and child of signs and symptoms of covert bleeding including joint pain, erythema, discolora-

tion, edema, and decreased mobility. Treat by application of cold, elevation, immobilization, and administration of blood factors as prescribed (each visit).

11. Instruct caregiver and child on administration of cryo-precipitate or factors VIII or IX for bleeding. Child may begin self-administration when ready, generally in late childhood or early adolescence (reinforce each visit). Include the following:

   - Prepare client including an explanation of treatment, emotional reassurance, taking pulse, and administration of prescribed antihistamine.
   - Provide selection of superficial vein, venipuncture technique, and aseptic technique and universal precautions.
   - Prepare blood product including checking expiration date, using plastic syringes, mixing diluents thoroughly and gently according to manufacturer's directions, and warming.
   - Slowly administer prescribed replacement factor (depending on weight of child, severity of disorder, and extent of bleeding), generally small amounts over 5 to 10 minutes.
   - Monitor hemostatic response.
   - Monitor for adverse reactions including febrile or allergic reactions. Notify physician immediately for increases in pulse or allergic symptoms. Have anaphylaxis kit available per direction.
   - Apply prolonged pressure to venipuncture insertion site after infusion.
   - Discard unused portion of drug; replacement.
   - Maintain therapy log or diary with date, time, indication for treatment, dose, response, and need for repeated infusions.

12. Instruct caregiver to immediately notify physician of signs and symptoms of internal or potentially life-threatening bleeding, including profound blood loss; head, chest, or abdominal injuries; headache; loss of consciousness; neck or throat swelling; difficulty swallowing; and dyspnea (first visit).

CAREGIVER/CHILD AND FAMILY INTERVENTIONS

1. Provides safe living environment.
2. Maintains healthy lifestyle to include appropriate diet, moderate activity, and regular medical and dental care.
3. Complies with safety precautions and encourages developmental skills.
4. Wears identifying medical information.
5. Informs babysitters, other caregivers, and teachers of condition, activity restrictions, and treatment protocol.
6. Recognizes signs and symptoms of covert and overt bleeding, intervenes appropriately, and notifies physician as needed.
7. Practices infusion preparation technique before treatment is needed. Notifies home care provider of questions and concerns.
8. Administers plasma extracts slowly, safely, and as directed during bleeding episodes.
9. Notifies physician of new or life-threatening signs and symptoms and transfusion reactions.

Nursing diagnosis

Pain

Related factors: bleeding, most frequently into joints, soft tissue, other confining body part

Defining characteristics: hemarthrosis, ill-defined feeling that something is wrong, verbal complaints, facial expression, irritability, guarding of affected area, refusal to move

OUTCOMES

Short-term
Decreased pain evidenced by statements; decreased redness/swelling of affected tissue; ability to rest/sleep (expected in 24 hours)

Long-term
Controlled pain evidenced by statements of well-being, relaxed posture, increasing mobility (expected in 48 hours)

NURSING INTERVENTIONS/INSTRUCTIONS

1. Assess for pain and pain behaviors. Assess affected site for redness, swelling, and limited mobility. Query regarding intensity using age-appropriate pain scale. Note precipitating/causative factors. After acute phase, assist in recognition and remediation of cause as indicated (each visit).
2. Monitor pain control measures (each visit).

   - Immobilize limb and align in functional position. Use splint as advised.
   - Elevate limb with pillows. Protect lower extremities by use of bed cradle.
   - Apply cold packs. If not readily available, use ice cubes in plastic bag and wrapped in towel. Thereafter, instruct on need for accessible supply of ice packs and not to use heat.
   - Administer oral analgesics, generally acetaminophen or acetaminophen with codeine as prescribed. Do not use aspirin or aspirin compounds.
   - Administer replacement factors per prescribed protocol.

3. Instruct on performance of passive range-of-motion exercises after acute phase has passed (generally 48 hours). Increase activity as symptoms abate (first visit, as needed).
4. Refer to physical therapist for rehabilitative program to prevent atrophy, contractures, and associated degenerative changes (first visit).

CAREGIVER/CHILD AND FAMILY INTERVENTIONS

1. Identifies unsafe environment or practices and corrects as appropriate.
2. Protects affected area from further injury and relieves pain through immobilization, positioning, cold packs, analgesia, and replacement therapy.
3. Keeps joints supple and functional through progressive passive and active range-of-motion and strengthening exercises.
4. Consults with physical therapist as needed for long-range rehabilitative services.

Nursing diagnosis

Ineffective family coping: compromised

Related factors: chronic nature of disorder; limited coping skills; genetic transmission of disease; distress of home infusion therapy; lack of emotional support, respite care

Defining characteristics: verbalization of inability to cope, maternal guilt; overprotective behaviors; difficulty in setting limits; inability/reluctance to perform medical therapy; anxiety about getting injured, developing AIDS

OUTCOMES

Short-term
Improved coping evidenced by caregiver's/client's appropriate limit-setting, increased social participation, receptivity to teaching of condition's cause/course (expected in 1 to 3 weeks)

Long-term
Optimal coping evidenced by participation in medical regimen, adaptation of lifestyle to facilitate physical/emotional growth, family well-being

NURSING INTERVENTIONS/INSTRUCTIONS

1. Assess family's strengths, cohesiveness, designation of roles, responsibilities, interactions, relegation of child care, sources of health care information, individual coping skills, and sources of support (each visit).
2. Establish trusting relationship. Involve entire family. Actively listen to questions, concerns, complaints, and misgivings. Draw on family's established strengths (each visit).
3. Provide accurate, current information about condition, treatment, and prognosis. Provide written information (each visit).
4. Assure family of assistance during crises. Provide agency telephone number and list of resources. Instruct on activation of Emergency Medical Service (EMS) system (each visit).

5. Instruct family on lifestyle modifications for child. Explore avenues for discipline, limit setting, fostering independence, self-reliance, and personal responsibility (each visit).
6. Be open, supportive, and nonjudgmental with adolescent client. Discuss interests, goals, career plans, and sexuality (whether HIV positive or not). Guide through career counseling and self-help groups (as needed).
7. Instruct family on need for regular medical follow-up and appointment with primary care physician, hematologist, physical therapist, dentist, and laboratory.
8. Refer to genetic counseling as needed (first visit).
9. Refer to specialty, self-help, and support groups; resource organizations; and social services for information, emotional support, and financial assistance (first visit).

CAREGIVER/CHILD AND FAMILY INTERVENTIONS

1. Develops trust in home health care provider and shares concerns about disorder and its impact on family and individual.
2. Identifies areas of need. Seeks assistance.
3. Assists and reinforces others in providing care.
4. Keeps telephone numbers for assistance and emergency services next to telephone.
5. Modifies lifestyle as indicated to enhance safety and well-being.
6. Keeps scheduled appointments for continuing health care.
7. Contacts National Hemophilia Foundation, church, school, and community and government agencies for assistance.

SAMPLE DOCUMENTATION INCLUSIONS

1. Specific assessment
   Assess age, weight, vital signs, developmental milestones, signs of overt/covert bleeding, diary of bleeding episodes, severity and duration of bleeding, replacement units needed, infusion technique, environmental hazards, and availability and accessibility of cold packs and fresh replacement factors.

2. Specific care/teaching
   Teach aseptic, venipuncture infusion therapy; signs and symptoms of bleeding; how to control bleeding and pain; when to contact physician; universal precautions; monitoring of response; and importance of laboratory and medical follow-ups.
3. General
   Note responses to care and teaching.
4. See "Documentation and Family Home Record Keeping" in Appendix for required documentation components for all home care visits.

 Hyperbilirubinemia

Hyperbilirubinemia refers to excess blood bilirubin levels that produce jaundice (icterus), the yellow discoloration of skin, sclerae, and mucous membranes that may indicate hepatic damage. Bilirubin is the insoluble by-product of heme degradation, and its accumulation may be the result of excessive RBC breakdown, decreased excretion, or altered metabolism. Jaundice becomes evident when bilirubin levels reach 5 to 7 mg/dl. Jaundice is a common occurrence in newborns and is frequently benign, as in physiologic jaundice or, less commonly, in breastfeeding-associated jaundice. Jaundice may be considered pathologic when bilirubin levels exceed parameters (e.g., 12 mg/dl in the full-term, formula-fed infant or 15 mg/dl in the full-term, breast-fed, preterm or low–birth-weight infant; when levels increase by 5 mg/dl/day; when direct bilirubin exceeds 1 mg/dl; or when jaundice persists past physiologic parameters). The pathologic condition is associated with erythroblastosis or congenital hemolytic disease; maternal diabetes, infection, or drug use; medications; enclosed hemorrhage; prematurity; sepsis; acidosis; polycythemia; hypoxia; hypoglycemia; or hepatocellular damage. Unconjugated bilirubin (indirect reacting) is neurotoxic, and its deposition in the basal ganglia and brain stem nuclei results

in encephalopathy (kernicterus). Conjugated (direct reacting) bilirubin, although not neurotoxic, may, in elevated levels, signal hepatic damage or biliary tract disease.
Cause is determined by careful history taking and clinical and laboratory assessments. Jaundice is best evaluated by blood bilirubin levels because its intensity is not related to severity.

Jaundice in the newborn period is of special concern in home health care because of early hospital discharge (frequently within 24 hours of birth) and limited or delayed follow-up. Physiologic jaundice results from developmental immaturity, peaks between 2 to 5 days after birth, and is generally self-limiting and without clinical consequences. Jaundice associated with breastfeeding is managed by temporary cessation of breastfeeding. Elevated bilirubin levels of 18 to 20 mg/dl in full-term infants (10 mg/dl in pre-term infants) are treated with phototherapy. Phototherapy, through a process of photoisomerization, renders bilirubin water soluble and excretable. Exchange transfusions may be necessary for pathologic, hemolytic, unconjugated hyperbilirubinemia occurring within 24 hours after birth or for high kernicteric risk based on bilirubin levels greater than 20 mg/dl, gestational age and weight, and clinical profile.

Home health care is primarily concerned with identification and assessment of jaundice, recognition of complications (neurologic manifestations or sepsis), instruction on home phototherapy for uncomplicated, nonprogressive disease, and caregiver support.

Nursing diagnosis

Knowledge deficit
Related factors: lack of information about underlying disorder; inadequate hospital discharge planning; lack of readiness to learn; complexity, rigor of home phototherapy; lack of assistance, support
Defining characteristics: request for information about disorder, its nature, course, implications; about infant care; phototherapy

OUTCOMES

Short-term
Adequate knowledge evidenced by caregiver's statements of symptoms, management of newborn, caregiver's demonstration of therapy protocols, precautions (expected immediately)

Long-term
Adequate knowledge evidenced by compliance with therapeutic protocols, uncomplicated course of therapy, optimal infant status (expected within 1 week)

NURSING INTERVENTIONS/INSTRUCTIONS

1. Assess caregiver's perception of newborn's condition, cause, course, resolution of disorder, readiness to learn, learning style, willingness to participate in therapy, ability to follow instructions, and sources of support and assistance (first visit).
2. Instruct caregivers about generally benign course of disorder and need for around-the-clock vigilance during phototherapy (generally 1 to 3 days). Repeat information as needed. Provide clear, written directions. Reassure. Provide agency telephone numbers (each visit).
3. Review maternal history of diabetes, infection, medication profile, and oxytocin-induced or traumatic delivery; sibling history of neonatal jaundice; and infant's gestational age, status at birth, history of infection, hypoxia, feeding schedule, blood bilirubin levels, hemoglobin, hematocrit, reticulocytes, and peripheral smear (first visit).
4. Assess all body surfaces of jaundiced infant in full, natural light. Depress skin surface and release and note color. Note color of sclerae, mucous membranes (especially on darker skinned infants), urine, and stool. Concurrently reassure caregiver that intensity of jaundice is not related to severity of condition (each visit).
5. Perform complete physical assessment (see specific assessments for guidelines). Note weight; gestational age; feeding method; temperature; neurologic status and Moro reflex; levels of alertness, irritability, and consolability; poor feeding; and vomiting (each visit).

6. Instruct caregivers on preparation of environment and handling of overhead light phototherapy unit (first visit, reinforce as needed).

   - Review manufacturer's instructions for specific phototherapy unit. Note local supplier's telephone number.
   - Place unit away from drafts, vents, and blowers.
   - Maintain room temperature at 72° F. Maintain optimal humidity.
   - Demonstrate crib probe for measurement of unit temperature and photointensity. Repeat until proficient.
   - Maintain, as indicated, high-intensity light source 30 inches from crib.
   - Maintain Plexiglas shield between infant and light sources to protect from ultraviolet rays and possible bulb breakage.
   - Maintain bedside log; every 2 hours, note room and crib temperatures, photointensity, light distance from infant, time of exposure, and body surface exposed.

7. Instruct caregivers on preparation and care of infant during prescribed overhead light phototherapy (first visit, reinforce as needed).

   - Depending on model type, apply eye patches over infant's closed eyes. Secure. Do not obstruct nose or mouth. Report any eye irritation or discharge to physician.
   - Position unclothed infant on side or abdomen and cover genitals with mini diaper.
   - Turn infant every 2 hours. Remove infant from unit for feedings or when fussy and remove eye patches, if used.
   - Change wet or soiled bedding frequently to prevent chilling or skin irritation. Reassure that loose stools are common occurrence and that green-brown stools and dark urine are evidence of desired excretion.
   - Delay bathing. Cleanse as necessary.
   - Take temperature, per physician's orders, every 2 hours until stabilized and then every 4 hours. Regulate room temperature accordingly. If infant is chilled, cover with blanket and retake temperature.

For sustained elevations or alterations, notify physician.

- Do not use lotions. Notify physician of marked erythema, blistering, or signs of dehydration. Reassure caregiver of transient and benign nature of maculopapular skin rash or bronzing.

8. Instruct caregivers on measures to promote hydration during overhead light phototherapy (first visit, reinforce as needed).

  - Feed frequently. Increase fluid intake up to 25% and supplement formula with water per physician's order. Calculation of fluid requirement is based on weight, body surface, and metabolic rate.
  - Breastfeed 8 to 10 times daily. Supplement with water per physician's recommendation.
  - Weigh daily.
  - Note number, color, and consistency of stools and number of diaper or padding changes (normally six or more wet diapers per day).
  - Notify physician of percentage of weight loss, decreased intake from pedetermined minimum, decreased output, and vomiting.

9. Instruct caregivers on establishment and maintenance of log to include 4-hour measurements or assessments of infant's temperature, position, time under light, eye protection, intake, feeding pattern, total output, and condition of skin (each visit).

10. Alternately instruct caregiver on prescribed use of fiberoptic device (Wallaby, Biliblanket) (binder-like appliance wrapped around infant and plugged into energy source). Include care of newborn, skin care, and safety precautions (first visit, reinforce as needed).

11. Perform heel stick for bilirubin and hematocrit as ordered. Correlate laboratory findings with assessment data and log review. Confer with physician (each visit).

12. Instruct caregivers on signs and symptoms to report to physician including spreading jaundice (cephalocaudal progression); fever; poor feeding; vomiting; lethargy; irritability; high, shrill cry; twitching; bleeding; and opisthotonos (each visit).

13. Instruct caregivers on need for regular follow-up health care visits. Should encephalopathy occur even after crisis resolution, child will need to be monitored for developmental delays, neurologic deficits, auditory and visual impairment, and learning disabilities (as indicated).

CAREGIVER/CHILD AND FAMILY INTERVENTIONS

1. Verbalizes cause of hyperbilirubinemia and rationale for treatment.
2. Verbalizes desire and ability to have home phototherapy. Seeks assistance when needed.
3. Enlists support and assistance of other caregivers to provide around-the-clock infant care and caregiver respite care.
4. Operates overhead light phototherapy unit safely and as directed.

   - Maintains equipment and care log.
   - Keeps infant in view at all times.
   - Monitors infant status every 2 to 4 hours and maintains safe thermal environment.
   - Provides appropriate eye and skin protection. Protects from fluid deficit.

5. Uses fiberoptic device safely and as directed.

   - Monitors infant status at least every 2 to 4 hours as indicated.
   - Keeps skin under appliance irritation-free.
   - Handles child appropriately for feeding and emotional nurturing.
   - Removes appliance for bathing and cleansing.

6. Notifies physician of signs and symptoms of light therapy-related hyperthermia, dehydration, or deteriorating neurologic status.

Nursing diagnosis

Risk for altered parent-infant attachment
Related factors: infant health status, phototherapy, caregiver fatigue

Defining characteristics: presence of ill/premature infant unable to initiate, sustain caregiver contact; physical barriers of phototherapy unit; verbalized, demonstrated caregiver anxiety

OUTCOMES

Short-term
Adequate attachment evidenced by compliance with physical/emotional components of therapy (expected immediately)

Long-term
Optimal emotional health and family interaction evidenced by positive bonding behaviors, increasing caregiver-infant attachment (expected ongoing)

NURSING INTERVENTIONS/INSTRUCTIONS

1. Assess family interactions (see "Psychologic and Family Assessments," pp. 25 and 41, for guidelines). Note bonding and attachment behaviors, influence of culture, coping abilities, and sources of assistance and support (each visit).
2. Query caregiver regarding experiences with sick children and established methods of positive parenting. Reinforce strengths. Assist with skill development as needed (each visit).
3. Instruct caregivers on measures to promote caregiver-infant attachment (each visit).

   - Talk, croon, and sing to infant when in unit.
   - Remove infant from unit for feedings. Remove patches and assess eyes. Encourage face-to-face contact, visual stimulation, touch, and body massage.
   - Encourage continuation of breastfeeding. If temporary cessation of breastfeeding is medically advised, instruct on expression of breast milk and its safe handling and storage.
   - Reassure caregiver of short course of therapy and benign nature of disorder.

CAREGIVER/CHILD AND FAMILY INTERVENTIONS

1. Uses past child-rearing experiences and coping strategies to effectively deal with sick infant and demands of therapy.

2. Provides safe care, comfort, and sensory stimulation to infant.
3. Demonstrates caregiver bonding and infant attachment.

SAMPLE DOCUMENTATION INCLUSIONS

1. Specific assessment
   Assess color of skin, sclerae, and mucous membranes; blood bilirubin and hematocrit; gestational age; weight; vital signs including temperature, developmental level, and neurologic status; level of alertness; feeding pattern; intake; output; type and model of phototherapy device used; evidence of dehydration; skin irritation, redness, blistering, bronzing; eye irritation, discharge; signs of progressive disease; adaptive capacity of family and bonding behaviors; compliance with safe use of photo-therapy unit; appropriate infant care; and care and equipment logs.
2. Specific care/teaching
   Teach care of overhead light phototherapy unit or fi-beroptic appliance; safety precautions; temperature con-trol for former; and infant care including feeding, posi-tioning, temperature regulation, cleansing, eye and skin precautions, sensory stimulation, recognition of com-plications, and need for follow-up.
3. General
   Note responses to care and teaching.
4. See "Documentation and Family Home Record Keep-ing" in Appendix for required documentation compo-nents for all home care visits.

Musculoskeletal system

 Congenital Hip Dysplasia

Congenital hip dysplasia, also known as *dislocation of the hip,* is an abnormality that presents at birth of one or both hips of various degrees of severity. The dislocation, more common in girls, ranges from mild lateral to complete displacement of the femoral head out of the acetabulum. It results from malpositioning of the fetus, arthritis, meningocele, and spastic or palsy neurologic conditions. Treatment of the condition for infants up to 6 months of age includes maintenance of the joint by splinting with an abduction device such as Pavlik harness, a brace, or double diapering. Traction can also be applied to slowly stretch the hip, followed by placement of a hip spica cast if stability cannot be attained. This cast is changed to adapt to the child's growth pattern. Treatment for children diagnosed at ages 6 to 18 months includes traction for reduction followed by cast application to immobilize and stabilize the joint. Open reduction followed by cast application to correct the abnormality and subsequent rehabilitation usually is performed if the diagnosis is made later, up to 6 years of age.

Home care is primarily concerned with assessment and teaching of long-term cast or brace/splint maintenance and appropriate skin care, ongoing comfort, and activity needs of the growing child.

Nursing diagnosis

Risk for injury
Related factors: internal physical factors of effects of corrective cast, brace, other appliance
Defining characteristics: unfamiliar with proper application of appliance, lack of safety precautions

OUTCOMES

Short-term
Risk for injury minimized evidenced by recognition, treatment of abnormality, proper hip joint maintenance (expected within 1 to 2 weeks)

Long-term
Restoration of normal hip joint physiology, function evidenced by successful long-term application of cast/device resulting in correction of displacement (expected ongoing)

NURSING INTERVENTIONS/INSTRUCTIONS

1. Perform complete physical assessment. Assess age and type of dislocation, treatment, and reduction device (cast or brace) (first visit).
2. Perform postoperative care if surgery was performed (see "Hospital Follow-up Home Care," pp. 370-375) (each visit).
3. Assess vital signs, instruct to assess cast for tightness, redness, musty odor, drainage, and pain indicating infection following surgery, and report complications (first visit).
4. Instruct on application of Pavlik harness, protective abduction brace, or splint continuously, as applicable, and if removal is permitted to ensure correction desired (first and second visits).
5. For infant, instruct on application of splint over diaper and use of disposable diapers or plastic pants (first visit).
6. Instruct to handle and position infant carefully to avoid any injury or displacement of device (first visit).
7. If cast is in place, instruct to protect cast from trauma, cracking, and soiling by covering with plastic during elimination, frequently changing diapers, cleaning with water and vinegar if not fiberglass cast, and not lifting cast (spica) by crossbar (first visit).
8. Instruct how to finance and acquire seats and other assistive aids designed for child with device in place. Suggest resources to acquire needed equipment (any visit).
9. Instruct to feed infant in supine position with head elevated and hip and leg supported on pillows, by holding infant in lap supported with pillows or with infant

seated in modified high chair or car seat (first and second visits).

10. Instruct caregivers on correct lifting methods (first and second visits).

CAREGIVER/CHILD AND FAMILY INTERVENTIONS

1. Maintains continuous and correct hip joint position by maintenance of splint or brace. Applies correct lifting and positioning techniques.
2. Protects apparatus or cast to keep dry and intact.
3. Provides child with appropriate assistance or assistive aids for safe care and basic needs of nutrition, stimulation, and elimination.
4. Reports signs and symptoms of infection to health care provider.
5. Secures or rents equipment and supplies.

Nursing diagnosis

Risk for impaired skin integrity
Related factors: external factors of pressure of cast, physical immobilization
Defining characteristics: irritation, redness, edema of skin at cast edges, bony prominences

OUTCOMES

Short-term
Minimal risk for skin breakdown evidenced by elimination of pressure from cast/splint with absence of pain, redness, irritation of skin (expected within 3 to 4 days)

Long-term
Optimal skin integrity at cast/splint site evidenced by skin intact in areas of bony prominences, integrity maintained (expected ongoing until device removed)

NURSING INTERVENTIONS/INSTRUCTIONS

1. Assess skin at edges of cast, splint, or appliance used to immobilize joint. Note redness, irritation, pain, or breaks in skin and instruct to report to health care provider (each visit).

2. Petal edges of cast/device with soft adhesive. Instruct on replacement of this petaling technique (first visit).
3. Instruct caregiver and child to avoid sticking things such as food or toys into cast that can cause friction or irritation (first visit).
4. Instruct on cleansing skin by giving sponge bath and massaging during bath (if device can be removed) or around cast, changing diapers frequently, tucking or fastening diaper or sanitary napkin beneath perineal opening, and using plastic wrap around perianal area of cast to prevent soiling and irritation of skin (first and second visits).
5. Instruct on padding shoulder pressure points if Pavlik harness is applied. Avoid using lotions and powders.
6. Instruct caregiver on need for frequent position change and methods of turning and positioning.

CAREGIVER/CHILD AND FAMILY INTERVENTIONS

1. Assesses skin daily at cast site or during removal of device if permitted.
2. Pads pressure points around cast edges and other areas if needed.
3. Prevents accumulation of irritants on skin by bathing, drying, and maintaining skin integrity under and around device.
4. Performs frequent position changes.

Nursing diagnosis

Risk for peripheral neurovascular dysfunction
Related factors: mechanical compression (spica cast, splint), orthopedic surgery
Defining characteristics: pallor or cyanotic color, coolness of skin at cast edges, change/loss of sensation proximal to cast edges, decreased peripheral pulses

OUTCOMES
Short-term
Neurovascular function preserved evidenced by temperature, color, sensation, pulse within normal parameters (expected within 3 to 4 days)

Long-term
Optimal benefit from cast/splint application without complications evidenced by maintenance of intact neurologic/ circulatory function until abnormality is corrected, immobilization device is removed (expected during length of immobilization)

NURSING INTERVENTIONS/INSTRUCTIONS

1. Assess child's feet or casted limbs for neurovascular complications. Instruct caregiver to assess for pain, tightness, color of digits (pallor, cyanosis), warmth or coolness at cast edges, numbness or loss of sensation, and movement of digits (each visit).
2. Assess and instruct to assess bilateral peripheral pedal pulses and capillary refill and to compare twice daily (first visit).
3. Instruct to report complications and any cracks or breaks in cast to physician (first visit).
4. Assess for edema and instruct caregiver to elevate extremity (as needed).

CAREGIVER/CHILD AND FAMILY INTERVENTIONS

1. Assesses neurovascular status of casted area every 2 hours or daily for changes in sensation, swelling, movement, or capillary refill time.
2. Maintains positioning, turning, and comfort to casted limbs. Avoids picking up or turning limbs by cast rod.
3. Reports neurovascular abnormalities to health care provider for corrective measures.

Nursing diagnosis

Impaired physical mobility
Related factors: musculoskeletal impairment, growth/development deficit with imposed immobilization
Defining characteristics: inability to purposefully move within physical environment, reluctance to move, imposed restriction of movement (cast, splint, appliance), constipation, joint deterioration viewed on radiography or tomography

OUTCOMES

Short-term
Maintains movement within environment evidenced by increased tolerance to activity within limitations (cast, splint), progressive ambulation (expected within 1 week)

Long-term
Maximizes movement evidenced by independent movement to fullest extent, participation in activities, absence of complications of immobility (expected within 1 month)

NURSING INTERVENTIONS/INSTRUCTIONS

1. Assess for movement restrictions such as limited weight bearing, splint, bivalved or full-cast, bed rest, or amount of movement in bed allowed (see "Musculoskeletal System Assessment," p. 21, for guidelines) (any visit as needed).
2. Assess for type of immobilization apparatus (Pavlik harness, abduction brace, or cast) (first visit).
3. Assess and instruct to assess for complications of immobility such as anorexia, bowel or urinary alterations, muscular weakness, and pulmonary infection (each visit).
4. Instruct to change position of infant frequently if movement is compromised or position properly if immobilizing apparatus is in place (first visit).
5. Discuss and collaborate on purposes of mobility, need for progressive healing, correction, planning for stimulation, motivation to move within environment, and placing child near safe window if immobile (first and second visits).
6. Assist to establish play/exercise program that complies with restriction in movement and encourages interaction with peers (any visit).
7. Perform range-of-motion (ROM) exercises to limbs when allowed. Instruct caregiver to perform this procedure daily (first visit, reinforce).
8. Instruct on positioning and supporting splinted or casted limb and using other extremities to perform self-care and to engage in play activities. Instruct on supervising safe movement with use of assistive aids (first and second visits).

9. Instruct to use crutches, if permitted, with single leg-hip spica cast (any appropriate visit).
10. Obtain order for rehabilitation referral for exercises and mobility and dietary inclusions of fiber, calcium, and juices if needed postoperatively (any visit).

CAREGIVER/CHILD AND FAMILY INTERVENTIONS

1. Schedules and assists or participates in daily activities as tolerated.
2. Avoids extremes in activity and allows for as much independence as possible. Increases activities daily as endurance and healing allow.
3. Establishes recreation, study, and exercise programs within identified restrictions as healing progresses.
4. Uses assistive aids or devices adapted for immobilization or ambulation if needed (wheelchair, crutches, scooter, or stroller). Protects affected limbs during activity.
5. Modifies environment for safe movement.
6. Selects play activities that can be performed in prone position, on floor, or in seats devised to protect casted or splinted extremities.
7. Follows recommendations of physical therapist to maintain mobility, muscle tone, and ROM.

Nursing diagnosis

Altered family processes
Related factors: situational crisis of infant with congenital physical abnormality
Defining characteristics: age of child; degree of dislocation; fear, anxiety about prognosis, providing care; family unable to meet physical/emotional needs of members and child; lack of information, knowledge about disability; possible future surgical correction; inability of child and family members to express/accept feelings, adapt to child's needs

OUTCOMES

Short-term
Beginning progress toward family acceptance of and adaptation to child with abnormality evidenced by

open communication among family members regarding understanding of abnormality; discussion of fears, concerns about child's special needs; ability to provide care; effect on family (expected within 1 to 2 weeks)

Long-term
Development and fostering of positive behaviors, attitudes, interactions that support child's, family members' lifestyle changes evidenced by demonstration of effective coping skills; confidence in child's and family's abilities; ability to set goals, plan care; early participation in care, problem-solving; seeks information, understanding, support (expected within 1 to 2 months)

NURSING INTERVENTIONS/INSTRUCTIONS

1. Assess level of development as family, stressors on family and extended family, effect of child's chronic illness on parents' and siblings' behavior (protective, nurturing, supportive, disruptive, neglectful, or use of coping mechanisms), and ability to adjust to diagnosis and participate in care planning (see "Family Assessment," p. 41, for guidelines) (first and second visits).
2. Assess feelings of family members and allow them to express their concerns (fears, anxiety, guilt, and grief) regarding responsibilities involved in providing care and support to one another (each visit).
3. Encourage open communication among family members and inform them of importance of maintaining own health and social activities and support from friends (first visit).
4. Discuss family's reaction to child and abnormality. Emphasize positive family relationships and coping mechanisms. Discuss child's positive abilities, potential, and limitations (each visit).
5. Suggest referral to family counselor, local agencies, support group, financial resources, or respite care. Introduce family to child with similar condition (any visit).

CAREGIVER/CHILD AND FAMILY INTERVENTIONS

1. Verbalizes feelings and concerns and resolves reactions and negative behaviors toward child and within family.
2. Identifies problems within family and role changes and types of assistance needed. Works together to solve problems as they arise (immediate and long-term).
3. Promotes and demonstrates adjustment and adaptation to diagnosis and its long-term implications.
4. Reduces own anxiety and negative feelings about abnormality and prognosis of condition.
5. Gains confidence in ability to cope with child's needs and effect on family harmony. Includes child in family activities.
6. Demonstrates positive growth-promoting behaviors in family and child by interacting with other families and seeking support from community resources.

SAMPLE DOCUMENTATION INCLUSIONS

1. Specific assessment
   Assess age, developmental status, verbal/nonverbal responses to immobilization, postoperative status, signs and symptoms of infection, type and effect of immobilization device, skin and neurovascular status, amount of independence in self-care, and growth/developmental needs.
2. Specific care/teaching
   Teach care of cast, appliance, and skin; expected responses to devices, immobilization, and positioning; comfort; limb protection; use of assistive aids (wheelchair, car seat, or crutches); nutritional requirements; and appropriate stimulating activities.
3. General
   Note responses to care and teaching, goal achievement, changes or modifications of plan, importance of medical follow-up, and contact with health care provider and community support groups.
4. See "Documentation and Family Home Record Keeping" in Appendix for general required documentation components for all home care visits.

Juvenile Rheumatoid Arthritis

Juvenile rheumatoid arthritis, also known as *juvenile chronic polyarthritis,* is a systemic chronic inflammatory disease of the joints, connective tissue, and organ systems. There is no known cause, but the disease is believed to be associated with immunodeficiency. It is characterized by remissions and exacerbations of the symptoms. It results in joint effusion, and its long-term nature causes erosion and eventual destruction of the cartilage of the joint surfaces. Three types exist based on manifestations of the disease and include systemic onset with pain, decreased mobility, temperature, rash, and organ involvement (heart, eyes, liver, spleen, and lymphatics). Monarticular or pauciarticular types involve one or up to five joints and include swelling, anorexia, poor weight gain, and low-grade fever. The polyarticular type involves more than five joints and includes pain and stiffness, involvement of large joints, tissue swelling, anorexia, fatigue, and a low-grade to high temperature.

Home care is primarily concerned with physical management and teaching to relieve signs and symptoms that affect the lifestyle of the child and family and the preservation of musculoskeletal function by preventing deterioration and deformity of affected joints.

Nursing diagnosis

Chronic pain
Related factors: physical injuring agents (one or more joints, organ involvement)
Defining characteristics: verbal/nonverbal communication of pain based on child's age (joint stiffness, pain, swelling, warmth at large and small joints, irritability, weakness, loss of movement) (see "Pain Management," pp. 398-402)

OUTCOMES

Short-term
Comfort with minimal pain evidenced by effective response to analgesic therapy; ability to move, engage in activities without pain (expected within 3 weeks)

Long-term
Optimal relief or control of pain evidenced by reduction in exacerbations of signs, symptoms of inflammatory process; ability to engage in rehabilitation; ROM exercises (expected within 4 weeks)

NURSING INTERVENTIONS/INSTRUCTIONS

1. Assess child's response to pain (see "Nursing Interventions/Instructions on Pain Management," pp. 400-401) (each visit, if needed).

2. Assess pain severity, joints or body parts involved, loss of movement, fever, other symptoms of active inflammation, known joint destruction, and joint deformities (when needed).

3. Instruct on administration of antipyretic and longterm analgesic therapy (nonsteroidal antiinflammatory drugs, slow-acting antirheumatic drugs, corticosteroids, or cytotoxic drugs) as prescribed, depending on individual responses and debilitation with dose, frequency based on responses of temperature, pain relief, and potential for compliance (see "Medication Administration and Teaching Guidelines," pp. 450-463) (each visit until all aspects of regimen completed).

4. Collaborate to plan and maintain anticipatory drug schedule and to coordinate medication for pain 30 minutes before activities. Instruct on signs and symptoms of toxicity and prevention of stomach irritation (first visit).

5. Instruct to position and protect affected joints to prevent additional pressure or injury (first visit).

6. Instruct on need to immobilize (splint) and avoid movement of painful joints, if ordered (first visit).

7. Provide and instruct on application of heat to joints such as warm soaks, wet packs, and tub baths in morning to treat painful areas (first and second visits).

CAREGIVER/CHILD AND FAMILY INTERVENTIONS

1. Maintains painful joints in position of comfort.
2. Administers correct analgesic. Complies with regimen based on planned schedule and pain assessment. Monitors for gastric irritation.
3. Institutes nonpharmacologic measures to relieve pain.
4. Performs heat treatments to painful areas.
5. Uses diversional activities during painful episodes.
6. Avoids environmental changes and overactivity that can affect joints.
7. Notes unrelieved pain and reports to health care provider for adjustment in regimen.

Nursing diagnosis

Impaired physical mobility
Related factors: pain, discomfort; musculoskeletal impairment; decreased strength, endurance
Defining characteristics: inability or reluctance to move, imposed restriction of movement, deterioration of joint function

OUTCOMES
Short-term
Maintains movement evidenced by increased tolerance to activity within limits (cast, splint), progressive ambulation, play, rest (expected within 1 week)

Long-term
Maximizes movement evidenced by independent movement to fullest extent; participation in activities based on age, developmental level; absence of complications of immobility (contractures, atrophy, joint dislocation) (expected within 1 month)

NURSING INTERVENTIONS/INSTRUCTIONS
1. Assess for movement restrictions such as altered weight bearing, splint, bed rest, or amount of movement in bed allowed; activity tolerance; endurance; muscle strength; and deformities (see "Musculoskeletal System Assessment," p. 21, for guidelines) (any visit as needed).

2. Collaborate with caregiver, child, and interdisciplinary team to assess and plan for progressive mobility, protection of joints from injury, and prevention of complication of iridocyclitis or spondyloarthropathy (first and second visits).

3. Instruct on importance of posture and body mechanics during rest and activity (first visit).

4. Instruct to incorporate exercises and regular rest periods into play activities to avoid fatigue (first visit).

5. Instruct to perform physical and occupational regimen such as passive ROM to joints when allowed and muscle strengthening exercises (first visit, reinforce).

6. Instruct on positioning and supporting affected areas to reduce possibility of deformity, to apply splints to prevent contractures, and to use sandbags or other immobilizing aids to maintain position during acute phases (first and second visits).

7. Instruct to encourage and supervise exercises and therapeutic play such as swimming in warm water, ball tossing, bicycle riding, walking, dancing, or other activities (first and second visits, if needed).

CAREGIVER/CHILD AND FAMILY INTERVENTIONS

1. Schedules and assists or participates in daily activities as tolerated.

2. Provides firm mattress for sleeping to maintain body alignment and electric blanket at lowest setting under sheet to provide heat, if appropriate. Monitors scrupulously to prevent thermal injury.

3. Applies splint or other appliances correctly. Uses crutches if weight-bearing is restricted.

4. Avoids extremes in activity and allows for as much independence as possible. Increases activities daily as endurance and disease status allow.

5. Establishes recreation, study, and exercise programs within identified restrictions and provides rest periods, as needed, to avoid overactivity.

6. Uses assistive aids/devices (wheelchair and splints) for immobilization or ambulation if needed to protect affected areas during activity.

7. Establishes self-care program within parameters recommended by physical therapist to maintain mobility, muscle tone, and ROM.
8. Attends school and advises school nurse and teacher to permit medications and limit activities if necessary.

Nursing diagnosis

Self-care deficit (bathing/hygiene, dressing/grooming, feeding, toileting)
Related factors: musculoskeletal impairment, pain, impaired mobility status
Defining characteristics: impaired ability to perform/complete bathing, dressing, undressing, eating meals, using bathroom; fatigue; limited energy

OUTCOMES

Short-term
Ability to perform self-care activities within imposed restrictions evidenced by participation in activities such as eating, personal hygiene, toileting, play, rest (expected within 1 to 2 weeks)

Long-term
Maximum capability, independence in achieving self-care activities during remissions of disease evidenced by full participation in activities without fatigue (expected within 3 weeks)

NURSING INTERVENTIONS/INSTRUCTIONS

1. Perform complete physical assessment. Assess movement capability, use of joints for daily routine activities within limitations or imposed restrictions, energy level, and tendency for fatigue (each visit).
2. Instruct on application of splints and when to use them for participation in activities (first visit, reinstruct as needed).
3. Instruct to revise daily routines, to modify plan to encourage participation, and to avoid activity during pain or acute phases (first visit).

4. Encourage optimal independence in activities of daily living (ADL) without fatigue (each visit).
5. Identify and instruct caregiver and child to note need and select assistive aids to allow for self-care activities with minimum pain (modified eating, personal hygiene utensils, use of tongs and handrails, modified clothing with fasteners to dress and undress, and toilet seat) (first visit).
6. Encourage and praise child for independent function (each visit).
7. Refer to occupational therapist as necessary (any visit).

CAREGIVER/CHILD AND FAMILY INTERVENTIONS

1. Modifies home environment to facilitate independence in self-care.
2. Provides necessary assistive and adaptive aids to encourage self-care. Supervises use of aids for safety and effectiveness.
3. Prevents injury to joints by restricting self-care. Provides assistance if needed for ADL.
4. Encourages and praises all efforts to perform self-care in daily routines.
5. Encourages child to interact with peers, family, therapists, and social worker.
6. Complies with plans for progressive ADL that prevent excessive strain on joints.
7. Participates in occupational therapy program.

Nursing diagnosis

Ineffective family coping/individual coping (child): compromised

Related factors: prolonged disease that exhausts supportive capacity of significant people, family disorganization

Defining characteristics: significant person's expression of inability to cope, feelings of fear, anxiety, guilt, anger, inadequate understanding of chronic illness, long-term care by family; inability of child to cope, ask for help; chronic fatigue, anxiety of child; changing roles, family relationships

OUTCOMES

Short-term
Family members demonstrate ability to plan, care for child evidenced by provision of normal environment; decreased anxiety, feelings of inadequacy; integration of information about family needs into care, support of child (expected within 1 to 2 weeks)

Long-term
Family coping, adaptation evidenced by optimal support, participation in care, maintenance of family relationships (expected within 1 to 2 months)

NURSING INTERVENTIONS/INSTRUCTIONS

1. Meet and collaborate with family members to assess stressors, coping mechanisms, and planning of care (first visit, repeat as needed).
2. Reinforce information to promote family understanding of illness, care needs, remissions, and exacerbations of disease (each visit).
3. Discuss and allow family to express feelings of guilt, anxiety, and depression. Promote communication among family members to verbalize feelings and expectations (any visit).
4. Instruct on methods to develop appropriate coping skills and to meet family's needs (medical, emotional, financial, food, respite care, supplies, and equipment) by referral to social or counseling services (each visit as needed).
5. Refer parent to Juvenile Arthritis Foundation for information and support (as needed).

CAREGIVER/CHILD AND FAMILY INTERVENTIONS

1. Displays decreasing anxiety and anger. Provides supportive family environment.
2. Develops trust in home care personnel. Collaborates in developing and modifying daily care.
3. Provides care and treatments effectively. Supports child during painful and restrictive periods or when feeling most vulnerable and not able to participate in daily routines with family or friends.

4. Avoids overprotection or rejection of child by caregiver or family. Encourages play activities to comfort level and promotes self-care activities.
5. Recognizes and assumes role changes. Maintains family integrity.
6. Develops coping mechanisms that have positive effect within family.
7. Identifies problem areas and obtains community or professional assistance or social services as needed.

SAMPLE DOCUMENTATION INCLUSIONS

1. Specific assessment
   Assess age, developmental status, verbal/nonverbal responses to pain, type and responses to medication regimen (analgesic, antipyretic, or sedative), responses to immobilization, type and effect of immobilization device, activity level, if chair-bound or bed-bound, amount of independence in self-care, growth/developmental needs, stressors of caregiver and child and their effect on treatment regimen, family and child coping ability to comply with long-term management, possibility of self-monitoring, and signs and symptoms of complications.
2. Specific care/teaching
   Teach disease; signs and symptoms; administration of medication regimen to include name, dose, frequency, route, times of day, special considerations based on form, side effects, and expected response; use and care of splints or other devices, and body part immobilization; positioning; comfort; protection of affected parts; use of assistive aids; varied heat treatments; nutritional requirements; and stimulation activities.
3. General
   Note responses to care and teaching; goal achievement; changes or modifications of plan, adaptation of caregiver, family, and child to long-term care and change in lifestyle; rehabilitation referrals; importance of medical follow-up; and contact with health care provider and community support groups.
4. See "Documentation and Family Home Record Keeping" in Appendix for general required documentation components for all home care visits.

Osteomyelitis

Osteomyelitis is an infectious process of the bone, most commonly the femur and tibia, caused by *Staphylococcus aureus, Haemophilus influenzae,* or *Salmonella* microorganisms. The infection leads to abscess formation and bone destruction, and pressure from the abscess causes spread into the subperiosteal space. The spread to the periosteum adds to the necrosis, and as granulation forms, sinuses appear that retain the infection for years, resulting in a chronic condition. It is acquired from exogenous (invasion from an outside open or penetrating wound) or hematogenous (existing infections involving organs or skin conditions) sources.

Home care is primarily concerned with assessment, administration and teaching of antimicrobial therapy, care to prevent extension of the infection and associated complications, wound care, cast care, if appropriate.

Nursing diagnosis

Pain
Related factors: biologic injuring agents (infection), physical injuring agents (surgical procedure)
Defining characteristics: verbal/nonverbal communication of pain (tenderness, edema, warmth, muscle spasm over affected bone area) (see "Pain Management," pp. 398-402)

OUTCOMES
Short-term
Comfort with minimal pain evidenced by cooperation/participation in routine activities such as play, eating, resting, movement within imposed limitations (expected within 1 to 2 days)

Long-term
Optimal relief/control of pain evidenced by effective pharmacologic/nonpharmacologic therapy, ability to engage

in rehabilitation (expected within 2 to 4 weeks or when infection subsides)

NURSING INTERVENTIONS/INSTRUCTIONS

1. Perform complete physical assessment. Assess child's responses to pain (see "Nursing Inverventions/Instructions
   in Pain Management," pp. 400-401) (each visit, if needed).
2. Assess pain on movement, position of limb in semi-
   flexion, muscle tenseness, affect on appetite, and possible
   dehydration associated with fever (each visit until pain
   is controlled).
3. Instruct on administration of antipyretic and analgesic as
   prescribed and to reduce dose and frequency based on
   responses of temperature and pain relief (first visit, second visit if needed).
4. Instruct to position and support affected limb and to
   move and handle gently to prevent additional pressure or
   injury to area (first visit).
5. Instruct on need to rest limb and methods to immobilize
   in proper alignment to prevent pain (use of pillows and
   splints) (first visit).

CAREGIVER/CHILD AND FAMILY INTERVENTIONS

1. Maintains affected limb in position of comfort.
2. Administers analgesic 30 minutes before treatment and
   antipyretic based on temperature and pain assessment.
3. Institutes nonpharmacologic measures to relieve pain.
4. Performs measures to prevent pain and injury to affected
   limb.

Nursing diagnosis

Risk for infection
Related factors: inadequate primary defenses (broken skin,
   traumatized tissue)
Defining characteristics: presence of open surgical wound;
   spread of infection with abscess formation; redness,
   swelling, pain, drainage at open wound site or site of
   drainage/medication instillation tubes; positive wound
   culture for infective agent; febrile status

OUTCOMES

Short-term
Prevention of wound infection evidenced by effective response to antibiotic therapy (afebrile state, reduction of signs, symptoms), progressive wound healing, reduction in drainage (expected within 1 week)

Long-term
Maintenance of infection-free state evidenced by absence of spread of infection, negative cultures, return of appetite, return to activities (expected within 1 month)

NURSING INTERVENTIONS/INSTRUCTIONS

1. Assess home living conditions for cleanliness, safety, and facilities (see "Environmental Assessment," p. 37, for guidelines) (first visit, second visit for additional modifications).
2. Assess wound and insertion sites for redness, swelling, pain, drainage, and healing process (each visit).
3. Assess presence of splint or bivalved cast or cast with open area for observation (immobilizes limb and prevents spread of infection) for color, heat, swelling, pain, and movement. Assess casted area for pain, sensation, circulation, and musty odor (each visit).
4. Demonstrate, instruct on and observe correct administration, maintenance, and monitoring of prescribed antibiotic therapy via intravenous (IV) line, heparin lock device, or closed-tube instillation directly into wound (see "Medication Administration and Teaching Guidelines," pp. 450-463) (first visit, reinstruct as needed).
5. Instruct on side effects of antibiotic, especially renal, hepatic, or otic damage; diarrhea; and sore mouth and affect on other mucous membranes (first visit).
6. Instruct on change to oral administration of antibiotic following IV therapy (any visit).
7. Instruct on temperature monitoring if changes in wound or child's behavior are noted (first visit).
8. Demonstrate, instruct on handwashing before care procedures, wound isolation techniques if drainage is present, dressing change technique, and disposal of dressings and other used articles using universal precau-

tions. Have caregiver repeat demonstration (first and second visits).

9. Instruct on importance of high-calorie fluids and foods of high protein and calcium content to aid in healing and new bone formation (first visit).

10. Instruct on importance of compliance to antibiotic regimen and follow-up visits with health care provider (any visit).

CAREGIVER/CHILD AND FAMILY INTERVENTIONS

1. Observes for changes in wound and tube sites. Reports to health care provider.

2. Assesses for signs and symptoms of continuing, exacerbation of, or extended infectious process.

3. Administers and monitors antimicrobial therapy via correct route as ordered.

4. Performs proper handwashing technique frequently, especially before and after caring for child. Uses clean or sterile technique as appropriate during care and procedures. Gently washes and pats dry affected area if no open wound is present.

5. Performs wound precautions with use of gloves and proper care of linens and other articles.

6. Changes dressings as needed. Properly disposes of all articles and supplies according to universal precautions.

7. Provides cast care. Assesses for circulatory or neurologic complications.

8. Provides nutrients and fluids high in calories to promote healing.

9. Has cultures for laboratory examination and laboratory test for white blood count as ordered.

Nursing diagnosis

Impaired physical mobility
Related factors: pain, discomfort; musculoskeletal impairment; decreased strength, endurance
Defining characteristics: inability to purposefully move within physical environment; reluctance to move; imposed re-

striction of movement (cast, splint); joint deterioration viewed on radiography, tomography

OUTCOMES

Short-term
Maintains movement evidenced by increased tolerance to activity within limitations (cast, splint), progressive ambulation (expected within 1 week)

Long-term
Maximizes movement evidenced by independent movement to fullest extent, participation in activities, absence of complications of immobility (expected within 1 month)

NURSING INTERVENTIONS/INSTRUCTIONS

1. Assess for movement restrictions such as altered weight bearing, splint, bivalved or full cast, bed rest or amount of movement in bed allowed, and skin integrity (see "Musculoskeletal System Assessment," p. 21, for guidelines) (any visit as needed).
2. Collaborate with caregiver and child to assess and plan for progressive healing and mobility (first and second visits).
3. Perform ROM to limbs when allowed. Instruct caregiver to perform this procedure daily (first visit, reinforce).
4. Instruct on positioning, elevating, and supporting affected limb and on use of other extremities to perform self-care and engage in play activities; supervise safe movement with use of assistive aids (first and second visits).
5. Assess limb for neurovascular complications and instruct to assess for pain, color, warmth, and movement of digits (each visit).
6. Obtain order for physical therapy referral for exercises and mobility if needed (any visit).

CAREGIVER/CHILD AND FAMILY INTERVENTIONS

1. Schedules and assists or participates in daily activities as tolerated.
2. Assesses for cast tightness, skin irritation, musty odor, color of digits, or pain. Reports complications to physician.

3. Protects cast from trauma and soiling. Avoids allowing child to put small articles in cast.
4. Avoids extremes in activity and allows for as much independence as possible. Increases activities daily as endurance and healing allow.
5. Establishes recreation, study, and exercise programs as healing progresses within identified restrictions.
6. Uses assistive aids or devices (wheelchair or crutches) for immobilization or ambulation if needed. Protects affected limb during activity.
7. Follows recommendations of physical therapist to maintain mobility, muscle tone, and ROM.

SAMPLE DOCUMENTATION INCLUSIONS

1. Specific assessment
   Assess age; developmental status; verbal/nonverbal responses to pain; type and responses to medication regimen; cast or splint integrity; possible complications; signs and symptoms of infection; condition and size of wound, if present; specific drainage (progress or deterioration); activity level, if chair-bound or bed-bound; and amount of independence in self-care.
2. Specific care/teaching
   Teach administration of medication regimen to include name, dose, frequency, route, times of day, and special considerations based on form, side effects, and expected response; use and care of devices or sites used to administer antimicrobial therapy; wound dressing change; wound precautions; handwashing technique; disposal of contaminated articles; limb immobilization, positioning, and comfort; protection of affected limb; use of assistive aids (wheelchair or crutches); and nutritional requirements.
3. General
   Note responses to care and teaching; goal achievement; changes or modifications of plan, especially antibiotic therapy; importance of medical follow-up; and contact with health care provider and community support groups.
4. See "Documentation and Family Home Record Keeping" in Appendix for general required documentation components for all home care visits.

Renal system

 ## Chronic Renal Failure

Chronic renal failure is a slow, progressive degeneration of kidney function. It occurs over a long period of time with symptoms occurring as function is reduced. It involves the deterioration of the glomerular filtration rate (GFR), renal blood flow, resorption ability, and tubule function. Causes include congenital and acquired renal disorders. Common symptoms include polyuria with an inability to concentrate urine that eventually leads to oliguria. Hypertension occurs when fluid is retained, and blood urea nitrogen (BUN) and creatinine levels increase as the kidneys lose function. All systems are eventually affected with acid-base balance disturbance, resulting in metabolic acidosis; erythropoietin production impairment, resulting in anemia; hyperkalemia, hypocalcemia, and hyperphosphatemia, resulting in electrolyte imbalance; and problems with calcium-phosphate metabolism, resulting in osteodystrophy. When medical regimens fail to maintain renal function, end-stage renal disease (ESRD) occurs and dialysis is used to replace renal function (see "Terminally Ill Child," pp. 415-421, for psychosocial implications).

Home care is primarily concerned with health maintenance that includes individualized assessment and teaching of dietary and fluid needs, medications, growth and psychologic development, and dialysis regimens (see "Peritoneal Dialysis," pp. 351-361).

Nursing diagnosis

Ineffective family coping/individual coping (child): compromised
Related factors: prolonged disease that exhausts supportive capacity of significant people, family disorganization

Defining characteristics: significant person's expression of inability to cope; feelings of fear, anxiety, guilt, anger; inadequate understanding of chronic illness, long-term care by family; inability of child to cope, ask for help; chronic fatigue, anxiety of child; changing roles, family relationships

OUTCOMES
Short-term
Family members demonstrate ability to plan and care for child evidenced by provision of normal environment; decreased anxiety, feelings of inadequacy by caregiver and child; integration of information about family needs into care, support of child (expected within 1 to 4 weeks)

Long-term
Family and child coping and adapting evidenced by optimal support, participation in care of child with life-threatening disease, progression of child toward self-care, maintenance of family relationships (expected within 1 to 2 months)

NURSING INTERVENTIONS/INSTRUCTIONS
1. Meet and collaborate with family to assess stressors, coping mechanisms, and planning of care (first visit, repeat as needed).
2. Reinforce information to promote family understanding of illness and its long-term care needs and progressive nature. Offer reading materials, visual aids, dolls, pictures, and play therapy to enhance knowledge of disease and care implications (each visit).
3. Discuss and allow family and child to express feelings of guilt, anxiety, depression, and fear. Promote communication among family to verbalize feelings and expectations (any visit).
4. Instruct on methods to develop coping skills and to meet family's needs (medical, emotional, financial, food, respite care, supplies, and equipment) by referral to social or counseling services (initiate on first visit, as needed).
5. Prepare family and child for hemodialysis or peritoneal dialysis and possible future kidney transplantation. Provide information to assist in making decision regarding these options (any visit).

CAREGIVER/CHILD AND FAMILY INTERVENTIONS

1. Displays decreasing anxiety and anger. Provides supportive family environment. Realizes that these are normal feelings in these circumstances.
2. Develops trust in home care personnel and collaborates in developing and modifying daily care. Maintains contact with home health care provider.
3. Provides care and treatments effectively. Supports child during restrictive periods or when feeling most vulnerable and unable to participate in daily routines with family or friends.
4. Avoids overprotection or rejection of child by caregiver or family. Encourages play activities suitable to limitations.
5. Recognizes and assumes role changes. Maintains family integrity.
6. Develops coping mechanisms that have positive effect within family.
7. Takes time away from child to attend to own needs. Seeks respite care.
8. Identifies problem areas and obtains community or professional assistance or social services as needed.
9. Contacts American Association of Kidney Patients or National Kidney Foundation for available services and information for families and children who have kidney disease.

Nursing diagnosis

Fluid volume excess
Related factors: compromised regulatory mechanism (renal)
Defining characteristics: edema; weight gain; intake greater than output; hypertension; increased BUN, creatinine levels

OUTCOMES
Short-term
Reduction in fluid volume excess evidenced by intake and output (I&O) ratio within baseline determination with adequate hydration, normal blood pressure (BP), decreasing edema, appropriate weight loss/gain with effective diuretic therapy (expected within 3 to 5 days)

Long-term
Fluid retention controlled evidenced by I&O balance, optimal weight, BP maintained; effective restricted dietary sodium intake (expected within 2 weeks)

NURSING INTERVENTIONS/INSTRUCTIONS

1. Perform complete physical assessment. Assess renal status and evaluate baseline weight, hydration, peripheral edema, BP, pulse, output trends, urine characteristics, and specific gravity (see "Renal and Urinary Systems Assessment," p. 22, for guidelines) (each visit).
2. Assess and instruct caregiver to assess and measure I&O every 8 hours, depending on status, and to estimate wet diapers for output (first visit, reinforce instruction on second visit).
3. Instruct on amount of fluids allowed, frequency to administer, and amount of sodium in dietary intake, if restricted. Allow child to select preferred liquids if possible (see "Altered Nutrition nursing diagnosis," pp. 335-337) (first and second visits).
4. Assess and instruct on taking and recording daily or more frequent weight measurements if fluid is retained, using same scales at same time of day and with child wearing same clothing (each visit).
5. Assess and demonstrate taking BP. Allow for repeat demonstration to monitor disease (first visit).
6. Instruct on administration of diuretic regimen as ordered and response to expect such as weight loss. Include medication dose, route, frequency, and side effects (first and second visits, reinstruct as needed).
7. Instruct on administration of antihypertensive medicine. Include dose, route, frequency, and side effects (first visit, reinforce as needed).
8. Instruct to observe and report edema, inappropriate weight gain, decreased urinary output, and increased BP to home health care nurse or physician (first visit).

CAREGIVER/CHILD AND FAMILY INTERVENTIONS

1. Monitors I&O by amount of feedings and fluid intake by measuring fluids, estimating number of diapers used, or weighing diapers every 8 hours or daily based on symptoms of fluid excess.

2. Weighs daily or more frequently based on persistent signs and symptoms of fluid retention (edema in extremities).
3. Maintains fluid restrictions within prescribed limits over 24-hour period. Restricts child's access to fluids.
4. Correctly administers prescribed medications in feedings or in proper form as ordered and assesses for side effects, primarily dehydration.
5. Offers low-salt diet with restrictions in adding salt and eating processed or canned foods, convenience foods, or snack foods.
6. Complies with ongoing dialysis treatments to remove accumulated fluid and electrolytes.
7. Reports fluid retention and adverse responses or reactions to medications to physician.

Nursing diagnosis

Altered nutrition: less than body requirements
Related factors: inability to ingest enough nutrients because of anorexia, refusal of special diet
Defining characteristics: inadequate food intake (protein), anorexia, nutritional anemia, retarded growth pattern

OUTCOMES

Short-term
Improved appetite with adequate basic nutritional intake by child evidenced by ingestion of planned special meals/feedings that include necessary restrictions, inclusions (expected within 1 to 4 weeks)

Long-term
Adequate nutritional status for optimal growth evidenced by nutritionally balanced food, prevention of dietary deficiencies; compliance with adjustments in protein, electrolytes in diet (expected within 1 to 3 months)

NURSING INTERVENTIONS/INSTRUCTIONS

1. Assess nutritional requirement for age and weight, needed caloric intake, growth deviation from standard for age, appetite and food preferences of child,

times of meals/feedings (see "Gastrointestinal Assessment," p. 16, for guidelines) (first visit).

2. Assess status of renal failure, if receiving dialysis, and effect of treatments on need to restrict dietary inclusions (first visit).

3. Inform caregiver and child of importance in complying with dietary regimen to ease or prevent symptoms (first visit).

4. Instruct and collaborate with caregiver and child on planning and administering high-calorie diet with restricted protein and electrolyte content and possibly vitamin and mineral inclusions (first and second visits).

5. Instruct on selection of foods that are preferred by child. Monitor protein restriction and include foods with high biologic value of protein. Monitor inclusions of carbohydrates and unsaturated fats to supply increased caloric need; restrictions of foods containing sodium, potassium, and phosphorus; and inclusions of foods containing calcium (if appropriate), folic acid, iron, and vitamins C and D. Offer food lists and sample menus to assist in meal planning (first, second, and subsequent visits as needed).

6. Instruct on selection and administration of low-protein, low-electrolyte infant formula and lower volume supplement inclusion as ordered (first visit).

7. Collaborate with caregiver and child to offer small feedings/meals of preferred foods of appropriate consistency and liquid supplement (commercial high-calorie, low-protein liquid) inclusion to meet additional caloric needs at normal feeding times (first and second visits).

8. Demonstrate and instruct caregiver to weigh child every 3 to 7 days or daily, if appropriate, using same scale at same time of day with child wearing same clothes to assess for losses and differentiate between fluid and actual weight losses (first visit).

9. Support participation and presence of caregiver and family at mealtime (each visit).

10. Initiate social services referral for assistance in obtaining food and nutritionist referral for diet planning if needed (appropriate visit).

CAREGIVER/CHILD AND FAMILY INTERVENTIONS

1. Plans and provides menus of food or formula that contains prescribed caloric, protein, carbohydrate, and fat intake with inclusions of supplements as needed.
2. Reads labels on foods to avoid those containing sodium. Notes caloric values of purchased foods and avoids fast foods.
3. Prepares nutritional foods and fluids of proper consistency and texture, finger foods, snacks, and other appealing selections for child. Offers foods at appropriate times and frequency and in proper amounts.
4. Restricts foods containing electrolytes (K, Na, P) such as cow's milk, bananas, citrus fruits, and dried fruits. Includes foods high in essential amino acids.
5. Promotes pleasant environment for child that can enhance intake. Integrates mealtimes into family routine. Allows for adequate rest.
6. Weighs child using same scale at same time of day with child wearing same clothes. Records and compares changes to determine weight gain or loss.

Nursing diagnosis

Altered growth and development
Related factors: environmental, stimulation deficiencies; effects of chronic illness, inadequate parental caregiving, prescribed dependence, nutritional deficit

Defining characteristics: altered physical growth from effect of chronic disease on ingestion of nutrients, depletion of protein, restrictive dietary intake; presence of anxiety, anger, depression; disruption in school, socialization caused by treatments; changes in body image caused by medications, anorexia

OUTCOMES
Short-term
Minimal growth/development deficits, delays, or regression evidenced by growth or functioning within limits imposed by illness (expected within 6 to 12 weeks)

Long-term
Maximum growth/development potential for advances, achievement of physical, emotional, social parameters within disease limitations (expected ongoing)

NURSING INTERVENTIONS/INSTRUCTIONS

1. Assess expected growth/developmental level and extent of deficits from expected patterns (see "Growth and Developmental Assessment," p. 31, for guidelines) (every visit).
2. Assess caregiver, family, and environment for stressful events and ability to provide love, caring, adequate stimulation, and play activities (each visit).
3. Assess for caregiver overprotection or negligence (each visit).
4. Instruct on normal growth/development patterns for child's age and possible lag in development, maturation, and physical changes caused by chronic illness (first visit).
5. Assist caregiver and family to develop goals and participate in care plan to achieve optimal development potential (ongoing).
6. Instruct to monitor difficulties in school and feelings of differences from peers in size, fatigue level, presence of shunt, and absence from school for dialysis. Arrange to meet with peers with same problems (first visit).
7. Provide encouragement and support for child's and caregivers' efforts (each visit).
8. Provide early referral to professional resources such as home tutor, psychosocial counselor, or financial and social workers to assist child in specific areas of need (any visit).

CAREGIVER/CHILD AND FAMILY INTERVENTIONS

1. Provides activities in quiet environment to enhance stimulation, independence, and developmental progression (physical and psychosocial).
2. Sets realistic goals for growth/developmental achievement.
3. Maintains consistent caregiver and schedule of activities.
4. Implements consistent encouragement, support, and appropriate inclusion in activities.

5. Provides organized and consistent program of daily activities that include mobiles, music, toys, books, swimming, painting, sandbox, and other diversion and learning tools.
6. Promotes school attendance and participation. Discusses need for flexible program with teacher or home teacher.
7. Provides time for talking and playing with other children and family members. Invites friends to visit and play. Involves child in social and physical activities within ability.
8. Provides opportunity to participate in self-care activities, including dressing, bathing, eating, and toileting with adaptations as needed.
9. Identifies and uses specialized services (physical therapy, occupational therapy, and social services) to assist with growth/developmental lags.

Nursing diagnosis

Risk for injury/knowledge deficit (management and care of child with chronic renal failure, prevention of complications)
Related factors: lack of exposure to or misinterpretation of specific information regarding disease, cognitive limitations, internal factor of regulatory dysfunction
Defining characteristics: verbalized request for information; misconceptions about disease; lack of readiness for learning; fear/anxiety about health status, performing therapeutic regimen; complications of anemia, osteodystrophy, pulmonary and urinary tract infections; lack of consideration for cultural, ethnic, religious needs

OUTCOMES
Short-term
Development of attitude conducive to learning; adequate basic knowledge, understanding of condition, treatment regimen evidenced by verbalizations of definition of chronic renal failure; participation in components of care plan; demonstration of administration of medications, exercise requirements, personal hygiene needs; recognition of risk for complications (expected within 2 weeks)

Long-term
Adequate knowledge, counseling, performance of complete therapeutic regimen evidenced by progressive self-care; adaptation to lifestyle changes; modification of plan as needed to achieve/maintain renal function, prevent long-term complications; participation in continuing education, routine monitoring by health care provider (expected within 2 to 6 months)

NURSING INTERVENTIONS/INSTRUCTIONS

1. Assess caregiver, family, and child for health beliefs, learning readiness, educational and developmental level, competency and comprehension potential for implementing therapeutic plan, and best methods and approach for teaching and learning the information required (first visit, as needed).
2. Assess home environment for living, learning, and space for storing medications; facilities for handwashing and cleansing and disinfecting supplies; food preparation; personal hygiene needs; and need for financial assistance (see "Environmental and Financial Assessments," pp. 37 and 42, for guidelines) (first visit).
3. Include child in all discussions. Begin by describing renal system using doll and in language level that child can understand. Define disease effect on health status and importance and benefits of maintenance of renal function (first visit, as needed).
4. Provide care plan and initially perform all procedures for family to observe. Instruct and allow for return demonstration. Collaborate with caregiver and family to develop realistic teaching plan (any visit).
5. Use language and content appropriate for level of learners. Allow time for learners to respond and ask questions for clarification (each visit).
6. Explain treatment regimen including medication administration, meal plan, fluid restrictions, activities that do not cause fatigue, how these are interrelated, influence on renal function, and complication prevention (first visit, as needed).
7. Instruct on medication administration (calcium [calcium carbonate], alkalizing agent [sodium bicarbonate], alu-

minum phospate binder [aluminum hydroxide], vitamin
C, iron), including drug name, action, times of day,
forms, and expected effects (see "Medication Administration and Teaching Guidelines," pp. 450-463) (each
visit until all medication administrations are taught).

8. Instruct on constipation prevention, if receiving alumi-
   num hydroxide, and offer stool softener as ordered
   (first visit).

9. Instruct on care and monitoring of shunt or fistula. Include avoiding wearing tight clothing or having purse
   tugging, pulling, or lying on affected arm. Check
   patency by auscultating for bruit over shunt site or pulsations (fistula) at site if receiving hemodialysis (each
   visit).

10. Instruct on importance of daily bathing and skin care
    (especially around shunt site) and periodic dental and
    oral examinations (first visit, reinforce on second visit).

11. Instruct on measures to prevent infection including
    handwashing technique, avoiding people with infec-
    tions, using sterile or clean technique in performing
    procedures, administering medicines, and monitoring
    for nephrotoxicity (first visit).

12. Advise to wear identification that notes condition and
    telephone numbers of caregiver or health care provider
    (first visit).

13. Provide follow-up plan for renal function laboratory
    testing; visits to health care provider; referral to nutri-
    tionist, social worker, and counselor; and contact with
    resources in community to provide in-depth continu-
    ing education such as support group or National Kidney
    Foundation (any visit).

CAREGIVER/CHILD AND FAMILY INTERVENTIONS

1. Participates in initial and ongoing teaching sessions in
   management of renal failure. Integrates total medical
   regimen into lifestyle.

2. Defines disease and cause. Explains medications, side
   effects, and dietary and activity components of treatment.

3. Plans, prepares, modifies, and provides proper dietary
   and fluid therapy as disease progresses.

4. Complies with medication regimen and evaluates responses to prevent complications.
5. Maintains daily program of activities within tolerance levels.
6. Uses measures to prevent any infection.
7. Maintains dialysis access site and reports deteriorating condition or complications. Complies with appointments for hemodialysis.
8. Performs consistent personal hygiene with daily bathing and mouth and dental care.
9. Maintains follow-up laboratory and physician appointments.
10. Allows child to progress to self-care as appropriate.
11. Informs all health care providers and prescribers of diagnosis and care regimen (dentist and surgeon).
12. Wears or carries identification information.

SAMPLE DOCUMENTATION INCLUSIONS

1. Specific assessment
   Assess general health, renal status, stressors of caregiver and child and effect on treatment regimen, family role strain and child's coping ability to comply with long-term management, possibility of self-care, dietary and fluid needs, signs and symptoms of complications, need for reinstruction of aspects of care, growth/development deficits, and need for referrals (counselor, financial advisor, and nutritionist).
2. Specific care/teaching
   Teach disease, signs and symptoms, preparation and administration of medications, dietary inclusions and exclusions, fluid restrictions, daily weights, vital signs including BP, measures to prevent infections, activity regimen, energy conservation, personal hygiene, dental and mouth care, shunt or fistula care, signs and symptoms of complications and interventions, dialysis, and follow-up appointments.
3. General
   Note responses to care and teaching; goal achievement; changes in plan; regression of health status; adaptation of caregiver, family, and child to diagnosis and implications (long-term care and change in lifestyle); griev-

ing process; self-care abilities; resources for acquiring medication, supplies, and equipment for care; and need for monitoring by health care provider.
4. See "Documentation and Family Home Record Keeping" in Appendix for general required documentation components for all home care visits.

 # Kidney Transplant

Kidney transplantation is performed to provide a healthy, functioning kidney. The recipient's kidney is left in place and the donor kidney is grafted into the anterior iliac fossa. It is anastomosed to arteries and veins with the ureter attached to the recipient's ureter or into the urinary bladder. The procedure is reserved for children with chronic renal failure who are otherwise physically and mentally healthy and can comply with the postoperative regimen. This procedure offers an opportunity for the child to live a reasonably normal life.

Home care is primarily concerned with monitoring signs and symptoms of infection and rejection and teaching to prevent rejection of the transplanted kidney that includes suppression of the immune response, general health needs, and support to the child and family to cope with the stressors and burdens of kidney transplantation.

Nursing diagnosis

Anxiety/fear (child, parent)
Related factors: change in health status, threat of rejection of transplanted kidney, threat to self-concept
Defining characteristics: apprehension, restlessness, uncertainty, fear of organ rejection, verbalization of significance of physical change caused by immunosuppressive therapy, fear of death, mood swings, regression

OUTCOMES

Short-term
Minimal anxiety about transplant rejection and side effects
of drug therapy evidenced by caregiver and child accepting donor kidney; understanding physical, cosmetic implications of drug therapy (expected within 1 to 4 weeks)

Long-term
Fear/anxiety at manageable level during change from sick to
healthy role evidenced by effective use of coping mechanisms to deal with physical, emotional challenges; adaptation to kidney transplant; daily life as free of anxiety as possible regarding rejection, drug therapy (expected within 1
month)

NURSING INTERVENTIONS/INSTRUCTIONS

1. Assess emotional and mental status of caregiver and
   child and their ability to adapt to and comply with
   regimen to prevent kidney rejection (see "Psychologic
   Assessment," p. 25, for guidelines) (first visit, as
   needed).
2. Provide information about kidney donor. Support child if
   concerned about origin of kidney and clearly inform family of survival rate of transplant patients (first visit).
3. Inform of therapy and possible side effects (acne, obesity,
   hirsutism, and facial changes of puffiness, coarseness,
   and ridges). Assess for effect on body image (each visit).
4. Maintain calm, quiet environment during assessment and
   interactions with child, caregiver, and family (every visit).
5. Provide emotional support and opportunity for caregiver
   and child to verbalize fears and concerns. Encourage acceptance of kidney transplant and compliance needed
   to minimize rejection (each visit).
6. Assist caregiver to reduce feelings of guilt and self-blame
   for child's condition (each visit).
7. Provide continuing information about successful kidney
   graft and progress to wellness. Explain that rejection episodes can occur but do not mean that kidney will be
   lost (any visit as needed).
8. Arrange for child to meet peers who have experienced
   transplant surgery (any visit).

9. Initiate referral to counselor and support group for families with similar experiences (any visit).

CAREGIVER/CHILD AND FAMILY INTERVENTIONS

1. Recognizes anxiety associated with transplant procedure and possibility of rejection.
2. Maintains calm, supportive environment and manageable level of anxiety. Develops coping strategies for possibility of rejection and effects of drug therapy on body image.
3. Manages side effects of drug therapy by modifying clothing and using make-up if applicable.
4. Seeks information and uses support resources that reduce anxiety.
5. Listens to child's concerns and allows for expression of feelings.

Nursing diagnosis

Risk for injury
Related factors: internal factor of regulatory dysfunction (kidney rejection), internal factor of abnormal blood profile (immunosuppressants, antiinflammatory agents)
Defining characteristics: signs and symptoms of kidney rejection, untoward effects of medication

OUTCOMES
Short-term
Risk for transplant rejection, undesirable side effects of medications minimized evidenced by compliance with immunosuppressive therapy, absence of immediate rejection (expected within 1 week)

Long-term
Optimal level of health and kidney function achieved with rehabilitation of chronic renal failure evidenced by freedom of signs and symptoms of kidney rejection; active participation in health care, compliance with total therapeutic regimen (expected within 6 months)

NURSING INTERVENTIONS/INSTRUCTIONS

1. Arrange for case conference and collaborate with colleagues, family, and child in planning home care (first visit, repeat as needed).

2. Inform that organ rejection can occur within weeks, months, or years following procedure. Discuss feelings about this possibility (first visit, as needed).

3. Perform complete physical assessment. Assess and instruct caregiver and child to assess for signs and symptoms of acute organ rejection including temperature elevation, pain and swelling over transplanted kidney area, reduced urinary output, increased BP or appetite, and periorbital edema. Report to health care provider immediately.

4. Instruct on taking temperature and BP, assessing I&O, and weighing child daily. Allow return demonstrations of these procedures (first visit, as needed).

5. Assess and instruct caregiver and child to assess for signs and symptoms of chronic organ rejection and progressive deterioration occurring 6 months or more after transplant. Assess fever, flank pain, fatigue, irritability, fluid retention, and other manifestations of chronic renal failure. Implement urinary and blood testing for protein levels and ongoing visits to physician (first visit, reinstruct as needed).

6. Assess caregiver's and child's understanding of procedure, therapeutic regimen to prevent organ rejection and maintain health, and type of measures to take and when to implement them to prevent complications (first and second visits).

7. Demonstrate and instruct on oral administration, maintenance, and monitoring of prescribed immunosuppressive agents, steroids, antacid therapy, including drug action, dose, frequency, methods, and possible interactions with foods and other drugs, especially if they contain alcohol (see "Medication Administration and Teaching Guidelines," pp. 450-463). Have caregiver repeat demonstration. Reinforce content as necessary (first visit, reinstruct as needed for length of therapy).

8. Instruct on side effects of drug therapy including gastrointestinal irritation and bleeding, hepatotoxicity, nephrotoxicity, cushingoid body changes, visual changes,

fluid and sodium retention, growth retardation, and leukopenia (each visit).

9. Instruct on progressive resumption of activity and allow for adequate rest periods. Emphasize avoidance of contact sports or any activity traumatic to operative site unless protective device is worn (first visit).

10. Instruct on dietary modifications to include high-caloric, low-sodium intake. Initiate referral to nutritionist, if needed (first and second visits).

11. Stress importance of compliance with treatment regimen and need for ongoing laboratory testing, physician monitoring and supervision, and routine examination of teeth and eyes (first visit).

12. Explain how and when to notify health care provider if questions or concerns arise (first visit).

CAREGIVER/CHILD AND FAMILY INTERVENTIONS

1. Verbalizes understanding of causes of graft rejection, complications, and signs and symptoms manifested.

2. Assesses urinary output, BP, temperature, and tenderness at operative site daily. Reports abnormalities.

3. Notes signs and symptoms of rejection and intervenes early to prevent/correct acute transplant rejection.

4. Complies with therapeutic medication regimen. Monitors for side effects to report.

5. Resumes recommended activity with restrictions that can cause trauma to kidney. Resumes recommended nutritional regimen.

6. Consults with health professionals for monitoring and regular health checks and advice. Complies with necessary laboratory testing.

7. Wears or carries medical identification for emergency information.

8. Communicates with school nurse and teacher regarding child's needs (medications and activity restrictions).

Nursing diagnosis

Risk for infection
Related factors: inadequate secondary defenses (immunosuppression, suppressed inflammatory response)

Defining characteristics: presence of infectious process (peritonitis, cytomegalovirus, or other viruses or fungal infections); positive culture for infective agent; fever; respiratory distress; cloudy, foul-smelling urine; swelling, redness, warmth, drainage at incision site

OUTCOMES

Short-term
Prevention of infection evidenced by afebrile state, negative culture, performance of preventive measures and safe personal hygiene practices (expected at time of discharge from hospital)

Long-term
Maintenance of infection-free state evidenced by absence of signs and symptoms of infection in any body organ or area (expected within 1 month)

NURSING INTERVENTIONS/INSTRUCTIONS

1. Assess home and living conditions for cleanliness, safety, and adequate facilities (see "Environmental Assessment," p. 37, for guidelines) (first visit, second visit for modifications).
2. Instruct on temperature monitoring if child experiences behavior changes, anorexia, pain, breathing changes, or abnormal characteristics in urine are noted (first visit).
3. Instruct on and demonstrate oral administration of antibiotic therapy including dose, frequency, form, and side effects. Instruct to complete administration of all prescribed drugs. Have caregiver repeat demonstration (any visit).
4. Instruct on technique for dressing change, if appropriate (first visit).
5. Instruct on handwashing of caregiver and child before care and eating and following use of bathroom and to avoid exposure to contagious diseases at school (first and second visits).
6. Instruct on importance of adequate dietary and fluid intake, high-calorie fluids, and rest to enhance and maintain health status (first visit).

CAREGIVER/CHILD AND FAMILY INTERVENTIONS

1. Assesses for signs and symptoms of onset or exacerbation of infectious process. Reports to health care provider immediately to prevent complications.
2. Administers and monitors medicine via correct route as ordered.
3. Performs proper handwashing technique frequently.
4. Provides nutrients, fluids, and opportunity for adequate rest to promote health.
5. Obtains cultures for laboratory examination as ordered.

Nursing diagnosis

Altered family processes
Related factors: situational crisis of kidney transplant
Defining characteristics: fear/anxiety about organ survival and complications of rejection; family unable to meet physical, emotional needs of members; lack of information, knowledge about therapeutic regimen; inability to express, accept feelings of child and family members and to adapt to child's needs; inability to investigate sources and accept assistance or support

OUTCOMES

Short-term
Progress toward family acceptance of, adaptation to child after organ transplantation evidenced by open communication among family regarding understanding of procedure; discussion of fears, concerns about child's special needs, financial responsibilities; ability to comply with therapeutic regimen (expected within 1 to 2 weeks)

Long-term
Development and fostering of positive behaviors, attitudes, interactions that support child and family; lifestyle changes evidenced by demonstration of effective coping skills; confidence in child's and family's abilities; ability to set goals, participate in care, solve problems; seeks information, assistance, understanding, support as necessary (expected within 1 to 2 months)

NURSING INTERVENTIONS/INSTRUCTIONS

1. Assess level of development as family stressors on family and extended family, impact of child's health on parents' and siblings' behavior (protective, nurturing, supportive, disruptive, neglectful, and use of coping mechanisms), and ability to adjust to unknown outcome of transplant and participate in care planning (see "Family Assessment," p. 41, for guidelines) (first and second visits).
2. Assess feelings of family and allow them to express concerns regarding responsibilities involved in providing care and support to one another (each visit).
3. Encourage open communication among family and inform them of importance of maintaining own health and social activities (first visit).
4. Discuss family's reaction to child and disease. Emphasize positive family relationships and coping mechanisms. Discuss child's positive abilities, potentials, and limitations (each visit).
5. Provide referral to family counselor, local agencies, hospital support group, respite care, or financial resources. Introduce to others with similar experience (any visit).

CAREGIVER/CHILD AND FAMILY INTERVENTIONS

1. Verbalizes feelings and concerns. Resolves reactions and negative behaviors toward child and among family.
2. Identifies problems within family and role changes and types of assistance needed. Works together to solve problems as they arise.
3. Promotes and demonstrates adjustment and adaptation to kidney transplant and its implications for family.
4. Reduces anxiety about child's health, therapies, and fear of future complications.
5. Gains confidence in ability to cope with child's needs and effect on family.
6. Demonstrates positive growth-promoting behaviors in family members and child by interacting with other families and by seeking support from community resources and appropriate referrals.

SAMPLE DOCUMENTATION INCLUSIONS

1. Specific Assessment
   Assess age; sex; renal status; growth/developmental sta-

tus and needs; responses to and stressors of medication regimen (anxiety and body image disturbance); amount of independence in self-care; family's and child's coping abilities; and signs and symptoms of rejection, infection, and other complications.

2. Specific care/teaching
   Teach source of donor kidney; signs and symptoms of rejection and infection; administration of medication including name, dose, frequency, route, times of day, special considerations, side effects, expected response, and cosmetic effects; nutritional and activity requirements; and risk for or presence of infection or organ rejection.

3. General
   Note responses to care and teaching; goal achievement; changes/modifications of plan; adaptation of caregiver, family, and child to change in lifestyle; importance of medical follow-up and contact with health care provider; prognosis for graft survival; community support groups; and financial support.

4. See "Documentation and Family Home Record Keeping" in Appendix for general required documentation components for all home care visits.

 Peritoneal Dialysis

Dialysis is a method of clearing excess fluid, toxic substances, electrolytes, and metabolic wastes from the body when the kidneys no longer function effectively (see "Chronic Renal Failure," pp. 331-343). This is accomplished by hemodialysis, peritoneal dialysis, or hemofiltration. Hemodialysis or peritoneal dialysis is used for those who need ongoing treatment. Hemodialysis requires regular visits of the child to a dialysis department but can be performed at home with proper training, equipment, and compliance of the child and family. Peritoneal dialysis is used most often for children in the home. It uses the abdominal cavity as a semipermeable membrane through which fluid and toxins are removed by osmosis (removal of solutes from blood to the dialysate by movement of solvent from a lower to a higher concentration) and diffusion (removal of solutes from blood to the dialysate by movement from a higher to a lower concentration). A surgically implanted Tenckoff catheter in the peritoneal cavity is used to instill and drain dialysate fluid. One method is continuous ambulatory dialysis (CAPD), which is performed while the child is awake. This allows for instillation of the dialysate, retention of the fluid, and drainage of the fluid into an empty container attached to the abdomen or placed in a pocket. Another method is continuous cyclic peritoneal dialysis (CCPD). With this method, a machine is used for 5 to 6 cycles of infusion and drains the dialysate during sleep; the child receives no daytime dialysis.

Home care is primarily concerned with performing and teaching the administration, monitoring, and prevention of complications associated with peritoneal dialysis and promotion of the welfare of the child and family.

Nursing diagnosis

Ineffective home maintenance management/knowledge deficit (parent/child)

Related factors: lack of information about disease, treatment regimen (peritoneal dialysis); insufficient planning, organization, finances, support system; altered lifestyle, self-concept of family/child

Defining characteristics: expression of need for information about disease, procedures, complications; health/emotional needs of child; expectations, responsibilities of caregiver; lack of necessary hygienic surroundings; inability to perform procedure correctly

OUTCOMES

Short-term

Adequate knowledge evidenced by verbalization of causes, progression, prognosis of disease; general principles, importance of dialysis procedures; nutritional, activity regimens; personal/family, environmental cleanliness (expected within 1 to 4 weeks)

Long-term
Adequate knowledge evidenced by compliance with effective
continuous peritoneal dialysis without complications; optimal lifestyle adaptations with maintenance of personal
hygiene, clean surroundings (expected within 1 month)

NURSING INTERVENTIONS/INSTRUCTIONS

1. Assess knowledge deficits of caregiver and family. Identify strengths and collaborate in instruction needed to
   manage dialysis and daily care routines (see "Family
   Assessment," p. 41, for guidelines) (first and second visits).
2. Instruct caregiver on reason for dialysis and status of
   renal disease. Relate information to care plan and
   clarify misconceptions and importance of cooperation in
   implementing long-term care (first visit).
3. Assess home environment and financial status for modifications needed to ensure supportive measures. Obtain
   equipment/supplies to perform peritoneal dialysis and
   enhance personal hygiene, nutrition, and follow-up care.
   Consider referral to social services for assistance (see
   "Family and Financial Assessments," pp. 41 and 42, for
   guidelines) (first visit, second visit if needed)
4. Review discharge care plan and teaching and training
   performed in hospital with caregiver and child before
   return home (first visit).
5. Collaborate with child and caregiver to incorporate
   teaching program and to implement procedures. Promote self-care and prevention of complications (first and
   second visits).
6. Instruct on use of face mask, handwashing, and sterile
   technique during CAPD/CCPD procedures (first visit).
7. Instruct on principles of peritoneal dialysis. Demonstrate and repeat demonstration of procedure, including set-up of bags of dialysate in prescribed amount and
   concentration; warming dialysate with heating pad; removing covering from bag spike; connecting tubing
   to bag and catheter; hanging bag in position; unclamping tube and allowing for inflow of solution at appropriate rate and time; closing clamp and leaving solution
   in abdomen, then clamping and folding empty bag and
   tubing connected to catheter in child's clothing; and

finally, when draining dialysate, opening clamp on tubing of empty bag and allowing dialysate to drain into bag placed on floor and discarding return flow in toilet (each visit until all aspects of procedure are completed with proficiency).

8. Instruct on attaching new bag of dialysate. Repeat procedure 3 to 4 times a day. Leave solution in peritoneal cavity overnight after last treatment of day (first and second visits, as needed).

9. Instruct, demonstrate, and repeat demonstration on use of cycler machine, including priming and threading of tubing to dialysate bags; allowing for 5 to 6 cycles during night (machine infuses and drains dialysate automatically); connecting tubing to container at base of machine for drainage, allowing final exchange solution to stay in peritoneal cavity during day; and then emptying at bedtime when cycler is again used. Inform and assist to review manual for machine operation, alarm system, and trouble-shooting activities (first visit, as needed).

10. Instruct, demonstrate, and repeat demonstration on daily insertion site care; dressing change, including gently removing existing dressing without pulling on catheter; assessment of site for signs and symptoms of infectious process; cleansing and rinsing around site with half-strength hydrogen peroxide; drying with gauze dressing; cleansing again with povidone iodine swabs; allowing to dry; and looping catheter and taping to secure with small gauze pad placed under catheter adaptor; follow with transparent bandage (first visit, as needed).

11. Include older child in instruction and performance of dialysis. Allow to perform procedures according to ability to gain control and independence (each visit).

12. Instruct on weekly weight measurement and dietary intake with prescribed modifications. Initiate referral to nutritionist if needed (first and second visits).

13. Instruct to record and maintain log for information related to dialysis procedure and responses (first visit).

14. Instruct and support daily routines of attending school, notifying school nurse, restricting contact sports and ex-

cessive activities, and setting aside time for rest (first visit).

15. Inform to report any leakage from catheter, cloudy dialysate, fever, abdominal pain, cramping, vomiting, or increased respirations (first visit, reinforce as needed).

CAREGIVER/CHILD AND FAMILY INTERVENTIONS

1. Collaborates with plan of care with reduced anxiety and constructive attitude about disease and treatments.
2. Describes disease process, importance of dialysis, and possible complications of continuous therapy.
3. Manages home environment to provide area for dialysis procedures and hygienic modifications for child as needed, including comfort, cleanliness, ventilation, and temperature.
4. Performs dialysis procedures safely and correctly. Allows self-care participation of child.
5. Performs site care and dressing changes daily using sterile technique.
6. Maintains optimal dietary, activity, and rest routines. Monitors weight and vital signs.
7. Maintains daily log of weight, vital signs, type and amount of dialysate inflow and outflow with characteristics, site assessment, medication mixed with dialysate, and responses to therapy.
8. Attends school or nursery school with instructions to school nurse and teacher.
9. Secures equipment/supplies to perform continuous peritoneal dialysis for long-term therapy.
10. Reports deviations from normal parameters to home care nurse or physician.
11. Complies with follow-up appointments with physician.

Nursing diagnosis

Risk for impaired skin integrity
Related factors: external factors of pressure, irritation at tube sites

Defining characteristics: tissue damage, disruption of skin at tube insertion site

OUTCOMES

Short-term
Skin at tube insertion site protected from irritation; minimal tube pressure to susceptible tissue sites evidenced by clean, dry, intact skin at tube insertion site; free of redness, irritation, pain (expected within 1 to 2 days)

Long-term
Intact skin evidenced by absence of discomfort, breakdown at tube insertion site (expected within 1 week)

NURSING INTERVENTIONS/INSTRUCTIONS

1. Perform complete physical assessment. Assess skin around tube site for redness, drainage, edema, rash, irritation, and tension or movement of tube. Use tape or dressing to ensure secure placement of tube (each visit).
2. Demonstrate and instruct to use only small amount of paper tape to secure looped catheter in place and prevent tube manipulation. Insert small 2 × 2 sponge under adaptor to prevent contact with skin when performing dressing change (first visit, reinstruct second visit).
3. Apply and instruct on use of ointment or creams (antimicrobial, corticosteroid) to tube site if ordered (first and second visits).
4. Instruct caregiver to report any irritation or soreness at tube insertion area to physician immediately (first visit).

CAREGIVER/CHILD AND FAMILY INTERVENTIONS

1. Assesses skin at insertion site daily.
2. Avoids excess movement or tension of catheter on tissues.
3. Applies ordered ointments to site. Applies gauze dressing over coiled catheter and tapes sparingly or secures in place with diaper.
4. Reports any reddened areas, drainage, swelling, or breaks in skin at tube site to physician.

Nursing diagnosis

Risk for infection
Related factors: inadequate primary defenses (broken skin, traumatized tissue), invasive procedure (contamination during dialysis)
Defining characteristics: presence of redness, swelling, pain, drainage at tube insertion site; abdominal pain; fever; cloudy dialysate; positive wound culture for infective agent; anorexia

OUTCOMES

Short-term
Site or peritoneal infection minimized evidenced by proper daily sterile technique, care to maintain clean tube insertion site, dialysis infusion procedure; effective response to antibiotic therapy (afebrile state, reduction of signs, symptoms) (expected within 2 to 3 days)

Long-term
Maintenance of infection-free state evidenced by absence of fever, signs, symptoms of site infection or peritonitis; negative cultures; return of appetite; interest in activities (expected within 1 month)

NURSING INTERVENTIONS/INSTRUCTIONS

1. Assess home and living conditions for cleanliness, safety, and facilities (see "Environmental Assessment," p. 37, for guidelines) (first visit, second visit for modifications).
2. Assess vital signs including temperature. Assess and instruct on assessment of insertion sites for redness, swelling, pain, and drainage and to report to health care provider (each visit).
3. Assess and instruct on assessment of abdominal pain, cloudy dialysate, and fever. Instruct to report to health care provider for early intervention to treat peritonitis (each visit).
4. Demonstrate and instruct on administration of prescribed antibiotic therapy to treat peritonitis by inserting medication into medication port of dialysate bag with syringe and needle or via oral route if infection is con-

fined to insertion site (see "Medication Administration and Teaching Guidelines," pp. 450-463) (first visit, reinstruct as needed).

5. Instruct on adding heparin to dialysate if fibrin clots occur as result of peritoneal infection (any visit as applicable).
6. Instruct on temperature monitoring if changes in site or child's behavior are noted (first visit).
7. Instruct caregiver and child on correct handwashing technique before and after care procedures, before eating, and after using bathroom (first visit).
8. Instruct on using sterile technique for dressing changes and instillation of dialysate and proper disposal of dressings and other articles according to universal precautions (first and second visits).
9. Inform of importance of compliance with antibiotic regimen and follow-up visits to health care provider (any visit).

CAREGIVER/CHILD AND FAMILY INTERVENTIONS

1. Observes for changes in skin around tube site. Reports to health care provider.
2. Assesses for signs and symptoms of peritonitis. Reports to health care provider. Monitors temperature for elevation.
3. Administers and monitors antimicrobial therapy as ordered.
4. Performs proper handwashing technique frequently, especially before and after caring for child. Uses clean or sterile technique as appropriate during care and procedures.
5. Changes dressings as needed, using sterile technique. Properly disposes of all articles and supplies according to universal precautions.
6. Obtains cultures for laboratory examination as ordered.

Nursing diagnosis

Caregiver role strain
Related factors: amount of caregiving tasks, duration of caregiving required, unpredictable illness course or insta-

bility in care receiver's health, infant/child with significant home care needs

Defining characteristics: worry about child's health, having
enough time, energy to provide care needed; conflict in
family about issues of providing 24-hour care, monitor-
ing/supervising child

OUTCOMES

Short-term

Identification of role strain evidenced by verbalization of
stress of daily dialysis schedules, interference with other important roles in life, loss of independence, need for assistance and support (expected within 1 to 2 weeks)

Long-term

Resolution of role strain by provision of continuous safe
care without compromise to caregiver's physical/emotional
needs, progression of older child to self-care (expected
within 1 to 2 months)

NURSING INTERVENTIONS/INSTRUCTIONS

1. Assess child's care needs and caregiver's ability and feeling of adequacy to perform role and care. Assess caregiver's feelings about demands and complexity of care (exhaustion and resentment) and feelings of guilt or
   inability to make decisions (first visit).
2. Assess relationship between caregiver and family and
   stressors placed on relationship, breakdown in family
   relationships, and role confusion or competing demands
   from family and care responsibilities (ongoing).
3. Assist caregiver to monitor continued ability to perform
   care and treatments. Assess needs to be changed or
   learned, changes in strains or stressors, maintenance of
   routines, and need for additional financial resources
   or help with care (each visit).
4. Provide time for caregiver and family to discuss frustration, anxiety, fear, and fatigue. Praise attempts and accomplishments in coping and providing care (each visit).
5. Encourage sharing of caregiver's roles and responsibilities among family, friends, and extended family to provide relief to immediate family and respite care from local agency or church (any visit).

6. Listen to family's feelings, concerns, expectations, and preferences for caregiving. Answer all questions (each visit).
7. Encourage older child to become independent and manage all or part of dialysis procedure with supervision and support (any visit).
8. Support caregiver's need for relief and social services (support group or summer camp) and counseling referral, if needed (any visit).

CAREGIVER/CHILD AND FAMILY INTERVENTIONS

1. Prepares for emotional changes associated with caregiving during discharge planning and teaching.
2. Develops ability to cope with caregiver role. Incorporates flexibility into day-to-day functioning.
3. Involves the older child (> 10 years of age) in progressive self-care as appropriate. Avoids overprotection and control of child's independence.
4. Explores and uses community resources (support groups) to provide physical and psychologic assistance and relief from role strain (respite care).
5. Maintains own health and well-being in caregiver role and as much independence and privacy as possible. Becomes involved in outside activities.
6. Develops new coping skills and strategies for role changes by family members needed to support and participate in care of child.
7. Preserves family relationships and minimizes stressors by sharing feelings, fears, and concerns with one another.
8. Caregiver and family members progressively adapt and accept dialysis.

SAMPLE DOCUMENTATION INCLUSIONS

1. Specific assessment
   Assess general health status; stressors of caregiver and child and effect on treatment regimen; need for home modifications, equipment, and supplies; family role strain and child's coping ability to comply with long-term management; type of peritoneal dialysis; amount instilled and drained; possibility of self-care; signs and symptoms of skin breakdown at insertion site; infection at site

or peritonitis; other complications; vital signs; weight, I&O balance; abdominal girth; and need for reinstruction of aspects of care or referrals (counseling or social services).

2. Specific care/teaching
   Teach procedures involved in peritoneal dialysis (site care, dressings, infusion, drainage, changing bags, and using cycling machine); signs and symptoms of complications and interventions; antibiotic therapy; nutritional inclusions; activity restrictions; and recording temperature, vital signs, and weight.

3. General
   Note responses to care and teaching; goal achievement; changes in plan; maintenance or regression of health status; adaptation of caregiver, family, and child to long-term care and change in lifestyle; community resources for support, assistance, supplies, and equipment for care; and need for monitoring by health care provider.

4. See "Documentation and Family Home Record Keeping" in Appendix for general required documentation components for all home care visits.

Special care plans

Nonorganic Failure to Thrive

Nonorganic failure to thrive (FTT) refers to malnutrition unexplained by any congenital or acquired physiologic disorder. It is generally evident by 6 to 12 months of age and is characterized by weight consistently below the 5th percentile on standardized growth scales, less than 80% of expected weight adjusted for age and height, or any sustained decrease from previously documented and expected growth curves. The syndrome may be attributed to caregiver ignorance, inexperience, neglect, or disturbed mother-child attachment. It is different from organic FTT, which is the result of or a symptom of an underlying physical disorder (e.g., central nervous system [CNS] abnormalities, chronic inflammatory or infectious states, or malabsorption syndromes). Organic FTT may occur at any age and treatment is directed at the underlying pathologic condition. FTT of mixed cause encompasses the complex interaction of physiologic condition and emotional response. In addition to a failure to gain weight or actual weight loss, clinical manifestations of nonorganic FTT may include a thin, frail, or short physique; apathy; flattened affect; social withdrawal; feeding/eating disorders; and developmental delays in speech, social, and motor development. Prognosis varies and is related to the length and the severity of deprivation, personality, and resources of the child. Most cases resolve by 5 years of age, although residual cognitive and behavioral problems may persist. Medical management is directed at reversing the malnutrition. Hospitalization may initially be warranted to evaluate the disorder and to provide nutritional support in a more nurturing environment.

Home health care is primarily concerned with assessment of the family's physical and emotional needs and resources; evaluation of infant status; instruction and reinforcement in nutrition and child care; facilitation of caregiver-child attachment process; and referrals for psychologic, emotional, and rehabilitative care.

Nursing diagnosis

Altered nutrition: less than body requirements
Related factors: inadequate caloric intake; nutritional, emotional deprivation
Defining characteristics: weight below 5th percentile or less than 80% of ideal weight, height/length less than expected per growth curve, eating/feeding difficulties, developmental delays, caregiver inexperience, limited income

OUTCOMES
Short-term
Adequate nutrition evidenced by intake of appropriate diet; minimum expected weight gain (e.g., 0 to 3 months, 1 oz/day) (expected in 1 week; ongoing until ideal weight is attained)

Long-term
Optimal nutrition evidenced by congruence with expected weight curve for age, height; appropriate developmental level (expected in 3 to 6 months)

NURSING INTERVENTIONS/INSTRUCTIONS
1. Before first visit, review hospital discharge plan and teaching caregivers received. Maintain link with departments and agencies also providing care. Assess for compliance with given instructions.
2. Perform complete physical assessment. Include general appearance and behavior, familial growth patterns, chronologic and developmental ages, weight, length or height, head circumference and shape, and condition of sutures and fontanels. Note any condition that might interfere with intake (e.g., poor suck or swallow reflex, cleft palate, respiratory difficulty, or activity intolerance related to cardiac compromise) (each visit).

3. Query caregiver about child's history of feeding problems, food retention, eating disorders, elimination, similar problems of siblings at comparable age and their resolution, and caretaker's perception of appropriate child intake. Include health beliefs, cultural/ethnic prescriptions, and financial ability (first visit).

4. Observe mother breastfeeding infant; note condition of breasts and nipples, positioning, ability of infant to latch on, length of time infant feeds at each breast, maternal or infant fatigue, recognition of infant cues, and discomfort. Encourage breastfeeding efforts. Instruct on self-care, positioning and technique, and other actual or perceived problems (each visit).

5. Observe mother bottlefeeding infant; note method of holding infant while feeding, mutual interest, child aversion behavior, amount and type of formula offered, amount taken, length of feeding, use of bottle propping, and recognition of infant cues (first visit).

6. Observe and query caregiver about toddler feeding. Include caregiver's knowledge of nutrition; types of food available, provided, and actually eaten; and interaction during feeding (first visit).

7. Based on observed need, instruct on feeding strategies and infant stimulation (each visit).

   - Recognizing hunger cues
   - Providing quiet time and place for feeding
   - Holding infant or young child for feeding; making eye contact
   - Talking to and soothing child
   - Feeding infant on demand; if there is no interest in feeding, then wake about every 4 hours; cuddle, provide oral stimulation, feed; be consistent and persistent
   - Establishing schedule for young child; offering appealing food and snacks with high nutritive value; praise; make food and eating priority, not issue

8. Query about and observe, if possible, formula preparation. Note selection of formula, interpretation of dilution requirements, attention to hygiene practices, actual milk supply, and maternal estimation of how long it will last (first visit).

9. Instruct on formula preparation and dilution and hygiene. Emphasize need to give proper dilution. Refer to supplemental food programs (e.g. women, infants, and children [WIC], for milk products) (each visit).

10. Instruct mother on nutrition (first visit).

    • Appropriate foods for age
    • Where to purchase food items
    • Average serving sizes
    • How to prepare high-protein, nutrient-dense foods per physician's recommendation (Supplementation or altered dilution of formula to yield more calories per ounce may be necessary to achieve the required increase in calories, i.e., approximately 150% of required kcal/kg ideal weight/24 hours.)

11. Instruct mother to keep food diary for 1 week and to include time, amount, interval of feeding, retention, actual food consumed, displayed preference, and special concerns. Review and teach as needed (each visit).

12. Instruct mother to weigh child once a week using same scale at same time with child wearing same clothing. Weigh child at each visit and plot on standardized graphs. Report failure to gain or actual loss to physician (each visit).

13. Instruct caregiver on nocturnal enteral feedings as appropriate (see "Alternate Feeding Management," pp. 205-215, for guidelines) (as needed).

14. Refer family to nutritionist as needed.

CAREGIVER/CHILD AND FAMILY INTERVENTIONS

1. Recognizes and responds to child's cues of hunger.
2. Breastfeeds on demand at least every 2 to 3 hours.
3. Prepares formula per recommendations, using clean technique.
4. Offers child frequent, nutrient-dense foods supplemented with MCT oil per recommendations.
5. Prepares age-appropriate, appealing, high-calorie, high-protein meals.
6. Provides warmth, affection, and nurturing before and during feedings.
7. After feedings, allows infant to sleep. Praises child.

8. Records weekly weight measurements and reports failure to gain or actual loss to health care worker.
9. Safely administers nightly nasogastric tube feedings.
10. Consults with nutritionist.
11. Uses supplemental food service programs.

Nursing diagnosis

Altered parenting
Related factors: lack of role models, inexperience, adolescent mother, immaturity, unwanted pregnancy, physical/emotional stressors, depression, financial instability, lack of support or resources
Defining characteristics: low self-esteem; apathy; disordered lifestyle; lack of recognition or response to infant's cries; disinterest in or aversion to child care; negative statements about child's appearance, needs, impact on lifestyle; minimal handling or looking at child; emotional distancing

OUTCOMES
Short-term
Improved parenting evidenced by recognition, positive response to at least one of child's needs weekly (expected by first week, ongoing)

Long-term
Positive parenting evidenced by positive maternal responses, increased maternal-infant attachment, demonstrated ability to provide appropriate child care, nurturing (expected in 3 to 6 months)

NURSING INTERVENTIONS/INSTRUCTIONS
1. Assign same nurse. Establish rapport and trust (each visit).
2. Perform family and social assessments (see p. 41 for guidelines). Include step-families and foster-families. Note evidence of physical/emotional illness, multiple responsibilities, financial problems, social isolation, family discord, domestic violence, and substance abuse (each visit).

3. Assess maternal life experiences and pregnancy history. Include mother's age, health, educational level, history of abuse, marital status, and perception of pregnancy and delivery; child's health and birth order; and condition of other children (first visit).

4. Observe parenting skills and characteristics. Consider ethnic/cultural beliefs and practices. Praise and encourage positive responses (each visit).

5. Encourage communication. Explore views on parenting. Refer to self-esteem workshops, support groups, vocational training, or family counselor as indicated.

6. Be open and responsive to family's needs. Avoid accusations or inferences of uncaring, blame, inadequacy, immaturity, or irresponsibility (each visit).

7. Enlist mother in child's treatment plan. Focus on child's needs, how child makes them known, and how they can best be met (each visit).

8. Be role model. Demonstrate physical care of child and incorporate emotional and nurturing components throughout (each visit).

9. Instruct on developmental milestones and appropriate activities. Assist in anticipating and responding to developmental issues (e.g., autonomy or emotional outbursts as child defines emotional capacity) (each visit).

10. Encourage caregiver to take time for self and family. Explore sources of support and respite care (each visit).

11. Explore option of temporary foster care if prolonged respite care or rehabilitative services are needed.

12. Immediately report any evidence of abuse or potential child endangerment to child protective services.

CAREGIVER/CHILD AND FAMILY INTERVENTIONS

1. Interacts openly with health care worker.
2. Observes demonstrations of child care and reads literature on parenting.
3. Identifies cues of child's needs and how to meet them. Learns new skill each week.
4. Feeds, bathes, grooms, and plays with child.
5. Increases eye contact, cuddling, and holding.
6. Identifies personal strengths and those in need of strengthening.

7. Uses respite services if available.
8. Participates in support groups as needed.

Nursing diagnosis

Altered growth and development
Related factors: environmental, stimulation deficiencies
Defining characteristics: aversion to touch, eye contact; vigilant
    manner; wariness; interactive with things, not people; un-
    pliable or limp body posture; lack of molding when being
    held; lack of spontaneity, fun, humor, responsiveness; de-
    creased range of feelings; later behavioral disorders

OUTCOMES
Short-term
Improved development evidenced by beginning or increased
eye contact, relaxing body language and responsiveness
(expected in 1 month, ongoing)

Long-term
Optimal growth/development evidenced by developmentally
appropriate activity, emotional responsiveness (expected
in 3 to 6 months)

NURSING INTERVENTIONS/INSTRUCTIONS
1. Assess developmental level and achieved milestones. Plot
   results on standardized record. Inform caregiver of activity and expectations (each visit).
2. Assess child's and caregiver's temperaments and interac-
   tional "fit." Note child's reaction to touch, gaze, demands for care and attention, irritability, consolability,
   and use of self-stimulation (e.g., rocking). Compare with
   caregiver's perception of child's appearance and behavior (each visit).
3. Recognize child. Talk to and include child in discussion
   as appropriate. Offer child positive reinforcement (each
   visit).
4. Reinforce child's needs for time, love, and attention and
   how best to satisfy these needs (review altered parenting) (each visit).

5. Encourage caregiver to provide emotional, environmental, and cognitive stimulation by singing, reading, listening to children's stories together, playing games, and providing toys (each visit).
6. Confer with stimulation specialist. Encourage enrollment in structured stimulation program (as needed).
7. Encourage educational placement in early or special programs (as needed).

CAREGIVER/CHILD AND FAMILY INTERVENTIONS

1. Observes developmental assessment.
2. Recognizes need for environmental stimulation and emotional nurturing for child's growth/development.
3. Focuses on child's needs.
4. Smiles, holds, looks at, and talks to child.
5. Offers appropriate sensory stimulation, praise, and positive feedback.
6. Participates in sensory stimulation and educational programs.

SAMPLE DOCUMENTATION INCLUSIONS

1. Specific assessment
   Child: Assess chronologic and developmental ages, weight, length/height, head circumference, feeding difficulties, vomiting, diarrhea, sleep disturbances, behavior, affect, developmental delays, and cognitive and behavioral problems.
   Mother: Assess social and family histories, previous experiences, perinatal events, current stressors, parenting skills, and coping and adaptive capacities.
2. Specific care/teaching
   Teach about nutrition; feeding; child care; nurturing; infant stimulation; and referrals for social, emotional, financial, and educational services.
3. General
   Note responses to care and teaching and child's physical and emotional health.
4. See "Documentation and Family Home Record Keeping" in Appendix for required documentation components for all home care visits.

Hospital Follow-up Home Care

Children discharged from the hospital after illness or surgery are provided with guidelines to prepare the family to manage the necessary care to restore the child's health or maintain a realistic level in the presence of chronic illness. Most children are discharged to home care without problems or need for home care visits and with the proposed regimen easily incorporated into the family routines. For those who return home with complex or special health needs, additional assessment, care, and teaching are coordinated and provided by home care visits from various professionals, depending on need. The number of visits depends on the child's condition (insurance companies frequently request an estimate of the number of home visits anticipated).

Home care is also concerned with the development of trust and rapport with the child and family; assistance to safely incorporate and follow the proposed regimen into their daily routines; encouragement of the child toward self-care; and the teaching of procedures, treatments, and the correct use of equipment needed to comply with the care plan.

Nursing diagnosis

Impaired home maintenance management
Related factors: lack of knowledge; surgical procedure (postoperative care); medical condition (posthospitalization care); insufficient planning, finances, support system
Defining characteristics: requests information, assistance with home care after discharge from hospital; lack of money, necessary equipment, supplies; inability to meet all needs of child

OUTCOMES
Short-term
Adequate knowledge for maintenance of progressive improvement in health evidenced by formulating and imple-

menting plan for home care that promotes safe, effective management of basic needs; return to optimal function after hospitalization (expected within 1 to 2 weeks, ongoing)

Long-term
Adaptation to home environment within maximum health parameters; independence in self-care evidenced by home modifications, compliance with personal hygiene needs, dietary/fluid/elimination requirements; safe activity regimen; correct medication regimen; return to school, former peer/social relationships (expected within 1 or more months, depending on reason for hospitalization)

NURSING INTERVENTIONS/INSTRUCTIONS

1. Arrange for predischarge conference to review discharge plan. Prepare written home care plan with time and frequency of visits.
2. Perform complete physical assessment. Inform caregiver and family of interruptions in sleep, temporary nightmares, withdrawal, and regressive behaviors after hospitalization (first visit).
3. Allow child to express feelings about surgery and changes in body image, use doll if appropriate (each visit).
4. Promote awareness of and suggest measures to continue growth/development, including stimulation; socialization; and in-home teaching, tutor, or schooling (any visit).
5. Review nutrition and fluid intake for balance and nutritional inclusions. Instruct caregiver to weigh child weekly for changes and to offer child diet high in protein and vitamin C to promote wound healing (each visit).
6. Initiate consultation with nutritionist for optimal growth/development (any visit).
7. Instruct to assess bowel pattern and need for stool softener, dietary change, and progressive activities to establish regularity (first visit).
8. Review, supervise, and demonstrate all medication administration instructions. Include method of administration, side effects, resumption of medication regimen for chronic medical conditions, and drug interactions.

Have caregiver repeat demonstration (each visit until all medications have been reviewed).

9. Supervise demonstration of treatments using equipment and supplies, including wound care; taking temperature, pulse, and blood pressure; and other procedures as appropriate. Allow for repeat demonstrations and verbalization of concerns (first and second visits).

10. Collaborate with caregiver and child in reviewing activity restrictions, safe physical play (refrain from rough play, pushing, pulling, and lifting) while conserving energy, time for rest and use of assistive devices as needed, and resuming school attendance or providing tutoring (first visit, second visit if needed).

11. Instruct to encourage self-care as condition improves. Reinforce handwashing technique and universal precautions to control infection (each visit).

12. Reinforce importance of follow-up visits to physician and scheduling at times that do not interfere with rest or meal times if possible (any visit).

13. Refer to community services for support, information, social, financial, respite care, or other assistance (any visit).

CAREGIVER/CHILD AND FAMILY INTERVENTIONS

1. Adapts to and cooperates with complete home care regimen.

2. Maintains written daily log to comply with posthospitalization home care that includes assessments and treatments.

3. Practices good personal hygiene and grooming that enhance self-image.

4. Child ingests fluids and nutrients. Offers child preferred foods and assists child in feeding when appropriate.

5. Participates in activities and play with reduced need for assistance; avoids activities that stress incisional area or cause pain or fatigue.

6. Schedules rest and activities based on needs and condition.

7. Establishes and maintains bowel and urinary elimination patterns.

8. Administers all medications accurately in most desirable form. Uses check-off sheet as reminder and to avoid errors.

9. Prevents infection by handwashing and using sterile technique for wound care and other invasive procedures. Avoids contact with others with infection.
10. Reports adverse effects of medications, treatments, temperature elevation, and signs and symptoms of infection or other complications to physician.
11. Arranges for follow-up appointments for monitoring health status and suture removal.
12. Returns to school and activities and participates in self-care and family routines.

Nursing diagnosis

Ineffective family/child coping: compromised
Related factors: situational crisis (discharge from hospital), family disorganization and role changes, lack of assistive or supportive behaviors
Defining characteristics: expression of inability to cope; feelings of fear, anxiety, inadequate understanding of posthospital care by family; inability of child to cope or ask for help; personal vulnerability; anxiety of caregiver or child

OUTCOMES

Short-term
Family members demonstrate ability to plan and care for child evidenced by provision of healthy environment; decreased anxiety, feelings of inadequacy; integration of information about family needs into care, support of child; able to ask questions, verbalize understanding of situation (expected within 1 week)

Long-term
Family coping, adaptation to home care of child after hospitalization evidenced by optimal support, participation in care, maintenance of family relationships (expected within 2 weeks)

NURSING INTERVENTIONS/INSTRUCTIONS

1. Meet and collaborate with family members to assess stressors, coping mechanisms, and effect on providing care (first visit, repeat as needed).

2. Reinforce information and teaching given during discharge planning to promote family understanding of child's condition and care needs (first visit, as needed).
3. Discuss and allow family to express feelings of anxiety. Promote communication among members to verbalize feelings and expectations with each other (any visit).
4. Instruct family members to encourage and allow child to progress to self-care and independence at own rate (each visit).
5. Instruct on methods to develop coping skills and to meet family's needs (medical, emotional, financial, food, supplies, and equipment). Refer to social worker or counselor (each visit as needed).

CAREGIVER/CHILD AND FAMILY INTERVENTIONS

1. Displays decreasing anxiety and apprehension. Provides supportive family environment.
2. Develops trust in home care personnel and collaborates in developing and modifying daily care of child until normal lifestyle is resumed.
3. Provides care and treatments effectively. Supports child during stressful times, when feeling most vulnerable, and when unable to participate in daily routines with family or friends.
4. Avoids overprotection or rejection of child by caregiver or family members.
5. Recognizes and assumes role changes during convalescence. Maintains family integrity.
6. Develops coping mechanisms that have positive effect within family.
7. Identifies problem areas and obtains assistance or social services as needed.

SAMPLE DOCUMENTATION INCLUSIONS

1. Specific assessment
   Assess age, individual and family developmental stage, reason for hospitalization, length of stay, discharge plan, teaching performed, care, complexity of regimens, responses to interventions, prescribed medications (dose, route, and frequency), responses to medication regimen, appearance of wound, wound healing or deterioration,

need for home modifications, child and family coping skills, and anxiety level related to home management.

2. Specific care/teaching
   Teach administration of medication regimen including name, dose, frequency, route, and times of day; special considerations based on form, side effects, and expected response; management of basic needs and comfort measures; imposed restrictions during convalescence; procedures to be performed; monitoring of essential components of care; use and care of supplies/equipment if used for care procedures; and recognition of signs and symptoms of complications that necessitate additional visits or reporting to physician.

3. General
   Note responses to care and teaching; goal achievement; changes/modifications of plan; abilities of caregiver and family to manage child's complete care; resources for acquiring medication, supplies, and equipment needed for therapy; and coordination among interdisciplinary team.

4. See "Documentation and Family Home Record Keeping" in Appendix for general required documentation components for all home care visits.

 Childhood Malignancies and Chemotherapy and Radiation Therapy

---

Cancer, although a leading cause of death in children, has a long-term survival rate of 50%. Types of cancers include leukemia (acute and nonacute), lymphoma (Hodgkin's and non-Hodgkin's), brain tumor (glioma, medulloblastoma, and cerebral astrocytoma), Wilms' tumor (nephroblastoma), bone tumor (osteogenic sarcoma and Ewing's sarcoma), muscle tumor (rhabdomyosarcoma), retinal tumor (retinoblastoma), and adrenal gland tumor (neuroblastoma).

Treatments include surgery, chemotherapy, radiation therapy, immunotherapy, and bone marrow transplantation. They are usually performed alone or in combination based on the diagnosis, tumor staging, child's age, and projected prognosis. The child is affected not only physically by the disease and treatment protocol, but also emotionally and developmentally. The psychosocial and financial impact is felt by parents, siblings, friends, and extended family members. The use of chemotherapy has become the greatest advancement in treating childhood cancer. Selection, dose, frequency, and method depend on the type of disease.

Combination chemotherapy affects the cells at different times in the cell cycle, reducing drug resistance by the cancer cells. Some drugs affect cell division, others act directly on the cell membrane to destroy the cell, and some interfere with RNA and DNA production by the cell. Therefore drugs are used in combination rather than as single agents. Specific drugs are toxic to various organs and organ structures. External radiation is administered alone or in combination with chemotherapy or surgery. It is used for local or regional control of the tumor, based on tumor sensitivity and the child's age. It acts by ionization that causes physical changes in the cell with subsequent chemical changes and disruption in the DNA strands of the cell, resulting in cell damage and death. Both healthy and malignant cells are affected and side effects include skin and mucous membrane reactions, fatigue, alopecia, vomiting, diarrhea, increased intracranial pressure, sterility, and bone marrow depression. Surgery can be diagnostic (biopsy for staging), palliative (tumor excision or nerve blocks), or curative (partial or total removal of tumor, body part, and nodes). Bone marrow transplantation is reserved for those with selected types of solid tumors or leukemia that have not responded to other therapy.

Home care by the home care nurse and other personnel is primarily concerned with care for the child through all phases of the disease, treatments, and provision of support to the child and family. The family needs many visits by home health providers to assist them in living to their fullest potential while facing a life-threatening illness or hospice care.

Nursing diagnosis

Altered growth and development
Related factors: effects of chronic illness; environmental, stimulation deficiencies; inadequate parental caregiving; prescribed dependence; nutritional deficit
Defining characteristics: delay/difficulty in performing skills; altered physical growth; inability of child to perform self-care, self-control activities

OUTCOMES
Short-term
Adequate growth/development behavior, activities evidenced by absence of deficits, delays, or regression of functioning; growth/development within limits imposed by illness (expected within 6 to 12 weeks)

Long-term
Progressive growth/development; achievement advances of normal physical, emotional, and social parameters (expected ongoing)

NURSING INTERVENTIONS/INSTRUCTIONS
1. Assess expected growth/developmental level for age and extent of deficits. Include fine and gross motor skills, language and social development, psychosocial and interpersonal skills, and cognitive development (see "Growth and Developmental Assessment," p. 31, for guidelines) (every visit).
2. Assess caregiver, family, and environment for stressful events and ability to provide love, caring, adequate stimulation, and appropriate play activities (each visit).
3. Assess for caregiver overprotection or negligence (each visit).
4. Instruct on normal growth/development patterns for child's age and possible lag in development caused by illness (first visit).
5. Assist caregiver and family to develop goals and participate in care to achieve optimal development potential (ongoing).

6. Instruct to monitor child's activity tolerance and collaborate to develop plan to provide visual, auditory, and tactile stimulation; gross motor skills of infant; and time with child for talking or playing and for self-care activities (ongoing).

7. Provide encouragement and support for efforts made by child and caregivers (each visit).

8. Provide early referral to professional resources such as speech or physical therapist, special education teacher, psychosocial counselor, or social worker to assist child in specific areas of need (any visit).

CAREGIVER/CHILD AND FAMILY INTERVENTIONS

1. Complies with activities to enhance stimulation, independence, and developmental (cognitive, psychomotor, and psychosocial) progression.

2. Sets realistic goals for growth/developmental achievement.

3. Maintains consistent caregiver and schedule of activities.

4. Provides organized and consistent program of daily activities that include mobiles, music, toys, books, and other learning tools.

5. Provides time for talking and playing with other children and family members.

6. Holds, rocks, and cuddles child to provide touch and loving care.

7. Provides opportunity to participate in self-care activities, including dressing, bathing, eating, and toileting with adaptations as needed.

8. Attends parenting classes for child stimulation, growth/developmental milestones, discipline, and expectations.

9. Identifies and uses specialized services to assist with growth/developmental lags.

Nursing diagnosis

Anxiety/fear (child and parent)
Related factors: change in health status (diagnosis of cancer); threat of death (life-threatening disease, poor prognosis); painful treatments (chemotherapy, radiotherapy, other interventions), procedures (diagnostic, surgery)

Defining characteristics: apprehension, restlessness, facial tension, uncertainty, regression, verbalization or lack of feeling of fear

OUTCOMES

Short-term
Minimal anxiety, reduction in fear evidenced by caregiver and child gradually accepting treatments for disease; expresses fear but demonstrates ability to remain calm and cooperate with planned protocol (expected within 4 weeks, possibly longer)

Long-term
Fear/anxiety at manageable level evidenced by effective use of coping mechanisms, ongoing support, adaptation to care requirements of disease with life as comfortable, free of fear/anxiety as possible (expected within 1 month)

NURSING INTERVENTIONS/INSTRUCTIONS

1. Assess emotional and mental status of caregiver and child and their ability to manage complex care and protocols (see "Psychologic Assessment," p. 25, for guidelines) (any visit as needed).
2. Provide information about disease, cause, meaning of metastasis, and prognosis in easily understandable language. Before treatments and procedures, inform parent and child of what will take place. Use visuals and dolls as appropriate (each visit).
3. Maintain calm, quiet environment during assessment and teaching (each visit).
4. Provide opportunity for caregiver and child to verbalize fears and concerns. Encourage acceptance of changes needed to comply with treatment modalities. Explain side effects to expect (each visit).
5. Suggest that caregiver stay with child during anxious times and provide support, especially during painful treatments (first visit).
6. Assess caregiver for feelings of guilt and self-blame for child's condition. Assist to reduce these feelings (each visit).

7. Provide accurate information about radiation therapy and chemotherapy. Dispel myths and fears associated with therapy (first visit).

8. Consider cultural and religious feelings of family and support their beliefs (first visit).

9. Inform of parent support group, if available, and community and national agencies such as American Cancer Society and Candlelighters (any visit).

CAREGIVER/CHILD AND FAMILY INTERVENTIONS

1. Recognizes anxiety associated with child's condition, unknown prognosis, and onset of behaviors associated with high level of fear.

2. Maintains calm, supportive environment and controls situation by remaining with, holding or hugging, and reassuring child during care. Prepares child before each aspect of treatment.

3. Child uses familiar relaxation techniques, diversion, and quiet play activities.

4. Involves child in helping with treatment such as holding pieces of equipment, taping dressing, and keeping records.

5. Uses appropriate support resources if needed.

Nursing diagnosis

Ineffective family/individual coping: compromised

Related factors: life-threatening disease that exhausts supportive capacity of significant people; family disorganization, role changes; frequent hospitalizations

Defining characteristics: expression of inability to cope; feelings of fear, anxiety, guilt, anger, denial, depression; child's expression of fear, lack of control; regressive behavior; inadequate understanding of disease, therapy, its side effects; complex care by family; inability of child to cope or ask for help; chronic fatigue, anxiety of family and child; marital conflicts; jealousy, anger of siblings; financial strain

OUTCOMES

Short-term

Family members demonstrate ability to plan, care for child evidenced by provision of normal environment; decreased anxiety, feelings of inadequacy; integration of information about family needs into care, support of child (expected within 2 to 4 weeks)

Long-term

Family coping, adaptation evidenced by optimal support, participation in care; maintenance of family relationships; demonstrates knowledge, understanding of treatments/ procedures involved in child's care (expected within 1 month)

NURSING INTERVENTIONS/INSTRUCTIONS

1. Arrange for case conference with total health care team (first week).
2. Collaborate with family members to assess stressors and coping mechanisms and to plan care (first visit, repeat as needed).
3. Reinforce information provided during discharge teaching to promote family understanding of disease and care protocol. Instruct on areas of knowledge deficit (each visit).
4. Explain and discuss treatments of chemotherapy and radiation therapy. Provide written schedule of treatments, tests, and procedures (all visits).
5. Explain side effects that can occur from chemotherapy or radiation therapy, reason for therapy, expected outcomes, and unfavorable responses to report to physician (first visit).
6. Assess parents for coping abilities; use of defense mechanisms, communication patterns, and stressors caused by relatives; and family members and family cohesiveness (any visit as needed).
7. Inform caregiver and family members that their reactions and behaviors affect child's perceptions of disease and create fear about outcome (first visit).
8. Assess potential family stressors such as financial problems, schedule to take turns giving care, other family ill-

ness, and potential strengths (support of family members, friends, relatives, and employer) (first visit, as needed).

9. Discuss and encourage family to express feelings of guilt, anxiety, and depression. Promote communication among family members to verbalize feelings and expectations with each other. Encourage to ask questions and speak openly about disease and treatments with health care provider (each visit).

10. Instruct on methods to develop coping skills and to meet family's needs (medical, emotional, financial, food, respite care, supplies, and equipment). Refer to social worker or counselor (first visit, as needed).

CAREGIVER/CHILD AND FAMILY INTERVENTIONS

1. Displays decreasing anxiety and anger. Provides supportive family environment. Openly verbalizes and discusses findings and child's needs with home health care provider and family members.

2. Develops trust in home care personnel and other professionals. Collaborates in developing and modifying care as needed. Answers child's and caregiver's questions honestly.

3. Provides care and therapy effectively. Supports child during stressful times or when feeling most vulnerable and unable to participate in routine activities.

4. Follows chemotherapy or radiation therapy protocol to ensure prescribed treatment.

5. Avoids rejection of child by caregiver or family members. Encourages siblings to verbalize feelings about disease and its effect on family.

6. Recognizes and assumes role changes. Maintains family integrity.

7. Develops coping mechanisms that have supportive effect within family.

8. Identifies problem areas. Obtains community or professional assistance or social services as needed.

Nursing diagnosis

Pain

Related factors: biologic injuring agents (chemotherapy/radiation therapy), physical (malignant process, procedures), psychologic (developmental, cultural)

Defining characteristics: moaning; crying; guarding behavior; lack of sleep; irritability; increased pulse, blood pressure; anorexia

OUTCOMES

Short-term

Decrease/control of pain evidenced by child verbalizing relief of pain; vital signs stable; behavior indicating pain relief 1 hour after analgesic therapy (expected within 1 to 2 days)

Long-term

Minimal or absence of pain evidenced by participation in activities, treatments performed without discomfort, able to rest or remain quiet, increased appetite (expected within 1 week)

NURSING INTERVENTIONS/INSTRUCTIONS

1. Perform complete physical and behavioral assessments (each visit).
2. Assess and instruct caregiver to assess for pain (anticipatory and actual) and need for analgesia; note effectiveness of medications in relieving pain (see "Pain Management," pp. 398-402, for guidelines) (each visit).
3. Assess for other possible causes of pain such as positioning, skin breakdown, or constipation and take appropriate measures to alleviate problem (each visit, as needed).
4. Administer analgesic as prescribed before activities that increase discomfort. Instruct caregiver about route, schedules, dosage, and side effects of medications; maintain drug level that ensures minimal pain; instruct on use and care of central venous catheter or other devices to ease discomfort of medication administration (see "Medication Administration and Teaching Guidelines," pp. 450-463) (each visit as needed).

5. Maintain environment free from noise and bright lights. Give analgesic during position changes. Avoid pressure on or abrupt movement of painful parts (each visit).
6. Teach older child various relaxation techniques (e.g., breathing, imaging, quiet diversion) (any visit).
7. Instruct to avoid any aspirin-containing products (first visit).

CAREGIVER/CHILD AND FAMILY INTERVENTIONS

1. Assesses child for pain using visual scale or behavior, possible reason for discomfort.
2. Formulates anticipatory schedule. Administers pain relief as prescribed via proper route.
3. Evaluates effect of analgesic and side effects of sedation.
4. Coordinates activities and treatments with analgesic administration. Changes position with gentleness and avoids painful positions or pressure on painful areas.
5. Provides nonpharmacologic measures to reduce pain.
6. Notifies physician if pain relief is not obtained or if side effects occur.

Nursing diagnosis

Altered nutrition: less than body requirements
Related factors: inability to ingest enough nutrients (anorexia, refusal of meals); digest, absorb nutrients (nausea, vomiting, diarrhea); increased caloric demand of malignant cells
Defining characteristics: inadequate food intake, stomatitis, nausea, vomiting, diarrhea, constipation, FTT, irritability during feedings/meals, taste alteration, dry oral cavity, weight loss

OUTCOMES

Short-term
Improved appetite with adequate nutritional intake evidenced by weight gain/minimal weight loss, improved oral daily intake of balanced meals by child, or feedings via alternate route, depending on extent/type of therapy (expected within 1 to 2 weeks)

Long-term
Nutritional status for optimal growth/development, increased metabolic need of child evidenced by acceptance of nutritional food, satisfactory weight maintenance or gains, control of gastrointestinal (GI) side effects of therapy, characteristics, activities that facilitate successful feeding (expected within 1 to 3 months)

NURSING INTERVENTIONS/INSTRUCTIONS

1. Assess nutritional requirement for age and weight; needed caloric intake; weight deviation from standard for age; appetite, food, and fluid preferences of child; and times of meals or feedings (see "Gastrointestinal Assessment and Nutritional Assessment," pp. 16 and 17, for guidelines) (first visit).

2. Assess and instruct to assess for side effects of therapy that affect nutritional intake (e.g., oral cavity for mucositis, dryness, tooth decay, nausea, and vomiting following therapy), anorexia from disease or therapy that results in taste alteration, stomatitis and esophagitis, nausea, decreased saliva, and neutropenia (avoid raw vegetables, fruits, and seafoods) (each visit).

3. Inform caregiver that appetite changes are normal and to avoid forcing child to eat (first visit).

4. Instruct and collaborate with caregiver in planning and providing high-caloric, high-protein, high-carbohydrate, and low-sodium foods that are tolerated and selected by child. Instruct to increase amounts as appetite increases (first and second visits).

5. Instruct caregiver to offer small feedings or liquids and allow snacks and preferred foods if desired; supplement with additional calories when possible; use local anesthetic to oropharyngeal area if ordered before meals; oral care as needed (first visit).

6. Instruct caregiver on providing oral care, administering antiemetic medicine before meals and therapy if nausea or vomiting occurs, and administering antidiarrheal medicine if diarrhea is persistent. Include instruction on dose and side effects (first and second visits).

7. Suggest calm, clean environment during meals and actions to minimize frustrations (allow rest periods and

avoid rushing during meals; place in position of comfort by holding infant upright and child in sitting position at table within easy reach of food; offer preferred foods and properly sized utensils) (any visit).

8. Demonstrate and instruct caregiver to weigh child every 7 days (infant more frequently) using same scale, with child wearing same clothing, at same time of day (first visit).

9. Support participation and presence of caregiver and family at feedings (each visit).

10. Administer nutritional intake by nasogastric tube or total parenteral nutrition as ordered (see "Alternative Feeding Management," p. 205-215) (any visit).

11. Initiate referral to nutritionist for diet planning if needed, especially if FTT is present (any visit).

CAREGIVER/CHILD AND FAMILY INTERVENTIONS

1. Plans and provides diet that contains calorie, protein, and carbohydrate intake with supplements as needed. Limits foods high in sodium if on steroid therapy. Restrict foods associated with neutropenia. Avoid milk and high-bulk foods for persistent diarrhea.

2. Allows child to participate in food selection and preparation and meal planning.

3. Prepares nutritional foods and fluids of proper consistency and texture, finger foods, and snacks for child and offers them frequently.

4. Administers antiemetic medication 30 minutes to 1 hour before treatment, oral care before and after meals if desired, and antidiarrheal medication if ordered. Identifies potential side effects to report to physician.

5. Feeds or assists with meals if needed to conserve energy and paces feedings according to appetite.

6. Promotes pleasant environment for child to enhance intake. Integrates feeding times into family routine, if possible, or offers food at times of optimal energy.

7. Obtains daily or weekly weight measurements using same scale, with child wearing same clothing, and at same time on specified days. Records and compares changes to determine weight gain or loss.

8. Reports weight loss, prolonged nausea, vomiting, and diarrhea to physician.

Nursing diagnosis

Risk for infection
Related factors: inadequate primary defenses (injury to skin), inadequate secondary defenses (immunosuppression, neutropenia, myelosuppression), invasive procedures (catheters, shunts, injections), insufficient knowledge of caregiver to avoid exposure of child to pathogens
Defining characteristics: temperature instability; irritability; lethargy; redness, swelling, drainage at catheter sites/incision site; diarrhea; oral candidiasis; changes in respiration, sputum characteristics

OUTCOMES
Short-term
Early detection of signs and symptoms of infection during chemotherapy or radiation therapy evidenced by absence of redness, edema, drainage at skin or mucous membrane sites; temperature stability; respiratory, bowel elimination status within normal parameters; reporting to physician for early interventions/treatments (expected with daily assessment)

Long-term
Adaptation to lifestyle that promotes clean, safe environment; actions to minimize risk for infection (ongoing)

NURSING INTERVENTIONS/INSTRUCTIONS
1. Assess home and living conditions (see "Environmental Assessment," p. 37, for guidelines) (first visit, follow-up for additional modifications).
2. Assess for signs of infection in area of radiation (redness, pain, and drainage) (each visit).
3. Assess for changes in respiratory rate, depth, and ease; change in color/odor of pulmonary secretions; and diminished breath sounds (each visit).

4. Assess and instruct to assess axillary temperature, changes in skin or oral/rectal mucous membranes, irritability, lethargy, and changes in feeding or elimination pattern. Have caregiver demonstrate temperature taking (each visit as needed).

5. Assess and instruct to assess central catheter sites and other invasive devices or surgical wound for redness, edema, drainage, and pain (each visit).

6. Instruct on administration of antibiotic or antipyretic medications in proper form. Inform about side effects to expect (first visit, reinforce).

7. Instruct caregiver to perform catheter care, dressing changes, and other procedures involving invasive devices using sterile technique (first and second visits).

8. Instruct on precautions to prevent infection such as washing hands, avoiding contact with those who have infection, and wearing mask and on importance of adequate nutritional intake and rest and maintaining clean environment (ongoing).

9. Instruct child to avoid contact with animal wastes. Instruct caregiver that child is not to receive immunizations without direction and supervision by oncologist; child should avoid people immunized with live viruses (first visit, reinforce).

10. Instruct caregiver to report any signs and symptoms of infection or if child has had contact with infected person (chickenpox, herpes zoster, or hepatitis) to physician (first visit).

11. Obtain sputum specimen for culture and laboratory testing for neutrophil count, if ordered, and notify physician of results (any visit).

CAREGIVER/CHILD AND FAMILY INTERVENTIONS

1. Takes temperature if signs and symptoms of infection are noted and reports elevation of >101° F. Avoids use of rectal thermometer. Assesses for cough or dyspnea, skin breakdown, or drainage in any area.

2. Observes for changes in behavior, assesses exposure to infection, and reports findings to physician.

3. Administers antibiotic therapy correctly for 7 to 10 days as prescribed by physician, until all medication is correctly taken.

4. Avoids possible exposure of child to family members or others with infections. Wears face mask if appropriate.
5. Performs proper handwashing frequently, especially before and after caring for child. Uses clean or sterile technique as appropriate during care and procedures.
6. Maintains environment that is free from respiratory contaminants and that is humidified and well-ventilated.
7. Properly disposes of articles and supplies used according to universal precautions.

Nursing diagnosis

Risk for fluid volume deficit
Related factors: excessive losses through normal routes (diarrhea, vomiting); altered intake of fluids; medications affecting renal, bladder function (chemotherapy)
Defining characteristics: oliguria, dysuria, hematuria, dry skin and oral cavity, weight loss, dehydration, thirst, sunken fontanelles

OUTCOMES
Short-term
Adequate fluids retained evidenced by absence of signs and symptoms of dehydration during therapy (expected within 2 to 3 days)

Long-term
Hydration maintained evidenced by freedom from fluid, electrolyte imbalances (expected ongoing)

NURSING INTERVENTIONS/INSTRUCTIONS
1. Assess intake and output (I&O) ratio and effect of losses from vomiting, diarrhea, and anorexia on fluid balance (each visit).
2. Assess and instruct to assess for dehydration including thirst, dry skin and mucous membranes, poor skin turgor, decreased urinary output, and weight loss (each visit).
3. Instruct on encouraging fluid intake following nausea, vomiting, and diarrhea. Offer child Pedialyte to replace electrolytes (each visit as needed).

4. Instruct caregiver to administer antiemetic medication 1 hour before chemotherapy (first visit).
5. Administer and maintain intravenous fluids if prescribed (any visit).
6. Instruct caregiver to weigh child daily for losses if vomiting and diarrhea are severe; use same scale, at same time, and with child wearing same clothing (first visit).

CAREGIVER/CHILD AND FAMILY INTERVENTIONS

1. Monitors I&O daily during therapy protocol.
2. Provides fluid intake of clear liquids when nausea and vomiting subside.
3. Administers antiemetic drug before therapy.
4. Avoids offering foods or fluids that increase vomiting or diarrhea.
5. Reports hematuria, urgency, back pain, and edema indicating effect of chemotherapy on renal function to physician.
6. Reports persistent fluid losses, weight loss, and signs and symptoms of dehydration.

Nursing diagnosis

Risk for impaired skin integrity
Related factors: external factor of radiation, internal factors of altered metabolic and nutritional states (emaciation), hyperpigmentation (chemotherapy/radiation therapy), medication (corticosteroid therapy)
Defining characteristics: rashes, acne, irritation, erythema, discoloration, sunburn, dryness, disruption of skin surface

OUTCOMES

Short-term
Minimal effects of therapy evidenced by appropriate care of skin problems as they occur (expected within 1 to 2 days)

Long-term
Compliance with skin protection, per physician's instruction, evidenced by integrity maintained during, after therapy (expected ongoing)

NURSING INTERVENTIONS/INSTRUCTIONS

1. Assess skin status for hyperpigmentation (bronzing) if radiation therapy is administered. If chemotherapy is administered, assess nail beds, teeth, gingiva, and veins. Assess acne from corticosteroids and irritated, dry skin from either type of therapy (each visit).
2. Instruct to cleanse skin daily using mild soap and to avoid any radiation markings (first visit).
3. Instruct to apply lubricating lotion to skin and lip ointment if dry and local antibiotic ointment, if ordered, for skin infection. Instruct to avoid applying creams or powders to irritated or itchy areas (first visit).
4. Instruct to wash perianal area and pat dry after each loose bowel movement, to apply protective ointment, if irritated, and to use Tucks and Puff tissues instead of toilet tissue (first visit).
5. Instruct to avoid exposure to sun because of photosensitivity. Suggest waterproof sunscreen and protective clothing to exposed areas (first visit, as needed).
6. Instruct to avoid direct exposure to hot or cold, or wearing tight clothing or rough fabric on affected area (first visit).
7. Assess patency of chemotherapy infusion site before, during, and after injection for extravasation (pain, swelling, and redness) (each visit).
8. Instruct to assess and treat infiltration of infusion by application of ice or warm compress as appropriate and elevation of extremity (any visit).
9. Instruct to assess and treat irritation of vein by applying warm, moist pack (any visit).

CAREGIVER/CHILD AND FAMILY INTERVENTIONS

1. Provides daily bath with warm water and mild soap without removing markings for radiation.
2. Applies moisturizing cream and antipruritic ointment to dry skin but avoids applying harsh soaps or powders to irritated areas. Applies petrolatum to perianal area if irritated from diarrhea.
3. Protects skin from sunlight and cold or hot applications. Provides hat and loose cotton clothing to protect exposed areas.

4. Applies antibiotic ointment to acne or skin infections as prescribed.
5. Assesses chemotherapy site for vein irritation, infiltration, or signs of inflammation and applies palliative treatment or reports to physician if severe.

Nursing diagnosis

Altered oral mucous membrane
Related factors: pathologic condition (radiation to head), chemical trauma (chemotherapy), ineffective oral hygiene, lack of salivation
Defining characteristics: stomatitis; oral pain, discomfort; desquamation; oral lesions, ulcers; gingivitis; dry mouth; pain on swallowing (esophagitis); hemorrhage

OUTCOMES
Short-term
Oral changes minimized evidenced by mucous membrane healing; reduced discomfort; ability to eat, drink within limits (expected within 1 week)

Long-term
Optimal condition of oral cavity evidenced by mucous membrane being intact, healed; oral ulceration, infection prevented; reporting to physician for early interventions, treatments (expected ongoing)

NURSING INTERVENTIONS/INSTRUCTIONS
1. Assess and instruct to assess oral mucous membrane for changes in appearance, including redness, bleeding, plaque, lesions, inflammation, ulceration, and candidiasis (each visit).
2. Instruct on providing mouth care with saline or baking soda solution mouthwash, soft toothbrush, swabs, or glycerin to lips and to avoid use of dental floss if platelet and neutrophil counts are low (first visit).
3. Instruct to administer nystatin as slush or frozen ice, mixed in water as mouthwash, or on lozenge and to

avoid drinking fluids for 1 hour after medication if prescribed (first visit).
4. Instruct to apply topical anesthetic to affected area, especially before eating. Suggest sugarless gum to increase saliva production.
5. Instruct to avoid spicy or acidic foods and fluids. Encourage cool, bland, soft, and moist foods and fluids if oral cavity is painful (first visit).

CAREGIVER/CHILD AND FAMILY INTERVENTIONS

1. Assesses oral and pharyngeal mucosa daily for redness and ulcers. Avoids taking oral temperatures.
2. Performs mouth care before and after meals, at bedtime, and every 2 hours if stomatitis is severe.
3. Administers topical local anesthetics to ulcerated areas, but limits application to 10 to 15 ml every 4 hours (to prevent throat, cheeks, or tongue from feeling numb and interfering with swallowing or increasing risk of injury).
4. Provides smooth, bland, and soft diet and avoids irritating foods and fluids. Uses straw to drink liquids. Offers complete nutritional supplement if necessary.

Nursing diagnosis

Altered protection
Related factors: abnormal blood profiles (leukopenia, thrombocytopenia, anemia), drug therapies (antineoplastics), treatments (surgery, radiation therapy), disease (cancer)
Defining characteristics: weakness, fatigue, anorexia, pallor, dyspnea, dizziness, headache, irritability, lethargy, altered clotting (bleeding from gums, bruising, petechiae, epistaxis, hematuria, blood in feces), decreases in platelet, hemoglobin (Hb) levels

OUTCOMES

Short-term
Hemorrhagic effects of therapy minimized evidenced by monitoring body fluids and areas for bleeding, platelet and Hb levels (expected during therapy)

Long-term
Prevention/control of bleeding episode evidenced by absence
of spontaneous bleeding from any area, no burning or dysuria (hemorrhagic cystitis) (expected ongoing)

NURSING INTERVENTIONS/INSTRUCTIONS

1. Assess and instruct to assess for signs of hemorrhage
   during chemotherapy, including bleeding from gums
   and nose, hemoptysis, hematemesis, hematuria, large
   bruises, petechiae, and platelet count of <5000 to
   $20,000/mm^3$ (each visit).
2. Assess and instruct to assess symptoms of anemia, including pallor, fatigue, anorexia, headache, dizziness,
   dyspnea, irritability, lethargy, and Hb of 10 g/dl or less
   (each visit).
3. Advise to avoid activities that can result in injury (running, rough play, skating, bicycles, and contact sports) if
   platelet count $<100,000/mm^3$ (affects platelets and
   metholrexate) (first visit).
4. Instruct to avoid over-the-counter medications, especially
   aspirin-containing products (affects platelets and metho-
   trexate) (first visit).
5. Instruct to apply pressure for 5 minutes to any area of
   bleeding and report bleeding that lasts more than 10
   minutes (first visit).
6. Instruct to report changes in behavior, abdominal pain,
   headache, bleeding from any route, pallor, fatigue, and
   lethargy (first visit).

CAREGIVER/CHILD AND FAMILY INTERVENTIONS

1. Assesses feces, urine, emesis, other substances or areas
   for color, volume, and presence of clots.
2. Modifies environment to prevent injury. Avoids contact
   play activities; wearing tight, restrictive clothing; and using hard toothbrush or flossing.
3. Takes appropriate steps to control/prevent bleeding from
   nose (pressure and ice with child in upright position),
   bowel (avoid straining and give stool softener), and
   mouth (soft brush, mouth rinses, and axillary temperature).
4. Reports any uncontrolled spontaneous bleeding or ooz-
   ing of blood from any site, bleeding at intravenous site,

presence of bruises and petechiae, and changes in neurologic status (level of consciousness and weakness).

Nursing diagnosis

Body image disturbance
Related factors: biophysical (effects of chemotherapy)
Defining characteristics: alopecia, moon face, change in mobility status (neuropathy), skin changes, weight changes, disfigurement, change in social involvement, negative feelings about body changes, fear of rejection by others

OUTCOMES
Short-term
Concerns for changes in body image reduced evidenced by use of clothing, head covering to enhance appearance; verbalizing temporary nature of changes (expected within 1 week)

Long-term
Adapts to changes in body image evidenced by coping with hair loss, cushingoid appearance, other changes (ongoing during therapy)

NURSING INTERVENTIONS/INSTRUCTIONS
1. Assess for hair loss and feelings about this and other changes in appearance (e.g., hyperpigmentation of nails and teeth, gingiva, skin rash, and acne) (each visit).
2. Inform child and caregiver what effects in body image to expect from specific therapy (first visit).
3. Allow expression of feelings about changes and effect on life. Arrange for child to meet peers who have had same experience (each visit).
4. Instruct to contact school officials, inform them of changes, and suggest educating peers about these changes to enhance child's acceptance (first visit).
5. Inform that hair will return; that scarf or hat will cover head; that facial changes are temporary and makeup and appropriate clothing can enhance appearance. Refer child to expert or volunteer in makeup, clothing, and scarf-tying (first visit).

6. Instruct on planning menus that restrict sodium if receiving steroid therapy (first visit).
7. Discuss physical disabilities (amputation or neuropathy), if appropriate, and therapy options for any impairments to attain optimal rehabilitation (any visit).

CAREGIVER/CHILD AND FAMILY INTERVENTIONS

1. Expresses feelings about coping with body image changes.
2. Supports and encourages child's and family's coping and acceptance of body image changes.
3. Meets with school teacher and nurse and enlists their support regarding changes that occur, child's limitations (physical and mental), preparation of peers for child's participation at school, and need for tutorial program.
4. Obtains needed physical, occupational, speech, or other rehabilitation therapy.

Nursing diagnosis

Anticipatory grieving

Related factors: perceived potential loss of significant other (parental), perceived potential loss of well-being (child), fatal illness

Defining characteristics: guilt; anger; sorrow; crying; expression of distress at potential loss; changes in sleep, eating, activity patterns

OUTCOMES

Short-term
Begin to adapt to possibility of potential death of child evidenced by verbalization of feelings about child's deterioration, consideration; openness to support services (clergy, social worker, nurse, physician, hospice, support group) (expected within 1 to 4 weeks [highly variable])

Long-term
Child and family progress through grieving process; provide care/support necessary to child, each other evidenced by

maintaining control of grief to perform daily care plan (expected ongoing)

NURSING INTERVENTIONS/INSTRUCTIONS

1. Assess feelings, fears, and wishes of child and family members about possibility of child's death (any visit as needed).
2. Encourage to openly and honestly express intensity of feelings in family (each visit).
3. Inform family of stages of grieving process (denial, anger, bargaining, depression, and acceptance); length of time involved in grieving; and movement within these stages. Clarify and provide information as requested (first visit, as needed).
4. Assist child and family to identify strengths and resources available to them that can assist in coping with disease and side effects of treatments (chemotherapy and radiation therapy) and other disease processes (each visit).
5. Encourage family to include siblings in conversations (first visit).
6. Allow for cultural differences in responding to potential loss and assist to arrange for spiritual support if requested (each visit).
7. Assist family to investigate hospice care if appropriate (any visit).
8. Provide continued contact and support to child and family in coping and moving through stages of grief (each visit).

CAREGIVER/CHILD AND FAMILY INTERVENTIONS

1. Discusses fears, anxiety, and other feelings. Shares concerns and needs based on stage of grieving.
2. Identifies stages of grieving and allows for individual members to accept possible loss.
3. Places emphasis on quality of life of child by providing supportive and caring environment.
4. Seeks resources for support (groups, friends, and peers).
5. Considers counseling (spiritual and psychologic) as needed.

SAMPLE DOCUMENTATION INCLUSIONS

1. Specific assessment
   Assess age, individual and family developmental stage, diagnosis, prognosis, discharge plan, response to teaching

performed, complexity of treatment regimens, responses to interventions, prescribed medication protocol and adverse responses to medication, pain, vital signs, weight, deterioration of condition, assistance needed to maintain basic needs, status in grieving process, need for home modifications, child and family coping skills, and anxiety level related to home management.

2. Specific care/teaching

    Teach disease and its progression; administration of medication including name, dose, frequency, route, times of day, special considerations based on form, side effects, and expected response; management of basic needs and comfort measures; procedures to be performed; monitoring of essential components of care; symptom control; nonpharmacologic pain relief measures; infection avoidance; use and care of supplies and equipment if used for care procedures; and recognition of signs and symptoms of complications or responses to therapy that necessitate additional visits or reports to physician.

3. General

    Note responses to care and teaching, goal achievement, changes/modifications of plan; abilities of caregiver and family to manage child's complete care; resources for acquiring medication, supplies, and equipment needed for therapy; and coordination among interdisciplinary team and hospice program care if appropriate.

4. See "Documentation and Family Home Record Keeping" in Appendix for general required documentation components for all home care visits.

 Pain Management

Young children experience pain physically and slowly develop a perception of psychologic pain as they move through later developmental phases. It is difficult for children to describe pain, and their perceptions are influenced by fear, fatigue, and environmental stressors. Pain is a subjective experience, and behavioral responses to pain are categorized according to developmental stages of children for the purposes of this plan. A thorough assessment of pain appropriate to the cognitive level of the child is most important in designing a pain management plan. Some sources of pain include surgical procedures, degenerative diseases, inflammatory disorders, fractures, malignancies, and medical procedures. Pain management includes the use of analgesic agents and nonpharmacologic strategies such as relaxation, diversion, positive approach and interactions, massage, and reward.

Home care is primarily concerned with ongoing pain assessment and administration of medications. Teaching of these assessments, procedures, and suggested measures to support the child in pain are provided. Care plans included in this book that are concerned with the nursing diagnosis of acute or chronic pain are cross-referenced with this plan.

Nursing diagnosis

Pain
Related factors: biologic, physical, psychologic injuring agents
Defining characteristics: verbal expression of pain, crying, moaning, screaming; nonverbal expression of guarding, protective behavior, body stiffening, restlessness, irritability, clinging, stalling, withdrawal, pointing; eating and sleeping pattern changes; increases in blood pressure, pulse, respirations

OUTCOMES
Short-term
Daily comfort with minimal symptoms, pain reduced to tolerable level evidenced by removal of factors that cause pain; effective administration of appropriate analgesic medicines, comfort measures; child becomes more cooperative, communicative, engages in play, rest, other routine activities (expected within 1 to 2 days)

Long-term
Optimal relief/control of pain evidenced by acceptance of
pharmacologic and nonpharmacologic therapy; awareness of
tolerance problems, side effects of long-term analgesic
therapy; ability of child and caregiver to cope with need for
continued pain control (expected within 1 week)

NURSING INTERVENTIONS/INSTRUCTIONS

1. Perform complete physical assessment (each visit).
2. Assess infant's responses to pain, including refusal to
   eat, crying loudly, thrashing, withdrawing from, resisting,
   or pushing away from stimulated area, and possible
   grimace expression of pain or irritability (all visits).
3. Assess older child's responses to pain, including screaming or crying loudly; restlessness; irritability; saying that
   something hurts, to stop it, or to wait until later;
   clinging; rigid muscles in limbs and body; gritting teeth;
   pushing away stimuli; and refusing to move or play
   (all visits).
4. Assess caregiver's and family's behavior when child has
   pain, feelings about child experiencing pain, and effectiveness of treatments (first visit).
5. Assess illness, pain that can be anticipated, and any factors that cause or increase pain. Note baseline vital
   signs (first visit).
6. Assess type, intensity, and site of pain by asking child to
   describe and by asking caregiver and family to describe
   behavior responses, child using pain scale to identify
   pain severity on continuum, and using pictures of different facial expressions to identify pain (each visit).
7. Instruct caregiver to assess pain and maintain log of
   signs and symptoms, medication administered, responses after therapy indicating pain reduction or control, and effect on respiration (first and second visits).
8. Administer and instruct caregiver to administer prescribed analgesic (especially 30 minutes before painful
   activities or procedures), opioids that act on central
   nervous system for severe pain, nonopiods that act on
   peripheral nervous system for mild or moderate pain,
   or a combination of both, in appropriate dosage, frequency, form, and route (see "Medication Administra-

tion and Teaching Guidelines," pp. 450-463) (first visit, until all aspects are taught).

9. Monitor and instruct caregiver on administration of bolus or continuous analgesic via intravenous, subcutaneous, patient-controlled, nasogastric, and use of infusion devices, if these routes are used (see "Medication Administration and Teaching Guidelines," pp. 450-463) (first visit, as needed).

10. Calculate and prepare medication for optimal relief and modify amount based on responses. Alter route from parenteral to oral gradually when appropriate (postoperatively), beginning with half dose given orally and half parenterally until able to discontinue parenteral route (any visit).

11. Collaborate with caregiver in planning strategies for nonpharmacologic interventions and 24-hour drug schedule to anticipate and prevent pain. Treat pain before it becomes severe (first visit).

12. Instruct caregiver to prepare child before administration of analgesic, preferably orally with avoidance of injections when possible (first visit).

13. Instruct caregiver on side effects to observe, including sedation, constipation, depressed respirations, personality changes, and possible signs of tolerance to analgesic and decrease in duration of pain relief (first visit).

14. Instruct on nonpharmacologic methods to control pain and assist child to participate in these methods, including distraction, diversion (playing, television watching, story telling, and singing), relaxation (holding, rocking, positioning, and breathing), imagery (real or imagined pleasurable events), stimulation (massage or pressure to area), and contracting (reward and privileges) (any visit as needed).

CAREGIVER/CHILD AND FAMILY INTERVENTIONS

1. Participates in planning and managing pain control.
2. Assesses for pain descriptors and identifies need for analgesic therapy throughout day and night.
3. Records all pertinent information regarding therapy and responses.

4. Remains with child until pain is relieved.
5. Administers correct medication dose via correct route when needed.
6. Prepares child for medication by using supportive statements (when pain relief can be expected in specific amount of time) and hugging when giving injections.
7. Avoids use of word "pain" and negative statements and uses other descriptive words to prepare child for medications.
8. Manages analgesic therapy via routes other than oral. Cares for site and devices.
9. Observes for side effects and lack of pain control and notifies health care provider.
10. Practices nonpharmacologic activities to reduce pain based on child's age.

SAMPLE DOCUMENTATION INCLUSIONS

1. Specific assessment
   Assess age, cognitive developmental stage (child, caregiver, and family), verbal/nonverbal responses to pain, cause of pain, acute or chronic condition, prescribed analgesic (dose, route, and frequency), responses to medication regimen, and child and family coping skills related to pain management.
2. Specific care/teaching
   Teach administration of medication including name, dose, frequency, route, and times of day; special considerations based on form, side effects, and expected response; risk of complications from regimen; comfort measures to relieve pain; and use and care of devices/sites if used for therapy.
3. General
   Note responses to care and teaching, goal achievement; changes/modifications of plan; abilities of caregiver and family to manage and control child's pain; symptoms and pain control in terminally ill child; and resources for acquiring medication, supplies, and equipment needed for therapy.
4. See "Documentation and Family Home Record Keeping" in Appendix for general required documentation components for all home care visits.

Premature/Low–Birth-Weight Infants

Neonatal maturity is classified by gestational age and birth weight. The full-term infant is born between 38 and 42 weeks of gestation. Birth weights range from 2500 to 4000 g (5 lbs, 8 oz to 8 lbs, 13 oz). Premature or pre-term infants are those born at less than 37 weeks of gestation regardless of weight. Low–birth-weight (LBW) infants weigh less than 2500 g; very low–birth-weight (VLBW) infants weigh less than 1500 g and are frequently pre-term. Extremely low–birth-weight (ELBW) infants weigh less than 1000 g. The term *small for gestational age (SGA)* refers to infants who weigh below the 10th percentile at any given week of gestation on an intrauterine growth chart. Gestational age is estimated by a graded assessment of neuromuscular and physical maturity of the neonate. It is a better indicator of status and outcome because it reflects organ system maturity. Prematurity is a significant factor in infant mortality and morbidity. Generally, the greater the prematurity/immaturity, the greater the risk to the infant. LBW is associated with a genetic component, congenital anomalies, infection, errors of metabolism, and maternal and placental factors. Prematurity is associated with multiple or closely spaced pregnancies, maternal disorders, malnutrition, infection, or drug use. Common to both are low socioeconomic status, inadequate prenatal care, and young gravida age, all of which affect long-term infant outcome. Prognosis depends on the severity and duration of the intrauterine insult, gestational age, weight, and presence of concurrent anomaly or illness. Premature infants are at risk for a myriad of disorders related to system immaturity. More common ones include respiratory distress syndromes, alteration in thermoregulation, chronic cardiac insufficiency, intraventricular hemorrhage, necrotizing enterocolitis (NEC), hyperbilirubinemia, hypoglycemia, anemia, and infection. Hospitalization is required until the medical disorders are resolved and organ system maturity is attained.

The infant is generally discharged when gestational age approximates full term, weight is 2000 g, thermoregulation is stabilized, and the infant is able to suck. Problems with apnea, cardiovascular insufficiency, seizures, and FTT may persist (see specific care plans). Normalization of growth and development may take up to 3 years. Some deficits may persist, and rehospitalization is not uncommon.

Home health care is primarily concerned with instruction on nutrition, feeding, and child care; use of monitoring equipment; prevention and management of common health problems associated with prematurity; facilitation of growth and development; and support of the caregiver.

Nursing diagnosis

Ineffective breathing pattern
Related factors: biochemical, mechanical lung immaturity; cerebral respiratory control immaturity
Defining characteristics: fatigue, decreased exercise/activity tolerance, irritability, poor feeding, tachypnea, labored breathing, increased bronchial secretions, increased susceptibility to infection, recurrent apnea of prematurity

OUTCOMES
Short-term
Adequate breathing pattern evidenced by rate, depth, regularity of respirations; clear breath sounds (expected immediately, ongoing)

Long-term
Optimal breathing pattern evidenced by maintenance of respiratory parameters, energy for activities associated with growth/development (expected ongoing)

NURSING INTERVENTIONS/INSTRUCTIONS
1. Before first visit, ascertain if caregivers know cardiopulmonary resuscitation (CPR); if feasible, coordinate with hospital discharge team to teach this before infant's discharge.

2. Collaborate with caregiver to develop emergency protocol; teach CPR to at least one other household member; leave infant alone only with trained caregiver (first visit, reinforce each visit).

3. Assess respiratory status when child is asleep or awake and not crying (see "Pulmonary System Assessment," p. 10, for guidelines). Include rate, depth, regularity, and effort of respirations; use of accessory muscles; and presence of nasal flaring, dyspnea, rales, rhonchi, grunting, and decreased or absent breath sounds. Report aberrations to physician (each visit).

4. Assess caregiver competency and confidence in temperature and apical pulse taking, apnea monitoring, administration of supplemental oxygen, and recognition and management of adverse signs and symptoms. Note immediate availability of suppliers' names and telephone numbers (first visit, reinforce as needed).

5. Instruct caregivers on previously mentioned techniques, using culturally, linguistically, and educationally appropriate language. Demonstrate and have caregivers repeat demonstration. Provide written instructions (each visit).

6. Instruct caregivers to position infant for optimal comfort on sides or on back with head of bed or mattress elevated (first visit).

7. Administer and assist/instruct caregiver on administration of humidified supplemental oxygen at dose and method prescribed. Include safe management of oxygen delivery (first and second visits).

8. Monitor oxygen saturation by pulse oximetry with portable unit, during rest and activity, and with and without supplemental oxygen. Monitor for hypoxic changes and report to physician as appropriate (each visit).

9. Demonstrate and reinforce instruction on percussion, vibration, and postural drainage with infant positioned on lap or bed (first visit, reinforce as needed).

10. Assess apnea monitor function and readings and proper belt attachment. Instruct caregiver on use of monitor (see "Apnea," pp. 57-63) (first visit, follow-up visit).

11. Instruct caregiver on infection prevention, including handwashing and avoidance of crowds and infected persons (first visit, reinforce as needed).
12. Instruct caregiver to report signs and symptoms of infection or deteriorating condition, including fever, poor feeding, irritability, discoloration, and rapid or labored breathing to physician (each visit).
13. Instruct caregivers on care during apneic episodes (each visit). Emphasize the following:

    • Gentle stimulation will usually revive infant.
    • Episodes diminish with time.
    • Emergency protocol, including CPR and activation of Emergency Medical Service (EMS), is in place.

CAREGIVER/CHILD AND FAMILY INTERVENTIONS

1. Becomes CPR certified. Places list of emergency activities and telephone numbers in strategic place for easy access.
2. Correctly administers humidified oxygen, using correct nasal prongs.
3. Follows safety precautions for oxygen use including the following:

    • Sign on front window or door stating, "oxygen in use"
    • No sparks
    • No open flames
    • No oil or grease
    • No smoking

4. Prevents infection by providing good handwashing technique and hygiene, adequate nutrition, periods of uninterrupted sleep and avoiding contact with people with coughs, fever, and upper respiratory infections.
5. Performs chest physiotherapy by use of pillows and positioning without fatigue to infant. Percusses only over rib areas. Frequency and time depend on need for mucus removal.
6. Performs postural drainage, aligns, positions, and supports.
7. Correctly applies apnea monitor and monitors cardiopulmonary status.

8. Identifies any deterioration in respiratory status and reports to physician.

Nursing diagnosis

Altered nutrition: less than body requirements
Related factors: inadequate energy stores, small stomach capacity, inability to ingest required nutrients because of respiratory compromise
Defining characteristics: lethargy, disinterest in feeding, ineffective sucking, failure to gain weight

OUTCOMES
Short-term
Adequate nutrition evidenced by positive responses to touch and feeding, adequate intake and retention of calories and nutrients (expected in 1 to 4 weeks)

Long-term
Optimal nutrition evidenced by steady weight gain and ultimate congruence with standardized weight curves for age and height (expected in 3 months)

NURSING INTERVENTIONS/INSTRUCTIONS

1. Assess nutritional status and GI function (see "Gastrointestinal System Assessment and Nutritional Assessment," pp. 16 and 17, for guidelines). Include chronologic and developmental ages; current, birth, and ideal weights; length; and head circumference (each visit).
2. Observe mother feeding infant. Note competency and confidence of mother; mutual interest in feeding experience; infant position; suck, swallow, and gag reflexes; coordination of breathing with sucking and swallowing; and amount of formula offered, consumed, and retained (each visit).
3. Assess/query about number and saturation of diapers wet and soiled daily. Relate to intake as well as cardiovascular, renal, and GI status (each visit).
4. Based on data assessment, instruct mother on measures to facilitate feeding (each visit).

- Recognize infant hunger, distress, and satiety cues.
- Provide positive emotional climate before and during feeding (e.g., cuddling, soothing, and talking to infant and allowing infant to sleep after feeding).
- Be consistent and persistent in feedings (i.e., feed on demand and at least every 3 hours around the clock).
- Stimulate disinterested or lethargic infant by cooling (take off socks and blanket) and movement and activity (talk to or gently rock or bounce infant). Use pacifier and oral stimulation between feedings.
- Separate feedings from procedures or treatments.
- Hold infant when feeding. Have infant's neck slightly flexed or at least neutral midline; do not hyperextend.
- Use soft, small, easy-to-suck nipple.
- Encourage and praise mother's efforts.

5. Encourage breastfeeding. Observe mother breastfeeding infant and, based on observations, instruct on technique. If feeding taxes infant greatly, instruct mother on breast pumping and bottlefeeding expressed milk (as applicable).
6. Observe formula preparation, noting especially clean technique and dilution of prescribed formula (first visit, reinforce as needed).
7. Based on observed need, instruct mother on formula preparation and feeding. Include need for correct use of recommended formula, calorie supplementation, small and frequent feedings, and gradual advancement of diet (each visit).
8. Instruct mother on administration of dietary supplementation per physician's recommendation.
9. Assess and instruct mother to report signs and symptoms of potentially dangerous disorders (i.e., respiratory distress, delayed gastric emptying, vomiting [especially early in feeding], abdominal distention, blood-tinged stools, increased lethargy, increased apneic episodes) to physician. Assess for bowel sounds and report loss of bowel sounds to physician (each visit).
10. As child progresses, instruct mother to add foods gradually and to supplement meals with nutrient-dense snacks.

11. Refer to community resources for assistance in obtaining food (first visit, as appropriate).

CAREGIVER/CHILD AND FAMILY INTERVENTIONS

1. Correctly follows instructions for mixing and refrigerating formula.
2. Provides ordered caloric intake (i.e., 20 cal/oz of standard formula, 24 cal/oz of preemie formula).
3. Supplements formula with lipids, vitamins, and minerals as prescribed.
4. Promotes pleasant environment to enhance intake and nurture child emotionally.
5. Positions child for comfort and safety.
6. Child eats at least every 3 hours, wets six or more diapers a day, and generally stools once or more daily.
7. Uses food supplementation programs (e.g., WIC to obtain milk, formula, and food staples).
8. Reports respiratory compromise during or after feedings, reflux vomiting, irritability, diarrhea, and signs of NEC (lethargy, abdominal distention, bloody stools, gastric retention, bile-tinged or bloody vomiting, and increased apneic episodes).

Nursing diagnosis

Knowledge deficit
Related factors: lack of information, lack of readiness to learn
Defining characteristics: verbalized need for child care information concerning handling, activity; tension, insecurity when handling infant

OUTCOMES

Short-term
Adequate knowledge evidenced by caretaker's more relaxed posture, statements identifying elements of child care (expected in 1 to 2 weeks)

Long-term
Adequate knowledge evidenced by caregiver competency, confidence in child care; optimal infant development (expected in 1 to 4 weeks)

NURSING INTERVENTIONS/INSTRUCTIONS

1. Assess caregiver's learning needs, styles, maturity, and receptivity. Provide information in appropriate manner (each visit).
2. Assess caregiver's understanding of discharge teaching, infant status, and infant's needs. Note coping ability, perceived and actual needs of infant, and sources of support and assistance (first visit).
3. Assess adequacy of physical home environment. Assist and refer for procurement of basic services and supplies. Demonstrate adaptive measures as necessary.
4. Continue to encourage feeding and optimal nutrition (each visit).
5. Observe infant being bathed and groomed. Based on observed need, instruct on necessity of skin care (first visit, reinforce on second visit).

   - Handling infant gently and securely, washing with warm water and mild soap
   - Using soft, not fluffy bedding
   - Turning to alternate side or repositioning after feedings

6. Assess infant's color, temperature, amount of clothing, and evidence of chilling or perspiration. Note ambient temperature. Based on observed need, instruct on thermoregulation including the following (first visit, as needed):

   - Maintaining neutral thermal environment with necessary humidification
   - Avoiding drafts
   - Dressing infant appropriately, avoiding overbundling

7. Instruct caregiver on measures to conserve infant energy, including providing uninterrupted periods of rest and feeding by alternate means if indicated (each visit).
8. Instruct caregiver on need for regular health care follow-up, including the following (each visit):

   - Regular well-baby visits with primary care physician or clinic
   - Immunizations

- Regular and long-term visual screenings
- Specialty clinics for pulmonary or neurologic problems

9. Refer to community resources for parent-infant education programs, support groups, and respite care (as needed).

CAREGIVER/CHILD AND FAMILY INTERVENTIONS

1. Obtains appropriate supplies and resources for infant care.
2. Maintains optimal nutrition through regular oral feedings; uses alternate feeding methods as indicated.
3. Handles infant safely, adeptly, and nurturingly.
4. Maintains optimal thermal environment.
5. Balances infant's rest requirement and energy conservation needs with nutrition requirements.
6. Bathes and handles infant to maintain skin integrity and prevent injury.
7. Keeps regularly scheduled health care appointments.
8. Obtains childhood immunizations on modified schedule for premature infants with history of early protracted hospitalization.
9. Child has regular eye care for residual effects of retinopathy of prematurity.
10. Explores informational sources and participates in support groups.
11. Secures respite care to minimize caregiver exhaustion.

Nursing diagnosis

Altered growth and development
Related factors: physical environmental, stimulation deficiencies (inadequate parental caregiving); nutritional deficit
Defining characteristics: delay/difficulty in performing skills (motor, social, expressive) typical of age group, altered physical growth

OUTCOMES
Short-term
Growth/developmental behavior, activities evidenced by absence of deficits, delays, or regression of functioning; perfor-

mance of age-appropriate growth/development (expected within 6 to 12 weeks)

Long-term
Progressive growth/development advances; achievement of normal physical, emotional, social parameters

NURSING INTERVENTIONS/INSTRUCTIONS

1. Assess expected growth/developmental level (see "Growth and Developmental Assessment," p. 31, for guidelines) (each visit).
2. Assess caregiver, family, and environment for stressful events and ability to provide physical care, love, and adequate stimulation (each visit).
3. Assess for caregiver overprotection or negligence (each visit).
4. Instruct on normal growth/development patterns for infant's age and possible lag in development caused by prematurity or concurrent deficit, anomaly, or defect (first visit).
5. Assist caregiver and family to develop goals and to participate in care to achieve optimal development (ongoing).
6. Instruct caregiver to monitor infant activity tolerance and collaborate to develop plan based on this information to provide visual, auditory, and tactile stimulation; gross motor skills for infant; and time with child for talking or playing (ongoing).
7. Provide encouragement and support for caregivers' efforts (each visit).
8. Provide early referral to professional resources such as speech or physical therapist, special education teacher, psychosocial counselor, or social worker to assist in specific areas of need (any visit).

CAREGIVER/CHILD AND FAMILY INTERVENTIONS

1. Provides activities to enhance stimulation and developmental (cognitive, psychomotor, and psychosocial) progression.
2. Sets realistic goals for growth/developmental achievement.

3. Maintains consistent caregiver and schedule of activities.
4. Holds, rocks, and cuddles infant to provide touch and loving care.
5. Provides organized and consistent program of daily activities that include use of mobiles, music, and other learning tools. Does not overstimulate child.
6. Attends parenting classes for infant stimulation, growth/developmental milestones, and expectations.
7. Identifies and uses specialized services to assist with growth/developmental lags.

Nursing diagnosis

Ineffective family coping: compromised
Related factors: prolonged hospitalization that exhausts supportive capacity of significant people, frequent rehospitalizations, family disorganization, role changes
Defining characteristics: expression of inability to cope; feelings of fear, anxiety, guilt, anger; inadequate understanding of condition, care by family

OUTCOMES

Short-term
Family members demonstrate ability to plan, care for infant evidenced by provision of normal environment; decreased anxiety, feelings of inadequacy; integration of information about family needs into care, support of infant (expected within 1 to 2 weeks)

Long-term
Family coping, adaptation evidenced by optimal support, participation in care, maintenance of family relationships (expected within 1 to 2 months)

NURSING INTERVENTIONS/INSTRUCTIONS

1. Meet and collaborate with family members in assessing stressors, coping mechanisms, and planning of care (first visit, repeat as needed).
2. Reinforce information to promote family understanding of prematurity and care needs (each visit).

3. Discuss and allow family to express feelings of guilt, anxiety, and depression. Promote communication among members to verbalize feelings and expectations with each other (any visit).
4. Instruct on methods to develop coping skills and to meet family's needs (medical, emotional, financial, food, respite care, supplies, and equipment) by referral to social worker or counselor (first visit, as needed).

CAREGIVER/CHILD AND FAMILY INTERVENTIONS

1. Displays decreasing anxiety and anger. Provides supportive family environment.
2. Develops trust in home care personnel. Collaborates in developing and modifying daily care.
3. Provides care and treatments effectively.
4. Recognizes and assumes role changes. Maintains family integrity.
5. Develops coping mechanisms that have positive effect within family.
6. Identifies problem areas and obtains professional assistance or services as needed.

SAMPLE DOCUMENTATION INCLUSIONS

1. Specific assessment
   Assess chronologic age, developmental status, birth weight, current weight, head circumference, vital signs, concurrent disorders or anomalies, intake, thermoregulation, skin integrity, need for assistive devices or equipment, environmental hazards, and adaptive capacity of family.
2. Specific care/teaching
   Teach feeding and nutrition; temperature regulation; bathing and handling; infection control; monitoring equipment and supplemental oxygen; what to report to physician; and referrals for follow-up, specialty clinics, supplemental food, support groups, and respite care.
3. General
   Note responses to care and teaching.
4. See "Documentation and Family Home Record Keeping" in Appendix for general required documentation components for all home care visits.

Terminally Ill Child

Care of the terminally ill child includes complete physical and emotional care and family support as death approaches. The decision of the parents to have their child home before death is one that should be respected and supported. A plan of total care should be formulated by the family with the assistance of the home health nurse as well as teaching of symptom management and indicators of change in condition. The plan should include the child's perception of and fears that are associated with dying. Hospice care is an alternative to hospitalization that includes compassion, concern, support, and skilled care for the terminally ill child. It involves physical, psychologic, social, and spiritual care by a medically supervised, interdisciplinary home care team of professionals and volunteers. It can be part-time, intermittent, and scheduled on a regular basis or on a 24-hour on-call basis. It is also concerned with the family needs during the dying process and bereavement for 1 year after the death of the child.

Home care is primarily concerned with control of symptoms and promotion of comfort through palliative care, as well as support for grieving before and after the death of the child.

Nursing diagnosis

Ineffective family coping: compromised
Related factors: situational crisis (terminal status of child) that exhausts supportive capacity of family members; family disorganization, role changes
Defining characteristics: family expression of inability to cope; personal feelings of fear of loss, anxiety, guilt, anger, denial, grief, lack of control, helplessness; unwillingness to let go; inability to cope, ask for help; chronic fatigue, anxiety of family

OUTCOMES

Short-term
Family members demonstrate ability to plan, care for child evidenced by provision of caring environment; control of anxiety, feelings of inadequacy; integration of information about family needs into 24-hour availability of home care team on behalf of child (expected within 1 to 4 weeks)

Long-term
Family coping/adaptation evidenced by optimal support, participation in care, maintenance of family relationships; demonstrates knowledge/understanding of home team function, imminent death process (expected until death of child)

NURSING INTERVENTIONS/INSTRUCTIONS

1. Meet and collaborate with family members to assess stressors, coping mechanisms, and planning of terminal care around family's needs (first visit, as needed).
2. Reinforce information provided during discharge teaching to promote family understanding of care protocol (each visit).
3. Provide information about goals and treatments of hospice care to include spiritual care and assist in decisions regarding this assistance (family feelings and financial ability) (first visit).
4. Assess parents for coping abilities, use of defense mechanisms, communication patterns, stressors caused by relatives and family members, and family cohesiveness (first and second visits).
5. Assess potential family stressors such as making funeral arrangements, scheduling to take turns giving care, caring for other ill family members, unresolved past issues associated with terminal illness, and potential strengths (support of family members, friends, relatives, and employer) (first and second visits).
6. Discuss and encourage family to express feelings of guilt, anxiety, and depression. Promote communication among family and patient to verbalize feelings and expectations with each other. Encourage family to ask questions and speak openly about imminent death of child and effect on siblings with health care provider (each visit).

7. Institute measures to keep child free of pain (see "Pain Management," pp. 398-402).
8. Instruct on methods to develop coping skills and to meet family's needs (medical, emotional, financial, food, respite care, supplies, and equipment) by referral to social worker or grief counselor (first visit, as needed).

CAREGIVER/CHILD AND FAMILY INTERVENTIONS

1. Provides supportive family environment. Openly verbalizes and discusses feelings and child's needs with home health care team and family members.
2. Develops trust in home health care personnel and other professionals. Collaborates in planning and modifying care as needed. Answers family's questions honestly.
3. Offers reassurance of support, love, and caring to child.
4. Recognizes and assumes role changes. Maintains family integrity.
5. Allows expression and use of coping mechanisms within family.
6. Verbalizes understanding of home team functions and availability.
7. Identifies problem areas and obtains professional assistance, clergy, or social services as needed.
8. Keeps child comfortable and allows child to choose activity as appropriate to ability.

Nursing diagnosis

Altered health maintenance
Related factors: terminal stage of child's illness, ineffective family coping, grieving of family members, lack of resources
Defining characteristics: difficulty in meeting needs of child in all areas; lack of supplies, equipment, financial, other resources; lack of adaptive behaviors to changes in health status of child; lack of knowledge regarding child's, family's needs (funeral preparation, will, organ donation)

OUTCOMES

Short-term
Adequate overall comfort evidenced by appropriate behaviors to control, implement total care of terminally ill child (expected upon decision to care for child at home)

Long-term
Optimal terminal care evidenced by effective symptom management of all systems (expected until death occurs; bereavement for 1 year after death)

NURSING INTERVENTIONS/INSTRUCTIONS

1. Inform family members of physical needs and process of impending death of child and what can and cannot be changed. Allow time for questions and clarification (any visit as needed).
2. Inform of home team functions, use of hospice services and volunteers, and 24-hour on-call services (first visit).
3. Instruct and assist to modify environment for easy access and safe, private care of child; optimal ambient temperature and ventilation; and removal of bright lighting (any visit).
4. Instruct on positioning child for comfort with loose, clean linens with protective pad, and pillows for support (any visit).
5. Instruct to limit care to palliative activities that promote comfort and rest (first visit).
6. Instruct on formulating pain management program to provide anticipatory pain relief over 24-hours as prescribed (first visit, as needed).
7. Instruct as needed on administration of medications by most comfortable form and route (each visit as needed).
8. Instruct on providing skin care by sponge bathing, backrub, and use of aids to prevent pressure on susceptible areas (first visit).
9. Provide and assist with elimination of urine and feces while avoiding fatigue. Assess for constipation and continence and initiate measures to provide care (use diapers and offer bedpan) (each visit).
10. Instruct to note changes in breathing pattern and to suction secretions and administer oxygen if appropri-

ate. Apply ordered scopolamine patch to reduce secretions if wet respirations occur (each visit).

11. Instruct that anorexia is common and allow any foods and fluids that child requests or prefers. Avoid rushing or insisting that child eats. Provide oral care (each visit).

12. Instruct on attention to and provision of any additional comfort measures (any visit).

CAREGIVER/CHILD AND FAMILY INTERVENTIONS

1. Accepts total physical care of all failing systems on continuous basis.

2. Conserves energy and preserves child's and family's physical/emotional status.

3. Elicits assistance from hospice home care team for symptom management and support before and after death of child.

4. Maintains maximum comfort and quality of life of child. Allows child to accept or reject care and procedures.

5. Plans for imminent death of child by deciding on legal will if appropriate and by preparing for funeral arrangements, organ donation, and autopsy permission.

Nursing diagnosis

Anticipatory grieving
Related factors: potential loss, near death of child
Defining characteristics: expression of distress at potential loss; high level of guilt, anger, sorrow, crying, interference with life (altered sleep, eating, activity pattern)

OUTCOMES

Short-term
Begins to grieve for death of child evidenced by verbalization of feelings regarding child's deterioration, consideration or openness to support services (expected based on anticipated death)

Long-term
Family progress through grieving process; provision of care, support necessary to child and each other evidenced by

maintaining control of grief to perform daily care plan (expected until grief is resolved)

NURSING INTERVENTIONS/INSTRUCTIONS

1. Assess feelings, fears, and wishes of family members about child's death (first and second visits).
2. Encourage family to express intensity of feelings in accepting, nonjudgmental environment (each visit).
3. Inform family of stages of grieving process; need for normal grieving; and possible length and movement within these stages, which varies with individuals. Clarify and provide information as requested (first visit).
4. Discuss death with child. Allow full expression of feelings. Use play therapy as appropriate.
5. Assist family to identify strengths and resources available to them that can assist in coping with loss of child (each visit).
6. Allow for cultural differences in responding to potential loss and assist to arrange for spiritual support if requested (each visit).
7. Provide continued contact and support to child and family in coping and moving through stages of grief (each visit).

CAREGIVER/CHILD AND FAMILY INTERVENTIONS

1. Discusses fears, anxiety, and other feelings. Shares concerns and needs based on child's needs and stage of grieving.
2. Identifies stages of grieving and allows for individual members to begin accepting loss.
3. Places emphasis on quality of life of family members in supportive, caring environment.
4. Meets own physical needs and comfort.
5. Seeks resources for support (groups, friends, and hospice care).
6. Considers family counseling as needed.

SAMPLE DOCUMENTATION INCLUSIONS

1. Specific assessment
   Assess verbal/nonverbal responses to child's terminal condition, discharge plan, needs and responses to medi-

cations and comfort care regimen, child and family coping skills related to symptom management and imminent death, knowledge of criteria and availability of hospice care team and selection before discharge from hospital, financial coverage, and stage of grieving.

2. Specific care/teaching

   Teach administration and provision of medications, procedures, and comfort measures with adjustments made as condition changes; possible changes in specific systems and modifications in care; use and care of devices/sites if used for therapy; and home care team functions and availability.

3. General

   Note responses to care and changes/modifications of care as needed; abilities of caregiver and family to manage and control symptoms in terminally ill child; resources for acquiring medication, supplies, and equipment needed for therapy; and using hospice care, community support, and professional referral services.

4. See "Documentation and Family Home Record Keeping" in Appendix for general required documentation components for all home care visits.

Appendices

Basic Life Support for Infants and Children

Basic life support is a critical technique for the resuscitation of children. It is required for all home health care workers and recommended for caregivers. The following charts outline one-rescuer and two-rescuer cardiopulmonary resuscitation of the infant, child, and adult. Management of foreign body airway obstruction is also included.

One-rescuer Cardiopulmonary Resuscitation

	Objectives	Actions		
		Adult (over 8 yr)	Child (1 to 8 yr)	Infant (under 1 yr)
A. Airway	1. Assessment: determine unresponsiveness.	Tap or gently shake shoulder.		
		Say, "Are you okay?"		Speak loudly.
	2. Get help.	Activate EMS.	Shout for help. If second rescuer available, have person activate EMS.	
	3. Position the victim.	Turn on back as a unit, supporting head and neck if necessary (4-10 seconds).		
	4. Open the airway.	Head-tilt/chin-lift.		
B. Breathing	5. Assessment: determine breathlessness.	Maintain open airway. Place ear over mouth, observing chest. Look, listen, feel for breathing (3-5 seconds).*		
	6. Give 2 rescue breaths.	Maintain open airway.		
		Seal mouth to mouth.		Mouth to nose/mouth.
		Give 2 slow breaths. Observe chest rise. Allow lung deflation between breaths.		

		b. Activate EMS.	
		c. Give 5 subdiaphragmatic abdominal thrusts (Heimlich maneuver).	c. Give 5 back blows.
			c. Give 5 chest thrusts.
		d. Tongue-jaw lift and finger sweep.	d. Tongue-jaw lift, but finger sweep only if you see foreign object.
		If unsuccessful, repeat a, c, and d until successful.	
C. Circulation	8. Assessment: determine pulselessness.	Feel for carotid pulse with one hand; maintain head-tilt with other (5-10 seconds).	Feel for brachial pulse: maintain head-tilt.
Cardiopulmonary Resuscitation (CPR)	Pulse absent: Begin chest compressions: 9. Landmark check.	Run middle finger along bottom edge of rib cage to notch at center (top of sternum).	Imagine line drawn between nipples.

Modified from Chandra NC, Hazinski MF (eds): *Textbook of basic life support for healthcare providers,* Dallas, 1994, American Heart Association.

*If victim is breathing or resumes effective breathing, place in recovery position: (1) move head, shoulders, and torso simultaneously; (2) turn onto side; (3) leg not in contact with ground may be bent and knee moved forward to stabilize victim; (4) victim should not be moved in any way if trauma is suspected and should not be placed in recovery position if rescue breathing or CPR is required. *Continued.*

EMS, Emergency Medical Service.

One-rescuer Cardiopulmonary Resuscitation – cont'd

Objectives	Actions		
	Adult (over 8 yr)	Child (1 to 8 yr)	Infant (under 1 yr)
10. Hand position.	Place index finger next to finger on notch:		Place 2-3 fingers on sternum. One finger's width below line. Depress ½-1 in.
	Two hands next to index finger. Depress 1½-2 in.	Heel of one hand next to index finger. Depress 1-1½ in.	
11. Compression rate.	80-100/min	100/min	At least 100/min
12. Compressions to breaths.	2 breaths to every 15 compressions	1 breath to every 5 compressions	
13. Number of cycles.	4	20 (approximately 1 minute)	
14. Reassessment.	Feel for carotid pulse.		Feel for brachial pulse.
	If no pulse, resume CPR, starting with compressions.	If alone, activate EMS. If no pulse, resume CPR, starting with compressions.	
Pulse present; not breathing. Begin rescue breathing.	1 breath every 5 seconds (12/min)	1 breath every 3 seconds (20/min)	

Two-rescuer Cardiopulmonary Resuscitation for Children (Continued)

Step	Objective	Actions
1. Airway	**One rescuer (ventilator):** Assessment: determine unresponsiveness.	Tap or gently shake shoulder.
		Shout, "Are you okay?"
	Call for help.	Activate EMS.
	Position the victim.	Turn on back if necessary (4-10 seconds).
	Open the airway.	Use proper technique to open airway.
2. Breathing	Assessment: determine breathlessness.	Look, listen, and feel (3-5 seconds).
	Ventilate twice.	Observe chest rise: 1-1½ sec/inspiration.
3. Circulation	Assessment: determine pulselessness.	Feel for carotid pulse (5-10 seconds).
	State assessment results.	Say, "No pulse."
	Other rescuer (compressor): Get into position for compressions.	Hand and shoulders in correct position.
	Locate landmark notch.	Landmark check.
4. Compression/ ventilation cycles	**Compressor:** Begin chest compressions.	Correct ratio compressions/ventilations: 5/1
		Compression rate: 80-100/min (5 compressions/ 3-4 seconds).

Modified from Chandra NC, Hazinski MF (eds): *Textbook of basic life support for healthcare providers*, Dallas, 1994, American Heart Association.

Note: Two-rescuer CPR for children ages 1 to 8 years can be performed similarly to that for adults with appropriate changes in chest compressions and ventilations.

EMS, Emergency Medical Service.

Continued.

Two-rescuer Cardiopulmonary Resuscitation for Children Over 8 Years Old — cont'd

Step	Objective	Actions
		Say any helpful mnemonic.
		Stop compressing for each ventilation.
	Ventilator: Ventilate after every fifth compression and check compression effectiveness. (Minimum of 10 cycles)	Ventilate 1 time (1½–2 sec/inspiration).
		Check pulse occasionally to assess compressions.
5. Call for Switch	**Compressor:** Call for switch when fatigued.	Give clear signal to change.
		Compressor completes fifth compression.
		Ventilator completes ventilation after fifth compression.
6. Switch	Simultaneously switch:	
	Ventilator: Move to chest.	Move to chest.
		Become compressor.
		Get into position for compressions.
		Locate landmark notch.
	Compressor: Move to head.	Move to head.
		Become ventilator.
		Check carotid pulse (5 seconds).
		Say, "No pulse."
		Ventilate once (1½–2 sec/inspiration).
7. Continue CPR	Resume compression/ventilation cycles.	Resume Step 4.

Foreign Body Airway Obstruction Management. Signs of Life-threatening Obstruction.

The truly choking child *cannot speak, becomes cyanotic, and collapses*

	Objectives	Actions		
		Adult (over 8 yr)	Child (1 to 8 yr)	Infant (under 1 yr)
Conscious Victim	1. Assessment: determine airway obstruction.	Ask, "Are you choking?" Determine if victim can cough or speak.		Observe breathing difficulty, ineffective cough, no strong cry.
	2. Act to relieve obstruction.	Perform up to 5 subdiaphragmatic abdominal thrusts (Heimlich maneuver).		Give 5 back blows. Give 5 chest thrusts.
	Be persistent.	Repeat Step 2 until obstruction is relieved or victim becomes unconscious.		
Victim who Becomes Unconscious	3. Position the victim: call for help.	Turn on back as a unit, supporting head and neck, face up, arms by sides. Call out, "Help!" Activate EMS. If second rescuer is available, have him or her activate EMS.		
	4. Check for foreign body.	Perform tongue-jaw lift and finger sweep.	Perform tongue-jaw lift. Remove foreign object only if it can be seen.	
	5. Give rescue breaths.	Open airway with head-tilt/chin-lift. Try to give rescue breaths. If airway is obstructed, reposition head, try to ventilate again.		

Modified from Chandra NC, Hazinski MF (eds): *Textbook of basic life support for healthcare providers*, Dallas, 1994, American Heart Association.
EMS, Emergency Medical Service.   *Continued.*

Foreign Body Airway Obstruction Management: Signs of Life-threatening Obstruction — cont'd

The truly choking child *cannot speak, becomes cyanotic,* and *collapses*

Objectives	Actions		
	Adult (over 8 yr)	**Child** (1 to 8 yr)	**Infant** (under 1 yr)
6. Act to relieve obstruction	Perform up to 5 subdiaphragmatic abdominal thrusts (Heimlich maneuver).		Give 5 back blows.
			Give 5 chest thrusts.
7. Be persistent.	Repeat steps 4-6 until obstruction is relieved.		
Unconscious victim			
1. Assessment: determine unresponsiveness.	Tap or gently shake shoulder. Shout, "Are you okay?"	Tap or gently shake shoulder.	
	If unresponsive, activate EMS.		
2. Call for help: position the victim.	Turn on back as a unit, supporting head and neck, face up, arms by sides.		
		Call out for help.	
3. Open the airway.	Head-tilt/chin-lift.	Head-tilt/chin-lift.	Head-tilt/chin-lift, but

Step	Action		
4. Assessment: determine breathlessness.	Maintain an open airway. Ear over mouth; observe chest. Look, listen, feel for breathing (3-5 seconds)		
5. Give rescue breaths.	Make mouth-to-mouth seal.		Make mouth-to-nose-and-mouth seal.
	Try to give rescue breaths.		
6. If chest is not rising, try again to give rescue breaths.	Reposition head. Try rescue breaths again.		
7. Activate the EMS system.	If airway obstruction is not relieved after about 1 minute, activate EMS as rapidly as possible.		
8. Act to relieve obstruction.	Perform up to 5 subdiaphragmatic abdominal thrusts (Heimlich maneuver).		Give 5 back blows. Give 5 chest thrusts.
9. Check for foreign body.	Perform tongue-jaw lift and finger sweep.		Perform tongue-jaw lift. Remove foreign object only if it can be seen.
10. Rescue breaths.	Open airway with head-tilt/chin-lift. Try again to give rescue breaths. If airway is obstructed, reposition head, try to ventilate again.		
11. Be persistent.	Repeat steps 8-10 until obstruction is relieved.		

Clinical Pathway Sample

Clinical pathways (critical pathways and care maps) are
an interdisciplinary health care tool and a component of
total quality management. They are a framework for
practice and may augment nursing care plans. Pathways
are process oriented and client centered. Their purpose
is the planning and, ultimately, the delivery of individualized health care that is specific, appropriate, timely, and
cost effective. Elements of this evolving care management system may include assessment data; patient problems and acuity; age-appropriate care standards; components of care (including nursing interventions);
treatments; patient activity and participation; and teaching, timelines, and desired or expected clinical outcomes.
Evaluation is ongoing and focal decision points may be
integrated.

The following is an example of a system approach, pediatric home care clinical pathways. It is intended only as a
guideline and must be tailored to the individual client's
clinical profile, needs, resources, and responses.

PEDIATRIC HOME CARE CLINICAL PATHWAY

System: *Pulmonary*
Physician: _____
Diagnostic code (DRG): _____
Anticipated number/range of visits/week: _____/_____
Cost estimate/type of reimbursement: _____
Anticipated outcomes
Established effective, stable respiratory pattern free from
respiratory distress via normal route or with assisted ventila-
tion (expected by _____)
Breath sounds intensity increased and adventitious sounds
diminished or absent (expected by _____)
Airway patency maintained via normal route or tracheos-
tomy (expected by _____)
Effective removal of secretions by chest physiotherapy,
coughing, and suctioning (expected by _____)
Adequate tissue oxygenation with or without use of supple-

mental oxygen (expected by _____)

Anxiety within management levels; uses appropriate coping behaviors (expected by _____)

Family demonstrates ability to meet physical, emotional, social, and security needs of its members (expected by _____)

Additional applicable outcomes _____

Homebound criteria: Severe respiratory distress with dyspnea associated with any movement, weakness, bedbound, chairbound, increased oxygen dependence, ventilator dependent

Possible Medical Diagnoses	Possible Nursing Diagnoses
Apnea	Ineffective airway clearance
Asthma	Ineffective breathing pattern
Bronchopulmonary dysplasia	Impaired gas exchange
Cystic fibrosis	Activity intolerance
Pneumonia	Risk for infection
Tuberculosis	Hyperthermia
	Anxiety
	Ineffective child, caregiver, and family coping

Home Care Clinical Pathway for Child with Pulmonary Condition

Intervention	Visit 1 (Date __/__/__)	Visit 2 (Date __/__/__)	Visit 3 (Date __/__/__)	Visit 4 (Date __/__/__)
Assessment and associated instruction	Disease process, status Risk factors associated with disease Discharge teaching review Respiratory rate, depth, ease Breath sounds, use of accessory muscles Cough/sputum amount, color, characteristics Skin color, cyanosis	Knowledge of disease/response to emergency Status of disease (respiratory, cough, sputum, breath sounds, skin color) Monitor for complications, fatigue level, sleep pattern Knowledge and compliance with previous teaching	Status of disease (respiratory, cough, sputum, breath sounds) Knowledge of teaching from previous visit Signs and symptoms to log, timely reporting to physician	Status of disease (respiratory, cough, sputum, breath sounds) Safety/home modifications needed

Caregiver/family support (assessment/ demonstrated)	Anxiety level Need for lifestyle changes Expectations of home care plan Written schedule for visits	Review care pathway with child, caregiver, family Ability to comply with written plan by participation in care Anxiety management, relaxation techniques	Coping skills of child, caregivers Adaptation to care of ill child, changes in lifestyle Caregiver, family participation in total care Effective relaxation, anxiety reduction	Use of effective coping skills Independent in providing home care Effective on family roles, cohesiveness Family intregrity (caregiver, parents, siblings)
Medications (instruction in action, dose, route, form, frequency, side effects) one medication/visit	Bronchodilator; orally, small volume nebulizer, measured dose handheld inhaler (cleaning of medication inhalation therapy equipment)	Bronchodilator compliance, effectiveness Instruct in corticosteroid, orally, measured dose handheld inhaler	Corticosteroid compliance, effectiveness Instruct in administration of antimicrobial, antipyretic, orally	Antimicrobial, antipyretic compliance, effectiveness Continue instruction as warranted by regimen to include expectorant, antitussive, antitubercular

Continued.

Home Care Clinical Pathway for Child with Pulmonary Condition — cont'd

Intervention	Visit 1 (Date ___/___/___)	Visit 2 (Date ___/___/___)	Visit 3 (Date ___/___/___)	Visit 4 (Date ___/___/___)
Treatment/ procedures (instruction/ demonstration as applicable)	CPR, emergency measures Weight Vital signs, axillary temperature Tracheostomy suctioning Positioning for comfort, optimal chest expansion, ease of breathing, aspiration prevention	Weight for gains, losses Axillary temperature, pulse for changes Postural drainage by gravity, breathing exercises, productive coughing Medical aseptic technique Tracheostomy patency, effective suctioning	Instruct to weigh and document in log Increase or change in vital signs Removal of liquefied secretions by coughing Comfort and sleep improved with positioning Instruct in I&O measurement Moisture to oral mucosa and nares	Chest physiotherapy to include vibration and percussion I&O ratio for fluid balance

Lines/tubes/devices (durable/nondurable) (instruction/demonstration as applicable)				
Safe, effective use of apnea monitor	Correct use, proper monitoring and troubleshooting, settings, alarms of ventilator	Continued effective use of ventilator, use of manufacturer's manual as appropriate	Procurement and storage of backup oxygen tank and other essential equipment
Safe, effective use of ventilator	Correct use, proper monitoring of apnea monitor	Continued effective use of apnea monitor	Periodic reduction in use of equipment if appropriate
Nasogastric, gastrostomy tube care	Effective oxygen use; knowledge of equipment and safety precautions	Continued effective use of oxygen administration and equipment	
Tracheostomy tube cleansing and change, tie and dressing change	Tracheostomy care procedures, tube removal and insertion, cleansing	Continued effective tracheostomy tube care	
Safe, correct use of oxygen, gauge, humidification, tubing, and care	Gastrostomy dressing, nasogastric tube taping	Continued effective feeding tube care	
Equipment, supplies needed	Cleaning of supplies, equipment	Precautions and disposal of used supplies	

Continued.

CPR, Cardiopulmonary resuscitation; *I&O*, intake and output.

Home Care Clinical Pathway for Child with Pulmonary Condition – cont'd

Intervention	Visit 1 (Date ___/___/___)	Visit 2 (Date ___/___/___)	Visit 3 (Date ___/___/___)	Visit 4 (Date ___/___/___)
Movement/ self-care (assessment/ instruction/ demonstration)	Bedrest, chair, ambulatory Activity tolerance, endurance Dyspnea with exertion Bathroom, commode Energy conservation	Advancement in activity, participation in self-care Methods to conserve energy, increase endurance Rest if short of breath during activity	Ability to perform ADL Aids to encourage self-care	Partial or full independence in activities and self-care Effective use of aids in ADL
Nutrition/fluids (instruction/ demonstration)	Fluid intake increased as allowed Increased calories/protein, small frequent meals Enteral feedings Feeding techniques (solid, formula, breast)	Dietary selection of preferred foods, fluids for calories, special diet Supplements to diet Tube feeding, preparation, technique, tolerance	Formulate sample menus Compliance in dietary/fluid intake	Daily adequate nutritional intake

Diagnostics (assessment as available)	Sputum culture Theophylline level Oximetry Chest x-ray	Obtain as ordered or review diagnostic tests, procedures as available	Obtain as needed Note changes and revise theophylline dosage as ordered	As appropriate
Referrals/ rehabilitation	HHA for ADL Social worker for community resources (equipment/ supplies, financial assistance, respite care)		Contact resources available for support, information Nutritionist for meal planning Physical therapist for breathing, musculoskeletal exercises	Contact physician for changes in condition to report Speech therapist
Discharge plan (as appropriate)				Complete or caregiver assisted self-care Remains homebound, needs skilled care Outpatient services Long-term care facility Hospitalization

ADL, Activities of daily living; *HHA,* home health aide.

Communicable Diseases and Recommended Immunization Schedules

Recommendations for infant and child immunization are developed by the Centers for Disease Control and Prevention (CDC), Altanta, Georgia and approved by the American Academy of Pediatrics, Advisory Committee on Immunization Practices, and the American Academy of Family Physicians. Schedules can be modified, depending on the age of initial immunization endemic areas and epidemics of a disease. As immunization schedules are revised frequently, the reader is advised to check with the CDC for the most recent immunization schedule (see p. 444).

 Documentation and Family Home Record Keeping

BASIC CONSIDERATIONS

1. Documentation of home care is included in criteria for agencies seeking to meet state certification and licensure requirements.
2. Documentation is basis for Medicare, Medicaid, and third-party payors. Information recorded determines billing statements to receive payment for care visits. Some payors require copies of nurses' notes with billing to receive reimbursement. It is advisable for agencies to request what services or types of care can be included in billing and to maintain ongoing communication with payment sources regarding documentation requirements during home care (see "Financial Assessment," p. 42.)
3. Documentation allows for continuity of planned care by providing communication to other professionals involved in care.

4. Records are considered legal documents and ensure that professional standards are followed in delivery of home care.
5. Documentation and maintenance of accurate record provide data for research and information for audits and payment review.
6. Documentation can include written narrative, flow sheets for checks, and notes related to frequent monitoring of equipment and physiologic function.
7. Documentation must be factual, objective, succinct, descriptive, and relevant; omit anything that is not essential information.
8. In home care, caregivers and older children are taught assessment procedures and how to use flow sheets or graphs to note daily monitoring information.

ESSENTIAL COMPONENTS

1. Health history and physical assessment with emphasis on systems related to child's medical diagnosis (list all medical diagnoses but document most acute one requiring skilled nursing care as principal diagnosis).
2. Qualified medical diagnoses when possible by inclusion of words such as *newly diagnosed, unstable, uncontrolled,* or *acute exacerbation.*
3. Identified nursing diagnoses with dates for each problem on care plan.
4. Goals or outcomes (long and short-term) (in collaboration with caregiver) and achievement with dates documented at least weekly; nursing interventions that achieved outcomes, frequency, and personnel responsible for activities.
5. Choices or alternate interventions to solve problems and implement goals developed by nurse and other professionals.
6. Documentation in care plan of exact services being provided that require nursing care and indication of other care needed.
7. Time frames in which care will be provided (number of times a week), depending on condition and insurance parameters; plans for more frequent visits at beginning of home care.

(*Text continued on p. 446.*)

Vaccine	Birth	1 Mo.	2 Mo.	4 Mo.	6 Mo.	12 Mo.	15 Mo.	18 Mo.	4-6 Yrs.	11-12 Yrs.	14-16 Yrs.
Hepatitis B[b]	Hep B-1									Hep B[c]	
		Hep B-2			Hep B-3						
Diphtheria and tetanus toxoids and pertussis vaccine[d]			DTP	DTP	DTP	DTP (DTaP at ≥15 mo)			DTP or DTaP	Td	
Haemophilus influenzae type b[e]			Hib	Hib	Hib	Hib					
Poliovirus[f]			OPV	OPV	OPV				OPV		
Measles-mumps-rubella[g]						MMR			MMR or MMR		
Varicella zoster virus[h]						Var			Var		

▨ Range of acceptable ages for vaccination   □ "Catch-up" vaccination[c, i]

[a] Vaccines are listed under the routinely recommended ages.

[b] **Infants born to Hepatitis B surface antigen (HBsAg)-negative mothers** should receive 2.5 μg of Recombivax HB (Merck & Co.) or 10 μg of Engerix-B (SmithKline Beecham). The second dose should be administered ≥1 mo after the 1st dose. **Infants born to HBsAg-positive mothers** should receive 0.5 ml hepatitis B immune globulin within 12 hours of birth, and either 5 μg of Recombivax HB or 10 μg of Engerix-Bat a separate site. The second dose is recommended at 1 to 2 mo and the third dose at age 6 months. **Infants born to mothers whose HBsAg status is unknown** should receive either 5 μg of Recombivax HB or 10 μg of Engerix-B within 12 hours of birth. The second dose of vaccine is recommended at age 1 month and the third dose at 6 months.

[c] Adolescents who have not received three doses of hepatitis B vaccine should initiate or complete the series at age 11 to 12 years. The second dose should be administered at least 1 month after the first dose, and the third dose should be administered at least 4 months after the first dose and at least 2 months after the second dose.

[d] The fourth dose of diphtheria and tetanus toxoids and pertussis vaccine *(DTP)* may be administered at age 12 months if at least 6 months have elapsed since the third dose of DTP. Diphtheria and tetanus toxoids and acellular pertussis vaccine *(DTaP)* is licensed for the fourth or fifth vaccine dose(s) for children aged ≥15 months and may be preferred for these doses in this age group. Tetanus and diphtheria toxoids, absorbed, for adult use *(Td)* is recommended at age 11 to 12 if at least 5 years have elapsed since the last dose of DTP, DTaP, or diphtheria and tetanus toxoids, absorbed, for pediatric use.

[e] Three *Haemophilus influenzae* type b *(Hib)* conjugate vaccines are licensed for infant use. If PedvaxHIB (Merck & Co.) *Haemophilus* b conjugate vaccine (Meningococcal Protein Conjugate) is administered at ages 2 and 4 months, a dose at 6 months is not required. After completing the primary series, any Hib conjugate vaccine may be used as a booster.

[f] Oral poliovirus vaccine *(OPV)* is recommended for routine infant vaccination. Inactivated poliovirus vaccine *(IPV)* is recommended for persons—or household contacts of persons—with a congenital or acquired immunodeficiency disease or an altered immune status resulting from disease or immunosuppressive therapy and is an acceptable alternative for other persons. The primary three-dose series for IPV should be given with a minimum interval of 4 weeks between the first and second doses and 6 months between the second and third doses.

[g] The second dose of measles-mumps-rubella *(MMR)* vaccine is routinely recommended at age 4 to 6 years or at age 11 to 12 years but may be administered at any visit provided at least 1 month has elapsed since receipt of the first dose.

[h] Varicella-zoster virus *(Var)* vaccine can be administered to susceptible children any time after age 12 months.

[i] Unvaccinated children who lack a reliable history of chickenpox should be vaccinated at age 11 to 12 years.

Use of trade names and commercial sources is for identificaton only and does not imply endorsement by the Public Health Service or the U.S. Department of Health and Human Services.

Fig. 3 Recommended childhood vaccination schedule—United States, January-June, 1996. (From Centers for Disease Control and Prevention: *Morb Mortal Wkly Rep 44:942, 1996.*)

8. Each notation must include why visit was needed. Use information from assessment to confirm medical necessity and specific care given.

9. *All* care that relates to medical diagnoses and physician orders; physician signature should appear on document according to agency and insurance requirements.

10. Unstable conditions or technology-dependent child who requires nursing care and response to changes in treatments or care; confirm that care matches diagnoses and physician's orders.

11. Exercise and other regimens to restore function lost because of illness and caused by the medical diagnosis; any obstacles to overcome to achieve optimal health.

12. Evaluation of goal fulfillment by changes in child's condition or need to modify care plan based on these findings.

13. All teaching to caregiver and family to develop ability to care for child, including disease-related information, assessments, strategies, demonstrations, and record keeping; note poor comprehension and lack of capability by caregiver and need for reteaching.

14. Referrals to professional personnel and community resources.

15. Discharge plan and instructions, summary to physician, and case closing date.

GENERAL DOCUMENTATION REQUIREMENTS FOR ALL CARE PLANS

The following list includes general documentation requirements to be used with those at the end of each care plan:

1. Date and signature of nurse preparing care plan.
2. Assessment data and child status in major areas affected.
3. Changes in child status.
4. Caregiver's and family's responses and adaptation to child's illness.
5. Care plan that includes problem identification, needs with expected outcomes, assigned interventions, and prescribed treatments.

6. Nursing activities including all assessments and teaching.
7. Child's response and need for further assessment, instruction, and referrals.
8. Plan and timing for next visit.
9. Readiness and plan for discharge from home care visits.
10. Dates and signature of all personnel performing care; evaluation when appropriate.
11. Have copy of plan available for caregiver.
12. Registered Nurse supervision of Nurse Aides.

 # *Energy Intake Recommendations*

Energy requirements translate into caloric requirements. The following chart delineates recommended energy intake based on age, gender, height, and weight.

Median Height and Weights and Recommended Energy Intake

Category	Age (yr) or condition	Weight (kg)	Weight (lb)	Height (cm)	Height (in)	REE* (kcal/day)	Average Energy Allowance (kcal)† Multiples of REE	Average Energy Allowance (kcal)† Per kg†	Average Energy Allowance (kcal)† Per day‡
Infants	0.0-0.5	6	13	60	24	320		108	650
	0.5-1.0	9	20	71	28	500		98	850
Children	1-3	13	29	90	35	740		102	1300
	4-6	20	44	112	44	950		90	1800
	7-10	28	62	132	52	1130		70	2000
Males	11-14	45	99	157	62	1440	1.70	55	2500
	15-18	66	145	176	69	1760	1.67	45	3000
	19-24	72	160	177	70	1780	1.67	40	2900
	25-50	79	174	176	70	1800	1.60	37	2900
	51+	77	170	173	68	1530	1.50	30	2300
Females	11-14	46	101	157	62	1310	1.67	47	2200
	15-18	55	120	163	64	1370	1.60	40	2200
	19-24	58	128	164	65	1350	1.60	38	2200
	25-50	63	138	163	64	1380	1.55	36	2200
	51+	65	143	160	63	1280	1.50	30	1900

Pregnant	1st trimester	+0
	2nd trimester	+300
	3rd trimester	+300
Lactating	1st 6 mo	+500
	2nd 6 mo	+500

From Recommended Dietary Allowances, Food and Nutrition Board National Academy of Sciences–National Research Council, Washington, D.C., 1989.

The data in this table have been assembled from the observed median heights and weights of children together with desirable weights for adults for the mean heights of men (70 inches) and women (64 inches) between the ages of 18 and 34 years as surveyed in the United States population (HEW/NCHS data). The energy allowances for the young adults are for men and women doing light work. The allowances for the two older age groups represent mean energy needs over these age spans, allowing for a 2% decrease in basal (resting) metabolic rate per decade and a reduction in activity of 200 kcal/day for men and women between ages 51 and 75 years, 500 kcal for men over 75 years and 400 kcal for women over 75 years. The customary range of daily energy output is shown for adults in parentheses and is based on a variation in energy needs of ±400 kcal at any one age, emphasizing the wide range of energy intakes appropriate for any group of people. Energy allowances for children through age 18 are based on medium energy intakes of children these ages followed in longitudinal growth studies. The values in parentheses are 10th and 90th percentiles of energy intake, to indicate the range of energy consumption among children of these ages.

*Resting energy expenditure.

†In the range of light to moderate activity, the coefficient of variation is ± 20%.

‡Figure is rounded.

Medication Administration and Teaching Guidelines

Medication administration by the caregivers to children in the home is the focus of these guidelines. A major responsibility of the home care nurse is teaching the family and caregiver to perform this procedure. Some of the more complex administration methods and routes require adequate or extensive instruction and practice time to ensure safe compliance to a medication regimen. Medications prescribed by the physician include those given orally, sublingually, topically, intramuscularly, subcutaneously, intravenously, by inhalation and feeding tube, and are scheduled for regular administration or in response to requests when needed. The following information provides helpful tips and actual procedures for nurses and caregivers to consider when administering medications.

TIPS FOR APPROACHING AND PREPARING CHILD

1. Offer explanation to child regarding medicine that is appropriate to age and level of development.
2. Maintain positive attitude with child about importance of and procedure for taking medications.
3. Let child express feelings about taking medication.
4. Involve child in choices when possible and within age limitations to enhance cooperation in taking medication.
5. Let child view and handle devices used in medication administration (dropper, syringe, and spoon).
6. Provide distractions or devise restraints if unable to administer medication because of fearful, uncooperative behavior.
7. Stay with child after administration of medications. Praise, hug, and soothe child for doing well and taking medicine.

TIPS FOR TEACHING SAFE ADMINISTRATION

1. Assess age, weight and drug allergies.
2. Assess compatibility with foods and other medications.

3. Assess cognitive and developmental level of child, caregiver's intellectual capacity, and level of understanding of drug administration.

4. Provide thorough instructions that include drug name, reason for use, dosage, frequency, route, form, length of time, expected effects, and adverse side effects to report or what actions to take. Nurse assesses if drug is within safe dosage range.

5. Preferable route is oral in form, most easily administered, depending on age of child and danger of aspiration if crying or uncooperative.

6. Offer or maintain written procedure and time schedules for administration of medication that comply with daily family routines.

7. Require repeat demonstrations until caregiver is competent and feels comfortable with procedure (especially for injections).

8. Inform child to take medicine only when given by parent, grandparent, or baby-sitter.

9. Never refer to medicine as candy because child may take overdose if opportunity arises.

10. Note expiration date; and store in cool, dry, locked cabinet with lid tightly closed, in original container, and labeled with written instructions. Refrigerate on a high rear shelf if medicine is to be kept cold.

ORAL MEDICATIONS

1. Check medication label for name, amount, and time to be administered.

2. Select device to give medication based on form and age of child.

   - Measuring cup or spoon, calibrated dropper, syringe, nipple with measured amount of liquid medicine
   - Pill crusher to crush tablets and juice, syrup, or soft food for mixing (avoid mixing in milk or formula)
   - Chewable tablets, if available, to preschool or school-age child

3. Administration to infant: Hold in semicircle position and place syringe or dropper with medication toward back of mouth to side of tongue. Administer slowly and

allow child to swallow. If medication is placed in bottle with nipple or nipple alone, mix with small amount of formula or other liquid and allow infant to suck until complete dosage is swallowed. Limiting amount will help ensure that full dosage of medication is ingested.

4. Administration to toddler: Inform child of what is to be done and how to help. Use cup or spoon with measured amount and allow child to swallow. Measuring spoon or dropper with measured amount can be placed in mouth, medication given, and time allowed to swallow.

5. Administration to preschooler: Explain reason for medication and how to help. Use cup, spoon, or any other measured device and allow child to hold and swallow liquid medication or crush tablet (if allowed) and mix with juice or applesauce and allow child to hold and drink or eat mixture. Offer reward for cooperation (stars or special treat and praise for helping).

RECTAL MEDICATIONS

1. Rectal route can be used if oral route is not possible.
2. Insert child-size and correct dosage suppository (removed from wrapper) into rectum 1 inch with smallest finger cot moistened with water. Hold buttocks together for about 5 minutes to prevent expulsion.
3. Place child in left side-lying position for medication administration by retention enema. Mix medication with small amount of water in container connected to child-size catheter. Insert into rectum; slowly allow solution to flow into rectum by gravity and hold buttocks together for 5 minutes to prevent expulsion.

EYE, EAR, NOSE MEDICATIONS

Administration by nose

1. Cleanse around nose and remove any accumulated secretion from nares with warm, damp cloth. Leave cloth in place if crusted secretions are present, until soft enough to be wiped away. Draw up medication into nose dropper.
2. Place child in supine position and gently tilt head back to rest on small pillow under neck, on lap, or over side of bed. If restraint is needed, swaddle infant in blan-

ket. For older child, place head between your legs and arms under your legs, or cross legs over child to prevent movement.

3. Place correct number of drops into each side of nose and retain head in tilted position for 1 minute. Avoid allowing tip of dropper to touch nose.

4. Wipe excess from nose and allow child to resume normal position.

Administration by ear

1. Warm bottle of medication in pan of water and check to assess warmth to avoid cold or hot drops. Draw up medication into ear dropper.

2. Cleanse outside of ears to remove any drainage with tissue or cotton tipped applicator. Avoid touching external ear canal.

3. Place child on side to expose ear to receive medication and then on other side to receive medication; if restraint is needed, follow procedure to hold head outlined previously.

4. Pull outer ear downward and backward for child less than 2 years old. Pull upward and backward for older child to straighten canal. Place correct number of drops in each ear toward side of canal. Avoid allowing tip of dropper to touch ears.

5. Maintain position of head for 1 minute after drops are inserted in each ear, and wipe away excess from outer ear if needed.

6. Place cotton ball in ears to prevent medication from leaking. Change cotton with each administration of drops to ears.

Administration by eye

1. Cleanse around eyes with warm, damp cloth to remove any secretions. Leave cloth in place if crusted material is present, until soft enough to be wiped away. Draw up medication into eye dropper.

2. Place child in supine position with head slightly tilted back and to side to expose eye to receive medication; if restraint is needed, follow procedure to hold head outlined previously.

3. Ask child to look up. Place wrist of hand holding dropper on forehead; gently pull lower lid downward with other hand and place correct number of drops into lower lid. Avoid allowing tip of dropper to touch any part of eye or skin.

4. Ask child to close eyes tightly and open again to disperse fluid. Wipe any excess medication from around eye with tissue.

5. For eye ointment, follow same procedure and squeeze ointment across inner aspect of lower lid from canthus to outer aspect of eye.

INHALATION MEDICATIONS

Administration by hand-held, small-volume nebulizer

1. Prepare nebulizer by attaching tubing and plugging into electric outlet with machine turned off.

2. Assemble nebulizer chamber by attaching mouthpiece or mask to piece that is connected to cap of chamber containing prescribed medication dose.

3. Place cap on chamber by turning clockwise and attach tubing from nebulizer (compressor) to chamber.

4. Check that all connections are tight. Turn machine on and note mist coming from mouthpiece/mask.

5. Place mouthpiece in child's mouth with lips around it and tell child to breathe through mouth. Use mask over nose and mouth or noseclip on infant.

6. Hold younger child to help feel secure during treatment.

7. Allow child to breathe slowly and deeply. Turn off machine to rest if fatigued. Continue when able until all solution is gone. Check pulse before and after treatment.

8. Turn machine off. Disassemble chamber and cleanse with mild detergent. Rinse with warm water and air dry on paper towel.

Administration by hand-held, metered-dose inhaler

1. Insert metal canister tightly into holder and shake well to mix medication with propellant.

2. Remove cap and ask child to exhale fully. Place inhaler in upright position and hold mouthpiece up to child's mouth or in mouth resting on lower teeth with lips around it.

3. Ask child to press on top of canister with finger and inhale slowly and deeply; then hold breath for 5 to 10 seconds or as long as possible.
4. Release finger and remove from child's mouth. Wait for 30 seconds and repeat procedure for second dose.
5. Perform as often as prescribed. Remove canister, rinse holder daily, and allow to dry on paper towel.
6. Instruct to rinse mouth after inhalation of medication if corticosteroids are prescribed.

ENTERAL TUBE MEDICATIONS

Indwelling tubes include nasogastric, orogastric, and gastrostomy types. They are placed in position for feedings when the oral route is not possible. Medications administered via these smallbore-feeding tubes are in the form of liquid or crushed tablets mixed in a small amount of liquid. They are administered by the gravity method as follows:

1. Place prescribed dosage in barrel of syringe. Unclamp tube end and connect barrel to tubing.
2. Check for placement of tube in stomach.
3. Allow liquid to flow into tube by gravity. When syringe barrel is almost empty, add 30 ml of water to clear tubing and to ensure that all medication has reached stomach.
4. Check patency of tubing for clogging if crushed or viscous medications are administered.

INTRAMUSCULAR AND SUBCUTANEOUS MEDICATIONS

Medication preparation
1. Wash hands.
2. Open proper-size packaged syringe and needle; assemble if needed.
3. Cleanse top of vial with alcohol swab or remove top of ampule.
4. Remove cap from needle. Draw in amount of air equal to amount of medication needed. Place needle into top of vial, inject air into vial, and withdraw amount of medication needed or place needle into ampule and withdraw amount of medication needed.

5. Remove needle from vial or ampule. Remove any air bubbles and replace cap loosely for easy removal when ready to administer injection.

Medication administration

1. Place child in sitting or lying position with site exposed. Have someone hold child if necessary (vastus lateralis muscle preferred for intramuscular [IM]; arm or thigh for subcutaneous [SC]).
2. Cleanse site with alcohol swab in circular motion from center outward. Allow to air dry.
3. Remove cap from needle. Hold skin firmly at appropriate site and insert needle at 90-degree angle (IM) or 45-degree angle with bevel of point facing upward (SC).
4. Pull plunger to check for blood. Remove and change needle if blood is present, or inject contents of syringe if no blood is present.
5. Quickly and smoothly withdraw syringe and gently swab area with tissue. Apply decorated bandaid.
6. Dispose of syringe and needle (without recapping or breaking needle) in waterproof, unbreakable container (covered coffee can or liquid laundry detergent bottle) for proper disposal of hazardous materials.
7. Hold, hug, and cuddle child for comfort and support after injection. Explain how medication will help child get well.

SYRINGE PUMP SUBCUTANEOUS MEDICATIONS

A syringe pump contains a battery powered motor that pushes fluid through the syringe in measured amounts and intervals for infusion of medication. It is usually used in children when continuous insulin administration is necessary to receive a more consistent insulin release. Gloves and sterile technique are used to perform syringe pump procedures.

1. With infusion tubing attached, fill syringe with prescribed amount of insulin and place in pump. Close cover while leaving tubing clamped and exposed on outside of pump.
2. Attach needle to tubing, unclamp, and prime. Insert into prepared abdominal or thigh site SC at 30- to 60-degree

angle. Secure a place with transparent dressing over needle and tubing to prevent dislodgement and to allow for site assessment.

3. Set program pump for continuous dose injections that are balanced with activities and dietary regimens.
4. Place pump in carrying case and attach to belt or place in pocket.
5. Perform pump alarm checks to determine malfunction. Alternate injection sites, change tubing and needle every 48 hours, and change batteries as needed.
6. Avoid exposure of site to water. Assess site for infection or abscess formation.
7. Instruct client to perform blood glucose and urine testing and report altered levels that indicate need for modification of insulin dosage or dietary regimen (see "Diabetes Mellitus," pp. 245-258).

HEPARIN LOCK INTRAVENOUS MEDICATIONS

A catheter is inserted into a vein and maintained over time to eliminate the need for multiple peripheral venipunctures to administer intravenous (IV) medication in the home. It is used for short-term IV therapy. Primary care involves maintaining and monitoring the tube for patency, placement, and safe medication administration and the injection site for infection.

Site assessment and protection

1. Note redness, edema, pain, and drainage at site daily.
2. Change sterile gauze dressing over heparin lock. Tape in place with capped end exposed. Gently wash around insertion site and avoid tube. Cover tube and area with plastic when bathing to protect from water.
3. Periodically change catheter according to policy or if problem develops.
4. Cover catheter site with clothing or other protection to prevent child from handling tube end or pulling catheter out.

Patency and use of heparin lock

1. Wash hands.
2. Prepare heparin and medication in separate syringes as outlined in IM and SC injections.

3. Flush catheter with specified amount of heparin solution at prescribed frequency and follow all medication administration guidelines. Use normal saline if heparin is not compatible with medication.
4. Cleanse heparin lock hub/cap with antiseptic. Insert needle of syringe with medication into hub/cap center and inject contents slowly over 3 to 4 minutes.
5. Remove needle from heparin lock and inject prepared heparin into hub/cap to ensure patency of device. Withdraw needle and cover catheter end for protection from trauma and dislodgement.

CENTRAL VENOUS CATHETER MEDICATIONS

An indwelling right atrial catheter is inserted through an incision in the right upper chest and directed through an SC tunnel into a deep vessel near the heart. A peripheral IV central catheter is inserted via a peripheral vein in the arm. They are inserted for continuous or intermittent IV administration of fluids, nutrients, and medications. Catheters commonly used include the Hickman/Broviac and, in some cases, Groshong.

Site assessment and protection
1. Through transparent dressing, note redness, edema, pain, and drainage at site daily or during dressing changes. Assess for temperature elevation.
2. Maintain transparent dressing to allow for visualization and anchoring of catheter in place, especially peripheral catheter.
3. Ensure that external central catheter is anchored to skin with tape.
4. Restrict activity during short-term therapy to prevent dislodgement. Avoid strenuous activity and contact sports with all types of central venous catheters.
5. Cover site with plastic when bathing to protect from water.
6. Cover site with shirt or clothing that opens in back to prevent child from handling or pulling out catheter.
7. Notify school nurse and teacher that catheter is present so assistance can be provided, if needed.
8. Report any signs of infection, damage, or occlusion to catheter and clamp if it is in place.

9. Dispose of all used articles and supplies according to universal precautions.

Patency and care of central catheters

1. Secure help to care for catheter if child has difficulty cooperating.
2. Palpate or examine area around catheter for tenderness.
3. Wash hands and use gloves and sterile technique for all central venous catheter care.
4. To remove or change transparent dressing (per policy or if soiled or loose), gently peel off dressing. Assess skin and site; hold catheter up and cleanse around insertion site with circular motion from center and moving outward using swabs with an iodophor solution. Allow to air dry; apply antiseptic ointment to site. Loop tube at insertion site with cap below area to be covered by dressing. Place window-frame type dressing on skin, gently pressing from top to bottom while eliminating any air bubbles. Secure cap area in place with tape for easy access and cover with clothing.
5. Site care should be performed by home care nurse because of risk of dislodgement when catheter is not sutured or secured in place.
6. To change gauze dressing follow same procedure as for transparent dressing. Apply antiseptic ointment around insertion site, position gauze dressing over site, loop catheter over gauze, and cover with another gauze dressing. Secure edges with tape and leave cap area exposed for easy access, but covered with clothing.
7. Prepare syringe with specified amount and concentration of heparin solution and 5 ml saline (Groshong) to flush catheter (as outlined for IM and SC injections). Use after all medication administrations and per schedule, depending on type of catheter (whether peripheral or right atrial catheter).
8. Cleanse injection cap or valve of catheter with antiseptic. Insert needle of syringe with flushing solution into cap center and slowly inject contents.
9. Remove needle from cap (Groshong). Last 0.2 ml of prepared heparin is injected in some types of catheters to ensure patency of device.

10. To replace an injection cap/valve (usually once or twice weekly), clamp tube in area between end of tube and skin. Cleanse around tip below cap with antiseptic swab. Remove old cap and attach new cap. Remove clamp if used.

Medication preparation and administration
1. Wash hands.
2. Prepare medication in syringe as outlined in IM and SC injections.
3. Cleanse cap with antiseptic. Insert needle of syringe with medication into cap center and inject contents slowly over 3 to 4 minutes.
4. Remove needle of empty syringe from cap. Insert needle of prepared heparin into cap and inject to ensure patency of catheter. Withdraw needle and cover catheter end with clothing for protection from trauma and dislodgement.

IMPLANTED INFUSION PORT CATHETER MEDICATIONS

A chamber containing an infusion port is surgically implanted in the chest wall or the antecubital space and sutured in place. It has a silicone-type catheter attached to the chamber (port) that is threaded through the SC tissue and into the central venous circulation. It can also be used to provide access to the peritoneum, epidural space, and hepatic artery. Various types of catheters are available and selection is based on need and physician preference. A catheter is used for long-term continuous infusion of medications or fluids and is often preferred by older children because it is less limiting and requires less care.

Site assessment and protection
1. Note redness, edema, and pain at site.
2. Note needle dislodgement during infusions if child is active.
3. Cover site with shirt or clothing if child desires.
4. Notify school nurse and teacher that catheter is present and of necessary activity restrictions.
5. Report any changes at port site or any difficulty in passage of needle through skin.

Patency and care
1. Prepare heparin solution in amount prescribed in syringe with small-gauge, nonboring needle.
2. Insert needle into port. Assess for blood return or easily injected solution with no signs of tissue infiltration. Inject solution. Heparinize after each use or once each month.

Medication preparation and administration
1. Wash hands.
2. Prepare medication in syringe as outlined in IM and SC injections.
3. Attach special Huber-point needle for entry via port.
4. Prepare skin at port site with antiseptic. Put on sterile gloves and insert needle through skin into port.
5. Check placement of needle in port by noting blood return, normal saline flush, and absence of tissue infiltration.
6. Administer medication and remove needle after injection. For continuous administration, secure in place. Attach longer tubing extension if intermittent medications are to be infused. Then attach to infusion pump controller, peristaltic pump, or ambulatory infusion device set at desired amount, rate, and time.
7. If needle is left in place for infusion therapy, place sterile gauze under needle to stabilize it. Cover with transparent dressing to allow for visualization of site.
8. Catheter can be left in place for continuous infusions instead of needle to provide more stability and prevent needle punctures. Same care is provided as if needle is used.

CHILD/CAREGIVER-CONTROLLED ANALGESIA
Controlled analgesia is a method of self-administering drugs that uses a programmable infusion pump for IV and SC routes intermittent doses at preset time intervals. Medication can be administered by initial bolus and then by continuous infusion.

Time between doses is known as the *lockout interval* and is the length of time needed for the drug to begin working. Infusion of medication is initiated by either the caregiver or child pushing a button when pain is felt.

EPIDURAL AND INTRATHECAL MEDICATIONS

Medication administration via epidural and intrathecal routes is usually reserved for terminal care. A catheter is inserted into the epidural or intrathecal space for intermittent or continuous infusion of analgesia. This provides consistent drug levels and a long-lasting effect by the direct action on receptors in the spinal cord.

INFUSION PUMPS FOR INTRAVENOUS MEDICATIONS AND FLUIDS

A variety of portable peristaltic pumps are available to deliver medications, fluids, or total parenteral therapy (TPN) via central venous lines (right atrial catheter and port catheter). The infusion pump controller is used when a sustained, slow flow rate is desired. Other infusion pumps deliver fluids at a high flow rate. Both types of pumps sound safety alarms when air gets in the line, when the line becomes occluded, or when the infusion is completed. Pumps are selected according to the type of infusion fluid, amount and rate of infusion, and route of administration. Depending on the model, pumps can deliver 1 to 400 ml/hr for 1 minute to 100 hours and can deliver two programs with one device for bolus, intermittent, or continuous infusion. The portable devices operate with battery power. The device and solution containers can be placed in a carrying case and hung over the shoulder or kept in the open for viewing.

Various brands of delivery systems are available for home use. Infusion pumps that control the amount, rate, and time of flow are preferred for home care over hand-regulated, gravity-drip methods unless simple, short-term intermittent therapy of a small amount of medication is to be administered.

Teaching guidelines
1. Threading infusion tubing through clothing to prevent pressure or dislodgement.
2. Wearing ambulatory pump.
3. Setting pump correctly and checking pump function; reading numbers on pump and checking if infusion is progressing.

4. Infusion bags, amounts, and monitoring decreases in amounts in bag and infusion rate.
5. Changing bags or flow rate and resetting pump as needed.
6. Knowledge of alarms, actions to take, and determining possible pump malfunction.
7. Safe bathing and activities when attached to infusion pump.
8. Changing and recharging batteries.
9. Maintaining of supplies needed.

*Nursing Diagnoses (NANDA)**

Activity intolerance
Activity intolerance, risk for
Adaptive capacity, decreased: intracranial
Adjustment, impaired
Airway clearance, ineffective
Anxiety
Aspiration, risk for

Body image disturbance
Body temperature, altered, risk for
Bowel incontinence
Breastfeeding, effective
Breastfeeding, ineffective
Breastfeeding, interrupted
Breathing pattern, ineffective

Cardiac output, decreased
Caregiver role strain

---

*From revised 1994 eleventh conference of official nursing diagnoses presented by the North American Nursing Diagnosis Association (NANDA).

Caregiver role strain, risk for
Communication, impaired verbal
Community coping, ineffective
Community coping, potential for enhanced
Confusion, acute
Confusion, chronic
Constipation
Constipation, colonic
Constipation, perceived
Coping, defensive
Coping, family: potential for growth
Coping, ineffective family: compromised
Coping, ineffective family: disabling
Coping, ineffective individual

Decisional conflict (specify)
Denial, ineffective
Diarrhea
Disuse syndrome, risk for
Diversional activity deficit
Dysreflexia

Energy field disturbance
Environmental interpretation syndrome: impaired

Family processes, altered
Family processes, altered: alcoholism
Fatigue
Fear
Fluid volume deficit
Fluid volume deficit, risk for
Fluid volume excess

Gas exchange, impaired
Grieving, anticipatory
Grieving, dysfunctional
Growth and development, altered

Health maintenance, altered
Health-seeking behaviors (specify)
Home maintenance management, impaired

Hopelessness
Hyperthermia
Hypothermia

Incontinence, functional
Incontinence, reflex
Incontinence, stress
Incontinence, total
Incontinence, urge
Infant behavior, disorganized
Infant behavior, disorganized: risk for
Infant behavior, organized: potential for enhanced
Infant feeding pattern, ineffective
Infection, risk for
Injury, perioperative positioning: risk for
Injury, risk for

Knowledge deficit (specify)

Loneliness, risk for

Management of therapeutic regimen, community: ineffective
Management of therapuetic regimen, families: ineffective
Management of therapeutic regimen, individuals: effective
Management of therapeutic regimen, individuals: ineffective
Memory, impaired
Mobility, impaired physical

Noncompliance (specify)
Nutrition, altered: less than body requirements
Nutrition, altered: more than body requirements
Nutrition, altered: risk for more than body requirements

Oral mucous membrane, altered

Pain
Pain, chronic
Parent/Infant/Child attachment altered, risk for
Parental role conflict
Parenting, altered
Parenting, altered, risk for

Peripheral neurovascular dysfunction, risk for
Personal identity disturbance
Poisoning, risk for
Post-trauma response
Powerlessness
Protection, altered

Rape-trauma syndrome
Rape-trauma syndrome: compound reaction
Rape-trauma syndrome: silent reaction
Relocation stress syndrome
Role performance, altered

Self-care deficit, bathing/hygiene
Self-care deficit, dressing/grooming
Self-care deficit, feeding
Self-care deficit, toileting
Self-esteem, chronic low
Self-esteem disturbance
Self-esteem, situational low
Self-mutilation, risk for
Sensory/perceptual alterations (specify) (visual, auditory,
    kinesthetic, gustatory, tactile, olfactory)
Sexual dysfunction
Sexuality patterns, altered
Skin integrity, impaired
Skin integrity, impaired, risk for
Sleep pattern disturbance
Social interaction, impaired
Social isolation
Spiritual distress (distress of the human spirit)
Spiritual well-being, potential for enhanced
Suffocation, risk for
Swallowing, impaired

Thermoregulation, ineffective
Thought processes, altered
Tissue integrity, impaired
Tissue perfusion, altered (specify type) (renal, cerebral, car-
    diopulmonary, gastrointestinal, peripheral)
Trauma, risk for

Unilateral neglect
Urinary elimination, altered
Urinary retention

Ventilation, inability to sustain spontaneous
Ventilatory weaning process, dysfunctional
Violence, risk for: self-directed or directed at others

 Specimen Collection

URINE SPECIMENS

Random specimens
Random specimens are collected for laboratory examination or immediate home testing by dipstick for specific constituent values. For some tests, the dipstick can be placed on the wet diaper and compared with a color chart to determine changes indicating positive or negative test results.

- **Male infant:** wash and dry genitalia and place penis and scrotum inside plastic collecting device. Apply lower adhesive portion to skin and then top half of adhesive. Press firmly to remove any wrinkles and prevent leakage. Re-apply diaper and monitor bag for specimen. Hold skin at bottom and peel from top to bottom to remove device. Place urine in clean container and label appropriately.
- **Female infant:** wash and dry as for male infant. Stretch perineum and apply lower half of adhesive portion of plastic collection device as flat as possible to perineum. Then remove top half of adhesive and press firmly in place toward symphysis. Remove bag by holding skin and peeling from top to bottom. Prepare specimen for laboratory as for male infant. Slight pressure to suprapubic area or stroking along spine to elicit reflex can initiate voiding in infants less than 6 months of age.
- **Preschool toddler:** offer preferred liquids and explain need to void. Remind to void in 30 minutes. Wash hands and allow to use own potty chair. Place receptacle in

toilet or hold container in place while child urinates. Praise child because procedure can cause confusion about voiding in place that has resulted in disapproval by parents in past.

- **School-age child:** explain reasons for specimen collection and what testing will be done with urine. Instruct child to wash hands and open container without touching inside or lid when preparing to collect specimen. Most children can void in clean plastic container held in place during urination. Specimen containers should be covered with lid, labeled properly, and taken to laboratory. Advise to refrigerate until taken to laboratory. Restrict amount of fluid to one glass because increased intake can interfere with test results.

Clean-catch specimens

- **Male child:** inform child of need to obtain urine specimen and collection procedure to follow. Wash hands and open specimen container without touching inside or lid. Cleanse tip of penis with wipe provided in kit or wash with soap and water and rinse. Pull back foreskin and wash and rinse if uncircumcised. Instruct child to begin voiding in toilet. Tell him to stop, position container, and continue voiding into cup. If child is unable to stop, place cup in flow to catch urine. Show child approval by praising him for successful collection of specimen. Place lid on container and label appropriately.
- **Female child:** inform of need to obtain urine specimen and collection procedure to follow. Wash hands and open specimen container without touching inside or lid. Spread labia apart with thumb and forefinger and cleanse with wipes or soap and water from front to back and rinse. Continue with procedure as for male child until specimen is collected and labeled for laboratory.
- Clean-catch specimens are collected for culture to determine urinary tract infections. Specimens that cannot be collected by proper cleansing and midstream flow to reduce contamination are still considered adequate for culture examination.

Twenty-four hour specimens

- **Infants and young children:** apply collection bag to infant or young child as described for random specimen collection. Empty bag of all urine hourly or as needed into large container from laboratory and refrigerate as directed. Reapply bag after each emptying. If collection base has collection tubes in place, connect these to container and monitor collection for duration of test.
- **Older children:** instruct child to notify caregiver of need to void. Collect urine in container for boys and bedpan in toilet for girls. Advise of importance to avoid contamination of urine with toilet tissue or feces. Place urine in large collection container from laboratory. If old enough, allow child to take responsibility for own collection. Refrigerate during collection time.

The 24-hour collection begins and ends with an empty bladder. The first voiding is discarded and the timing begins; the timing ends with the last voiding 24 hours later. The container is properly labeled and taken to the laboratory at the conclusion of the test.

FECES SPECIMENS

- **Infant:** apply urine device to avoid contamination of specimen by urine. Collect feces from diaper with tongue blade; place in clean, plastic, covered container; and label container appropriately. Remove urinary collection device.
- **Child:** advise child to urinate in toilet first and flush toilet. Place bedpan in toilet and ask child to defecate in bedpan. Remove feces from bedpan; place in clean, plastic, covered container; and label container appropriately. Document date and time on labels if series of specimens are collected.

Store specimens in a refrigerator unless the test requires that it be taken to the laboratory immediately. Immediate testing can be performed for occult blood.

BLOOD SPECIMENS

- **Capillary sample:** collect blood from heel of infants or from finger or earlobe of children by lancet penetration. Cleanse skin and perform puncture at appropriate site. Saturate test tape with blood, apply pressure, and apply adhesive strip when bleeding stops. Compare tape with color chart or analyze by Glucometer depending on test to be performed.

A specimen obtained by puncture may not provide enough blood for some tests. Inform the child that removing a small amount of blood is not a threat and that more blood is produced by the body. Also explain that no additional blood can leak from the puncture after the site is bandaged.

RESPIRATORY SPECIMENS

Sputum

- **Infants and young children:** obtain specimen by suctioning of trachea and place specimen in sterile container for culture examination. If tracheostomy is present, attach collecting device to suction device to obtain specimen. Label container and take to laboratory.
- **Older children:** Instruct child to cough up deep secretions, preferably in morning, and to expectorate into sterile container for culture examination. Label container appropriately and take to laboratory.

Nasal and throat secretions

- **Younger and older children:** obtain culture tube containing medium (Culturette). Place child in supine position for nasal swab or sitting position for throat swab. Remove cotton-tipped applicators and swab each naris for nasal culture. Swab back and sides of throat in nasopharyngeal and tonsillar areas for throat culture. Place applicators in tube's medium, slightly crush to cover material on applicators, and replace top on tube. Label tube appropriately and take to laboratory.

Throat swabbing is contraindicated in a child with suspected acute epiglottitis because this can result in edema, leading to severe respiratory distress.

Universal Precautions and Guidelines for Control of Body Substances

Universal precautions are used to prevent or minimize transmission of blood-borne and other infections between children, caregivers, and family members. Special guidelines were developed by the Centers for Disease Control and Prevention (CDC) to protect caregivers from contact with the child's blood, body fluids, and tissues. Universal precautions apply to blood, semen, vaginal secretions, cerebrospinal fluid, synovial fluid, pleural fluid, peritoneal fluid, pericardial fluid, and amniotic fluid. These do not include feces, urine, sweat, saliva, tears, nasal secretions, sputum, wound drainage, vomitus, and possibly other fluids unless they contain blood. Universal precautions do not generally apply to breast milk or saliva, although health care workers may be advised to use them in select circumstances. The care of young children in the home is usually confined to contact with urine, feces, vomitus, and occasionally blood, precautions need be taken.

All body fluids, secretions, and excretions are potentially pathogenic and should be handled accordingly. The precautions involve a combination of controls or safeguards in hand protection, personal protective clothing, and handling of equipment and supplies. The judgement of what protection safeguards to use depends on the type and degree of exposure.

Home care should include current information regarding latest guidelines and new technology to promote safer equipment, therapy techniques, and local regulations related to hazardous waste disposal. The following guidelines are outlined for use by the home care nurse and are taught to the caregiver for implementation.

HAND PROTECTION

- Wash hands with soap and water (count to 10). Then rinse with water and dry after all care, especially after diaper change if hands contact feces or urine.

- Wear gloves if cuts or open areas are present on caregiver's hands or if added protection is needed for handling body fluids such as when changing diapers with loose feces, suctioning secretions, cleaning up vomitus or blood, caring for superficial breaks in skin (cuts, abrasions, bites), obtaining capillary blood samples or other specimens for testing or for examination, if applicable.
- Wash hands after removal of gloves if used for care.

PROTECTIVE WEAR

- Wear disposable plastic apron or cover chest and shoulder with cloth when feeding infant to protect from vomit or spitting up when burping.
- Wear gowns or aprons during central intravenous catheter procedures and care.

EQUIPMENT AND SUPPLIES

- Gloves should not be washed, disinfected, and reused.
- Discard gloves in leak-proof bag with used disposable diapers, cleansing tissues, used dressings, and other disposable supplies for proper disposal.
- Wash soiled linens and clothing in hot water with detergent, rinse, and dry well for reuse.
- Dispose of lancet used in blood sampling, syringes, and needles (uncapped, intact, with no bending or shearing) and store in hard container (coffee can) until half full. Label for future disposal of hazardous materials.
- Take special precautions against needle sticks.
- Use needleless intravenous equipment if possible. Medical waste (tubing and dressings) contaminated with blood or body fluids should be double-bagged.

DISINFECTION

- Work areas should be cleansed with alcohol, bleach solution, or soap and water. If not, cover with waterproof protective barrier such as pad or towel.
- Suction catheters, tracheostomy tubes, and other reusable supplies should be rinsed with cold water and placed in jar filled with hot soapy water. Rinse with hot running water. Submerge in commercial solution diluted according to instructions for 10 minutes.

Then rinse well and place on clean paper towel to air
dry.

SPILLED LIQUIDS

- Cleanse liquids that spill such as vomitus, loose feces, and
  blood by putting on gloves and wiping with paper towels.
- Prepare and pour solution of bleach and water (1:10
  to 1:100, depending on amount of organic material) onto
  area. Wipe clean with paper towels.
- Place used towels in waterproof bag with gloves and other
  used articles for disposal.

 Vital Signs

Normal Respiratory Rates for Children

Age	Rate (breaths/min)
Newborn	35
1-11 mo	30
2 yr	25
4 yr	23
6 yr	21
8 yr	20
10 yr	19
12 yr	19
14 yr	18
16 yr	17
18 yr	16-18

From Wong DL: *Wong and Whaley's clinical manual of pediatric nursing,* ed
4, St Louis, 1996, Mosby.

Normal Blood Pressure Readings for Children (Boys)

Systolic Blood Pressure Percentile					Age	Diastolic Blood Pressure* Percentile				
5th	10th	50th	90th	95th		5th	10th	50th	90th	95th
54	58	73	87	92	1 day	38	42	55	68	72
55	59	74	89	93	3 days	38	42	55	68	71
57	62	76	91	95	7 days	37	41	54	67	71
67	71	86	101	105	1 mo	35	39	52	64	68
72	76	91	106	110	2 mo	33	37	50	63	66
72	76	91	106	110	3 mo	33	37	50	63	66
72	76	91	106	110	4 mo	34	37	50	63	67
72	76	91	105	110	5 mo	35	39	52	65	68
71	76	90	105	109	6 mo	36	40	53	66	70
71	76	90	105	109	7 mo	37	41	54	67	71
71	75	90	105	109	8 mo	38	42	55	68	72
71	75	90	105	109	9 mo	39	43	55	68	72
71	75	90	105	109	10 mo	39	43	56	69	73
71	76	90	105	109	11 mo	39	43	56	69	73
71	76	90	105	109	1 yr	39	43	56	69	73
72	76	91	106	110	2 yr	39	43	56	69	73
73	77	92	107	111	3 yr	39	42	55	68	72
74	79	93	108	112	4 yr	39	43	56	69	72

					Age					
76	80	95	109	113	5 yr	40	43	56	69	73
77	81	96	111	115	6 yr	41	44	57	70	74
78	83	97	112	116	7 yr	42	45	58	71	75
80	84	99	114	118	8 yr	43	47	60	73	76
82	86	101	115	120	9 yr	44	48	61	74	78
84	88	102	117	121	10 yr	45	49	62	75	79
86	90	105	119	123	11 yr	47	50	63	76	80
88	92	107	121	126	12 yr	48	51	64	77	81
90	94	109	124	128	13 yr	45	49	63	77	81
93	97	112	126	131	14 yr	46	50	64	78	82
95	99	114	129	133	15 yr	47	51	65	79	83
98	102	117	131	136	16 yr	49	53	67	81	85
100	104	119	134	138	17 yr	51	55	69	83	87
102	106	121	136	140	18 yr	52	56	70	84	88

From the Second Task Force on Blood Pressure Control in Children, National Heart, Lung and Blood Institute, Bethesda, Md. Tabular data prepared by Dr. B. Rosner, 1987.
*K4 was used for ages <13; K5 was used for ages 13 and over.

Normal Blood Pressure Readings for Children (Girls)

Systolic Blood Pressure Percentile					Age	Diastolic Blood Pressure* Percentile				
5th	10th	50th	90th	95th		5th	10th	50th	90th	95th
46	50	65	80	84	1 day	38	42	55	68	72
53	57	72	86	90	3 days	38	42	55	68	71
60	64	78	93	97	7 days	38	41	54	67	71
65	69	84	98	102	1 mo	35	39	52	65	69
68	72	87	101	106	2 mo	34	38	51	64	68
70	74	89	104	108	3 mo	35	38	51	64	68
71	75	90	105	109	4 mo	35	39	52	65	68
72	76	91	106	110	5 mo	36	39	52	65	69
72	76	91	106	110	6 mo	36	40	53	66	69
72	76	91	106	110	7 mo	36	40	53	66	70
72	76	91	106	110	8 mo	37	40	53	66	70
72	76	91	106	110	9 mo	37	41	54	67	70
72	76	91	106	110	10 mo	37	41	54	67	71
72	76	91	105	110	11 mo	38	41	54	67	71
72	76	91	105	110	1 yr	38	41	54	67	71
71	76	90	105	109	2 yr	40	43	56	69	73
72	76	91	106	110	3 yr	40	43	56	69	73
73	78	92	107	111	4 yr	40	43	56	69	73

					Age					
75	79	94	109	113	5 yr	40	43	56	69	73
77	81	96	111	115	6 yr	40	44	57	70	74
78	83	97	112	116	7 yr	41	45	58	71	75
80	84	99	114	118	8 yr	43	46	59	72	76
81	86	100	115	119	9 yr	44	48	61	74	77
83	87	102	117	121	10 yr	46	49	62	75	79
86	90	105	119	123	11 yr	47	51	64	77	81
88	92	107	122	126	12 yr	49	53	66	78	82
90	94	109	124	128	13 yr	46	50	64	78	82
92	96	110	125	129	14 yr	49	53	67	81	85
93	97	111	126	130	15 yr	49	53	67	82	86
93	97	112	127	131	16 yr	49	53	67	81	85
93	98	112	127	131	17 yr	48	52	66	80	84
94	98	112	127	131	18 yr	48	52	66	80	84

From the Second Task Force on Blood Pressure Control in Children, National Heart, Lung and Blood Institute, Bethesda, Md. Tabular data prepared by Dr. B. Rosner, 1987.

*K4 was used for ages <13; K5 was used for ages 13 and over.

Pulse Rates at Rest

Age	Lower Limits of Normal (per min)		Average (per min)		Upper Limits of Normal (per min)	
Newborn	70		125		190	
1-11 mo	80		120		160	
2 yr	80		110		130	
4 yr	80		100		120	
6 yr	75		100		115	
8 yr	70		90		110	
10 yr	70		90		110	
	Girls	Boys	Girls	Boys	Girls	Boys
12 yr	70	65	90	85	110	105
14 yr	65	60	85	80	105	100
16 yr	60	55	80	75	100	95
18 yr	55	50	75	70	95	90

From Behrman RE (ed): *Nelson textbook of pediatrics,* ed 14, Philadelphia, 1992, WB Saunders.

Water Requirements

Range of Average Water Requirements of Children at Different Ages Under Ordinary Conditions

Age	Average Body Weight (kg)	Total Water (ml) in 24 hr	Water (ml) per kg Body Weight in 24 hr
3 days	3.0	250-300	80-100
10 days	3.2	400-500	125-150
3 mo	5.4	750-850	140-160
6 mo	7.3	950-1100	130-155
9 mo	8.6	1100-1250	125-145
1 yr	9.5	1150-1300	120-135
2 yr	11.8	1350-1500	115-125
4 yr	16.2	1600-1800	100-110
6 yr	20.0	1800-2000	90-100
10 yr	28.7	2000-2500	70-85
14 yr	45.0	2200-2700	50-60
18 yr	54.0	2200-2700	40-50

From Behrman RE (ed): *Nelson textbook of pediatrics,* ed 14, Philadelphia, 1992, WB Saunders.

Bibliography

Ahman E: *Home care for the high-risk infant,* Gaithersburg, Md, 1986, Aspen.

American Heart Association: *Basic life support for the infant and child victim,* Dallas, 1993, American Heart Association Scientific Publishing.

Behrman RE et al (eds): *Nelson textbook of pediatrics,* ed 14, Philadelphia, 1992, WB Saunders.

Betz CL, Poster E: *Mosby's pediatric nursing reference,* ed 2, St Louis, 1992, Mosby.

Centers for Disease Control and Prevention: *Caring for someone with AIDS: information for friends, relatives, household members and others who care for a person with AIDS at home,* inventory #498, 1993.

Centers for Disease Control and Prevention: 1994 Revised classification system for human immunodeficiency virus infection in children less than 13 years of age, *Morb Mortal Wkly Rep* 43/RR-12, 1994.

Centers for Disease Control and Prevention: 1995 Revised guidelines for prophylaxis against *Pneumocystis carinii* pneumonia for children infected or perinatally exposed to human immunodeficiency virus, *Morb Mortal Wkly Rep,* 44/RR-4, 1995.

Centers for Disease Control and Prevention: USPHS/IDSA guidelines for the prevention of opportunistic infections in persons infected with human immunodeficiency virus: a summary, *Morb Mortal Wkly Rep* 44/RR-8, 1995.

Dee-Kelly PA, Heller S, Sibley M: Managed care: an opportunity for home care agencies, *Nurs Clin North Am* 29(3): 1994.

Dombi W: Home care coverage through HMOs, *Caring* 12(6):1993.

Dumas A, Bissonnette A (eds): Community health nursing and home health nursing, *Nurs Clin North Am* 29(3): 1994.

Edelstein S: *Nutrition and meal planning in child-care programs: a practical guide,* Chicago, 1992, American Dietetic Association.

Engel J: *Pocket guide to pediatric assessment,* ed 2, St Louis, 1993, Mosby.

Evans CJ: Postpartum home care in the United States, *J Obstet Gynecol Neonatal Nurs* 24(2):180, 1995.

Gingerich BS, Ondeck DA: *Clinical pathways for the multidisciplinary home care team,* Gaithersburg, Md, 1995, Aspen.

Giuliano K, Poirier C: Nursing case management: critical pathways to desirable patient outcomes, *Nurs Management* 22(3):52, 1991.

Gorski L: *High-tech home care manual,* Gaithersburg, Md, 1994, Aspen.

Haddad AM, Kapp MB: *Ethical and legal issues in home health care,* East Norwalk, Conn, 1990, Appleton & Lange.

Ignatavicius DD, Hausman KA: *Clinical pathways for collaborative practice,* Philadelphia, 1995, WB Saunders.

Marrelli TM: *Handbook of home health standards and documentation guidelines for reimbursement,* ed 2, St Louis, 1994, Mosby.

McCoy PA, Votroubek WL (eds): *Pediatric home care,* Gaithersburg, Md, 1990, Aspen.

Morrison BB: Home health care: staying safe in dangerous times, *Nursing 95* 25(10):49, 1995.

Mosher C et al: Critical pathways, *Am J Nurs* 92(1):41, 1992.

North American Nursing Diagnosis Association: *Official nursing diagnoses: proceedings of the eleventh conference,* St Louis, 1994, North American Nursing Diagnosis Association.

Novak RS: *National pediatric home care data base,* Shawnee Mission, Kan, 1995, Child Health Corporation of America.

Rudolph AM (ed): *Rudolph's pediatrics,* ed 19, Norwalk, Conn, San Mateo, Calif, 1991, Appleton & Lange.

Schmitt BD: *Instructions for pediatric patients,* Philadelphia, 1992, WB Saunders.

Selekman J: *Pediatric nursing,* ed 2, Springhouse, Penn, 1993, Springhouse.

Shield JE, Mullen MC: *Developing health education materials for special audiences: low-literate adults,* Chicago, 1992, American Dietetic Association.

Sigardson-Poor KM, Haggerty LN: *Nursing care of the transplant recipient,* Philadelphia, 1990, WB Saunders.

Smith DP et al: *Comprehensive child and family nursing skills,* St Louis, 1991, Mosby.

Whaley LF, Wong DL: *Clinical manual of pediatric nursing,* ed 4, St Louis, 1996, Mosby.

Wong DL: *Whaley and Wong's nursing care of infants and children,* ed 5, St Louis, 1995, Mosby.

Woodyard LW, Sheetz JE: Critical pathway patient outcomes: the missing standard, *J Nurs Care Qual* 8(1):51, 1993.

Index

Page numbers followed by *t* indicate
tables.